MOMMIES, DADDIES, DONORS, SURROGATES

DATE DUE

D0089829

MOMMIES, DADDIES, DONORS, SURROGATES

Answering Tough Questions and Building Strong Families

Diane Ehrensaft

THE GUILFORD PRESS
New York   London

© 2005 The Guilford Press
A Division of Guilford Publications, Inc.
72 Spring Street, New York, NY 10012
www.guilford.com

Printed in the United States of America

This book is printed on acid-free paper.

Last digit is print number: 9   8   7   6   5   4   3   2   1

Library of Congress Cataloging-in-Publication Data

Ehrensaft, Diane.
  Mommies, daddies, donors, surrogates : answering tough questions and
building strong families / Diane Ehrensaft.
      p. cm.
  Includes bibliographical references and index.
  ISBN 1-59385-179-0 (trade cloth)   ISBN 1-59385-133-2 (trade paper)
  1. Human reproductive technology—Psychological aspects. 2. Surrogate
motherhood—Psychological aspects. 3. Parenting—Psychological
aspects. 4. Parents—Counseling of. 5. Family psychotherapy. 6. Parent
and child. I. Title.
  RG133.5.E42 2005
  618.1′7806—dc22
                                                                        2005008205

*To my granddaughter, Satya, who is
growing up in this fertile new world*

Contents

Preface

On November 9, 2004, Aleta St. James, three days short of turning fifty-seven, gave birth to twins. She is reported to be the oldest woman in America to do so. She did this by using donor eggs and in vitro fertilization. Her remarkable story made front-page news all over the globe. Yet, while she shocked the world with her postmenopausal motherhood, thousands of other mothers and fathers have been quietly making their own news by discovering new ways to have families using egg donors, sperm donors, and surrogates.

I wrote *Mommies, Daddies, Donors, Surrogates* for a simple reason. As a developmental and clinical psychologist who works with children and parents, I was seeing more and more families in my office who had brought their children into the world in "new-fangled" ways. They came to me not because I hung up a shingle saying I specialized in work with families formed using assisted reproductive technology. They came just like any other family comes to me—because they were struggling with the problems of raising healthy children. But the more years that went by, the more I realized they also came with their own set of worries and concerns—tough questions no one had really thought about, like "How do you bring up a healthy child and build a strong family when your child was born with the help of a sperm donor, an egg donor, or a surrogate?" So I took it upon myself to start thinking and kept thinking over the past two decades, until I felt ready to share what I've learned about the hard questions, the moving but sometimes painful experiences, and the good outcomes for the children and for the mommies, daddies, donors, and surrogates in this fertile new world.

Acknowledgments

I would like to start by acknowledging all the people who must remain anonymous—the mothers, fathers, sons, and daughters who have opened up my thinking and inspired me to write *Mommies, Daddies, Donors, Surrogates*. To all of you who have so generously shared your lives with me as you have built your families with the help of assisted reproductive technology, I want to extend my deepest gratitude.

There are several people who have been my readers, my muses, and my mainstays as I went through the journey of writing this book. First, I would like to thank Barbara Waterman, who, with painstaking care, has read every word I have written and tended to both the sense of my ideas and all the dotted *i*'s and crossed *t*'s with the expertise of a professional and the love of a close friend. Toni Heineman, my close colleague who shares so much of both my professional and personal life, has read chapter drafts, sat with me on panels, traded manuscripts, and generously offered her own mind in thinking with me about our experiences working with children and families who are made in these new ways. She has truly helped me germinate this book. To Ron Elson, also my close friend and colleague, I extend my deepest thanks for bringing the lens of psychiatry and a male voice to the reading of chapter drafts and for guiding me in thinking about mommies, daddies, donors, and surrogates from every side of the elephant. There is a very special place for Lillian Rubin. More than a friend, more than a colleague, Lillian is a part of me and the main support of my writing since we first met over coffee more than twenty-five years ago. My hardest critic, she is also my deepest muse. And to Jim Hawley, my husband, I want to also thank you for reading every word I wrote, but we'll come back to that later.

There are other people who were not my readers, but who infused this book with their minds and hearts. To Anne Bernstein, whom I can hardly remember ever not being part of my life, I want to extend special thanks for her own inspiring work on families using assisted reproductive technology and for all of our discussions and shared work about alternative families over the past three-plus decades. To the members of my consultation group, Eileen Keller, Bonnie Rottier, and Stephen Walrod, I owe special gratitude for helping me think through my experiences and giving me the opportunity to share with them what I have learned about working with "alternative to the stork" families. To Gloria Lawrence, my close friend and suitemate, special thanks for bringing our clinical minds together, standing by my side through this process, and just being next door. Last, there are no words I can find to acknowledge the depth of my appreciation for the woman who has been not only my colleague, but my sister through most of my adult life. But I will try. To Joanna Levine, thank you for your mind, your spirit, your love, and your understanding as I went "underground" to write.

And now I want to turn to the people at The Guilford Press. I would like to thank Sarah Smith for her seamless guidance through the details and procedures for moving this project from a file in my computer to a book with a cover. I don't think anyone could have been luckier in editors: Chris Benton is not only a miracle worker as an editor; she also has a wealth of wonderful ideas, a generosity of encouragement, and a way of being both direct and positive at the same time that has made this book what it has become. Kitty Moore is more than just an editor—she has been a main supporter of my writing and intellectual work for almost a decade and one of the most intelligent and kindest women I have had the good fortune of working with. To both Chris and Kitty, the words "thank you" will never be enough.

I want to end with the people without whom this book would never have been written—my family. My mother and father, Edith and Morris Ehrensaft, bought me my first pencil and have continued to support my writing every step of the way. My granddaughter, Satya, lights up a room and reminds me that growing our children well is what it's all about. My daughter, Rebecca Hawley, is a living testimonial to building strong families, both her own and the families she works with, and my son, Jesse Ehrensaft-Hawley, is my muse in showing me all the ways we can think and thrive outside the box. And now I want to come back to my husband, Jim Hawley. He has not only read every word I have written, but also shared his fine mind, cheered me on, and stood next to me every step of the way. And loved me, as I do him. I would guess he'd be the first to say, "I'm glad it's finished."

MOMMIES, DADDIES, DONORS, SURROGATES

Beware Gifts Bearing Children

> Mommy, Mommy, when I grow up, I want to be a mommy just like you. I want to go to the sperm bank just like you and get some sperm and have a baby just like me.
>
> —Six-year-old Emily, dreaming of motherhood

You go to the sperm bank and become a mommy. No storks showing up at the doorstep with a bundle. No birds-and-bees sex scenes. Emily knows a new story—the story about parents who very much want a child and have found a new way to have one with the help of assisted reproductive technology. To Emily, it is such a good story that someday she wants to be one of those mothers, just like her mommy. I want to continue Emily's story and invite all of you to come with me as I tell what I have learned about women and men who have become parents with the help of sperm donors, egg donors, or surrogates and all I have learned about the children as well. I might be telling your own story, or maybe your story-to-be.

For everyone, parenthood today is an extremely stressful endeavor. As I open this story, you may already be imagining how much more stressful it can become if you're a parent or a child in a donor or surrogate family. And not just stressful, but complicated. These "new-fangled" methods of making babies are here to stay, and each week we read about a revolutionary new way to get a baby using reproductive science. Doctors can now mix an infertile mother's egg with someone else's egg to create a viable egg and then a fetus genetically related to both women. With future scientific advances, an adult skin cell may be able to be substituted for a sperm or an egg, meaning two women could create a baby genetically related to both of them, and so could two men. What next?

Forget about what's next; even with what's right now you may be faced with many complex questions: Do these techniques pose any risks? How do I (or will I) feel about the child who was made by me and someone else? How do I (or will I) feel about the child who was made by my partner and someone else? How will my child feel about me? Will it affect how I feel about my partner (if I have one)? How do I feel about the someone else (the donor or surrogate)? Where does that person fit into my family? How will I talk to my child about his or her beginnings? Will I tell other people? If I do, what will I tell them? Is my child okay? For any parent, these are daunting questions, and up until now you may have been left to sort them out on your own. I'd like to offer what help I can.

And not just to parents—donors and surrogates need help; friends, family, colleagues, and lovers need help; professionals need help; policymakers need help; the communities and the society in which your children grow need help as well. So I am enlisting all of us to come together as a village to ensure the health and well-being of the children and the parents who are members of the new swell of "alternative to the stork" families.

In both the wisdom and innocence of their youth, Emily and the children around her have already begun to tell the story that I want to tell, maybe even better than I can. Seven-year-old Andy has two mothers. He is out on the playground. Two boys stop him. They taunt him: "Andy, you can't have two mommies. You have to have a mommy and a daddy." Andy, glaring at them, hurls his retort: "Stupid, haven't you ever heard of donor insemination?" Jade, the six-year-old daughter of a single mother, ran up against a similar taunt. She offered a simple response: "Well, a man helped us." Her friend quickly rallied to her defense reminding Jade's taunters of yet another classmate. "And Lilly, she was made from a dish."[1]

Sylvie is eight years old and in love with life, with its theme of different strokes for different folks. She tells me what she's figured out—none of her friends live with their father; she's the only one who does. She goes into her litany: Jennifer has two moms, Mandy's parents are divorced and her father lives far away, and her friend Katy, "Well, she has a mom—and . . . and . . . [with an arching wave of her arm] and a father somewhere else." In fact, Katy has no father. Her mom has always been a single mother. Katy was conceived with the sperm from an anonymous donor, something Katy has known since she was a tiny child.

The children tell us their stories—of mommies going to the sperm bank, babies made in a dish, boys with two mommies, fictive fathers who float somewhere in the universe. Now it is time for *us* to tell a story—to our children and to ourselves. It is time for a story that will make sense of the new advances in reproductive technology and the families that are born of them.

Emily, Andy, Jade, and their classmates are universes away from the playground prose of my childhood, "Johnny and Susie sitting in a tree, k-i-s-s-i-n-g," where standard fare was fantasies of heterosexual couples kissing, marrying, and making babies. Sylvie negotiates the new vagaries of reproductive technology by making up a father for Katy because nothing else made sense to her. Every day on the playground, in living rooms, in bedrooms, and in doctors' offices, all of us, not just Emily, Sylvie, Andy, and Jade, are trying to make sense of these radical new situations where children are conceived with the help of donated sperm, eggs, or wombs. We make up stories, we get our facts mixed up, but most of all we experience waves of worry and angst that often render us helpless or incapacitated in our thinking about the topic or in our actions, both at home and out in the world.

THE FERTILE NEW WORLD

If we think about it, it is as though we are just emerging from the Dark Ages into a Renaissance as we rub our eyes and try to comprehend the profound changes in biological, psychological, family, and social life that have been ushered in by the new reproductive technologies. We have hardly begun to digest the new possibilities:

Donor insemination—the oldest form of assisted reproductive technology—a process whereby sperm is introduced into the female reproductive tract through the use of an artificial device.

Egg (ovum) donation—the process by which ova are extracted from one woman and joined with sperm through in vitro fertilization to be carried by another woman who will gestate the child.

Surrogacy—the process by which a woman carries a child conceived (through donor insemination or in vitro fertilization) with her egg or an egg donor's egg and a man's sperm, to be raised by that man alone or by that man and his male or female partner.

Gestational care—the process by which a woman gestates a baby for another individual or couple by means of an embryo transfer conceived by that couple or from another woman's egg and donated sperm.

Embryo adoption—the process whereby an embryo, created through in vitro fertilization from the egg of a woman and the sperm of a man, is gestated in the womb of another woman to be raised by her alone or by her and her partner, individual(s) who have not provided the gametes (eggs or sperm) and have no genetic ties to the child.

We may readily accept the story of Zeus birthing Athena from his head, yet that doesn't protect us from getting overwhelmed by the real reproductive technologies that allow people to have babies in ways only dreamed about in ancient myths. And before we have a chance to get our heads around the possibilities of borrowed eggs, sperm, and wombs, sensational media headlines both intrigue and trouble us with announcements of even newer miracles that already render these routes to parenthood obsolete or mundane. Soon we may be able to clone ourselves.

Baby boomers are believed to be the driving force behind this mad rush into the future. Baby boomers—a large, affluent generation born in the aftermath of World War II with the belief that the world was their oyster, a generation that typically postponed parenthood, a generation growing up in an ecologically polluted environment suspected to be interfering with fertility—were not going to be stopped short when they encountered problems with having babies. They would reach for whatever means possible. Not God, but technology is on their side. Yet whether we are baby boomers, the parents before them, or the next generation, we are all stumped. If we cannot even get into focus the reality of a child with up to five parents (sperm donor, egg donor, gestational carrier, legal parents), how are we to fathom a child who has three genetic parents or only one genetic parent or might be his own grandpa?

The story I would like to tell is a "strange bedfellows" story. More than a century ago, when the first reported donor insemination baby was recorded, Western medicine broke ground for infertile heterosexual couples to have a baby of their own. To this day, assisted reproductive technology is a boon to those couples or individuals unable to conceive a baby because of problems with their reproductive system or because of illness or disease that would contraindicate either carrying or conceiving a child. But now all of these men and women are joined by a whole other group of people wanting a child and celebrating that they can have one—people who have nothing wrong with their reproductive systems but are gay, lesbian, or single and, therefore, need some outside help to have a genetically related baby of their own.

The strange bedfellows don't always share the same emotional experiences. Those turning to assisted reproductive technology after confronting infertility often find themselves working through a sequence of desire, frustration, disappointment, and mourning. Single people and gay and lesbian families who discover in donorship or surrogacy a revolutionary new opportunity to become parents more likely find themselves traversing from desire to excitement to appreciative anticipation. So our story must weave together the experience of those who thought they never could but now discover they can have a child of their own and the experience of those who once thought they could and now discover that they cannot. Such an intricately woven story must inevitably be one of both sadness and celebration. It must be a story with many beginnings and many endings, but a single story nonetheless: the story of parents who raise a child who was brought to them not by the stork but with the help of another person—an egg donor, a sperm donor, or a surrogate.

This is not a brave new world, but a fertile new world. Right up to the present we seem to exclusively link assisted reproductive technology with infertility. We have books like *Beyond Infertility: The New Paths to Parenthood*[2] that itemize all of the assisted reproductive techniques to help a couple get a child of their own once they have confronted their inability to conceive. No mention is made of gay, lesbian, or single people who have no problems with their fertility. Yet increasing numbers of prospective single, gay, or lesbian mothers and fathers are availing themselves of these new paths to parenthood. For individuals in same-sex couples and for single people, the problem is not that their bodies do not work, but that they do not have another's body to work with. So in our new fertile world of reproductive technology, we might want to take the emphasis off the problem of infertility and put it on the solution—a solution that embraces not just problems with an individual's reproductive system but also the choice to have a child without the traditional male–female coupling. I suggest we just start thinking of this whole new world of possibilities as "assisted conception." This replacement is a twofer. "Assisted conception" removes the stigma and negative connotations historically associated with the word "infertility" while simultaneously including fertile gay, lesbian, and single people who avail themselves of these new options for parenting.

Entrance into the twenty-first century has brought with it a sea change not just in baby making but also more broadly in the definition of family. Over the past few decades we have watched increasing divorce rates result in new families with a mix of biological and nonbiological ties. We have also witnessed the increased acceptance of adoption, the trend for many to become parents first and choose partners later, and the technological advances that create myriad new combinations of biological and nonbiological parenthood. These transformations shake up our belief that blood is thicker than water and replace it with the sensibility that family ties are built more on love than on blood. Those of you who are using sperm donors, egg donors, or surrogates to build your families are our trailblazers. You are also part of the new generation of parents that increasingly accepts that "somebody else's child" can also be your child. Just as people no longer raise an eyebrow when a man pushes a baby stroller, your experience in your own families forecasts a time when no one will think twice about "yours and somebody else's" as they peek into the stroller.

BLOOD AND WATER

Culture affects family and family alters culture in round-robin ways. We used to have the biological versus the social family (adoptive families, for example). Now we have the new hybrid—the *biosocial* family. With the advances of reproductive technology, we have three kinds of parents: genetic, social, and gestational. So a child conceived with a sperm donor can have a genetic mommy and a nongenetic daddy, known as a social father. A mommy using an egg donor and her husband's sperm can have a little girl who is biologically but not genetically linked to her mommy (a gestational mother) and genetically linked to her daddy. Any of these mothers and fathers can qualify as the *legal* parent of the child.

In our culture, blood is still thicker than water. But what about when blood and water commingle? In families using donated gametes or borrowed wombs, we have both blood and water. Max is Julie's biological son. Jordan is his daddy and Julie's husband, but not Max's biological father. Sperm donor #143 from the local sperm bank holds that position. Will

Max be as strongly attached to Jordan as he would be to a biological dad? Will Julie think Max is more her child than Jordan's? Will Jordan feel he has a thinner relationship with Max because Jordan is "water" rather than "blood"?

And what about when two different forms of "blood" commingle? Marilyn and Phyllis have been a couple for ten years. They both have a strong urge to have a child. They know how hard it is to adopt as a lesbian couple. They also would like to have a child with biological ties to both of them. They are in their thirties, and both women are healthy and fertile. They decide to turn to assisted reproductive technology but are worried about an inequality in their maternal relationships with their child-to-be if only one of them has a biological tie to the baby. So they decide to extract eggs from Marilyn, fertilize them in vitro with an anonymous sperm donor, and implant the embryos in Phyllis's womb. This way each will have a biological link to their child: one as genetic mother, one as gestational mother. But how will Phyllis feel about a child who will never have any physical resemblance to her? And how will Marilyn feel about never having carried or birthed her child, never knowing the child from the inside out? And how will their child perceive each of them? Will one or the other of her mothers, the mother who carried her or the mother who conceived her, feel more like her "real" mom?

When we introduce a sperm donor, egg donor, or surrogate into family building, we have difficulty shaking the anxiety stirred up by all these questions. How can a sperm donor not be a daddy if a child is produced with his sperm? How can the surrogate not be a mommy if she grew the child in her womb? The challenge to our traditional beliefs about the saliency of blood relations and the relationship between blood and bonding gets to the core of the issue of assisted reproductive technology that we will be exploring in the pages of this book: Who is the mommy? Who is the daddy? How will the children see it? How will the parents feel it? What do the donors and surrogates have to say about it?

FACING UP TO OUR FEARS

I have invited us to come together as a village to support the families in this fertile new world. It is not only the health of individual families, but also the larger social and psychological ramifications of the new advances in reproductive technology that should be of concern to all of us as a society. Important issues get raised: What is a family? Who holds the parental rights? Are there social or moral limits to the advances in reproductive technology (as in the present controversy about human cloning)? And so forth. But it is you parents who are on the front lines, carrying the banner for all of us, struggling in your daily lives to find answers to the bigger questions that affect us all. It doesn't matter if you are a heterosexual couple, a lesbian couple, a gay couple, or a single lesbian, gay, or heterosexual person. The story I am about to tell, a tale of anxiety trumping clear thinking and the journey toward clarity and calm, is a story for all of you. Each of you will have your own individual and idiosyncratic experiences, but all of you share the thrills and challenges of creating a baby with a "someone else" who is not your lover or spouse. You all have experienced a deep desire to have a child or you live with a person who has, and all of you have turned to assisted reproductive technology to help you. And for all of you, within yourselves, between the two of you when there are two, and between you and the culture surrounding you, the risk that anxiety will cloud clear thinking seems to come with the territory.

Let us zoom in on the culture for a moment. People often malign parents who use donors or surrogates. Headlines about exorbitantly priced searches for the perfect egg donor with a high IQ, beauty, and physical prowess don't just inform, they also reinforce—even stimulate—our discomfort and judgment about affluent people in market pursuit of designer children.[3] But such parents are rare exceptions. Most parents using assisted reproductive technology do so because they strongly desire to have and to love a child and find this the best or only way to have one.

Regretfully, this doesn't protect parents from taking fire. With anger and hurt, a father described the response from one of their closest friends when he and his wife shared their decision to use an egg donor to have a baby after discovering the wife had no viable eggs: "Why would you want to do that?"[4] Some people consider giving away eggs or sperm as tantamount to giving away a child callously, similar to the aspersions cast on parents who place their child for adoption. Donating gametes or lending wombs generates a wholesale policy of purposely separating children from their genetic or gestational parents in order to hand them over to someone else, a terrible thing, some people say. Others feel that putting a price tag on sperm or eggs is equivalent to turning people into property, putting them up for sale. And still others just think the whole thing is creepy.

Parenting brings out people's stereotypes and generates strong emotional reactions. These feelings are not static but can often shift with expo-

sure and education. We've witnessed this in the dramatic change in acceptance of single mothers and single parenting. When I was growing up in the
1950s and 1960s, an unwed mother might just as well have worn a scarlet A.
She was either forced to marry the father or shamefully, secretly shipped off
to a home for unwed mothers. Now the unwed mother appears on the cover
of *Time* magazine[5] as a positive icon of the "new woman" with a proud message to her child: "Once upon a time, there was a very happy lady named
Marianne who had one thing missing from her life. She wanted a baby. But
since Marianne didn't have a husband, she went to a doctor, who gave her
seeds from a kind and generous man called a donor. Nine months later, out
popped a beautiful baby boy named Sam."[6]

Marianne is not only a single mother. She's the mother of a child conceived with the aid of an anonymous sperm donor. Pride, not shame, ema-
nates from her story to her son about his single-mother family and his donor-
insemination conception. Although we don't yet know how Sam will react
to this story, Marianne's proud tale replaces the tawdry image of designer
babies for sale with a positive picture of loving and conscientious mother-
ing. Her story pushes us to re-examine our negative attitudes and stereotypes
of narcissism gone mad in parents turning to borrowed wombs or donated
eggs or sperm to have a child.

Yet we'll need more than cover stories to remedy the negativity or
skepticism about the new paths to parenthood stirred up in so many of us.
Genevieve is a single woman in her early forties. For a number of years she
has been in desperate search of a husband, not just so she can walk down
the aisle but also so she won't miss the chance to have a baby. No eligible
bachelor has surfaced. With the biological clock ticking loudly, Genevieve
has worked through mourning the marriage that is not to be and has turned
her attention to the motherhood that still can. She had been exploring the
possibility of donor insemination until she heard an interview with a
young adult on a local radio talk show. This young woman talked about her
great pain and suffering as a child conceived with the aid of donor insemination because she never felt like she knew her roots and always felt weird
and different. That single radio broadcast was enough to make Genevieve
flee from the sperm bank and sprint to the nearest adoption agency. Fortunately, with the help of her therapist, Genevieve was able to slow down,
even with the clock ticking, and more thoughtfully weigh the pros and
cons of adoption versus donor insemination as a means to motherhood.
But for a moment her anxiety got the best of her, and she was off and run-

ning toward a more traditional road to parenthood on the basis of very little information.

Using my tools as a clinical and developmental psychologist who has spent many years working with children and parents in families formed with assisted conception, I am writing you a story in defense of and as a support to parents who are contemplating or have already embarked on the process of having a baby with the aid of assisted reproductive technology. I am writing a story that I hope will supplant stereotypes and negativity with acceptance and support. At the same time, I do not want to throw the baby out with the bathwater, so to speak, by avoiding the hard questions. Are there problems or issues for the children? Are there problems for the parents? Are there problems for the donors or surrogates? It will help no one if we attempt to dispel anxiety and negative biases by blindly insisting that everything is just fine.

Just as an example, many people, like Marianne, describe the donor as a kind, generous, or nice person wanting to help someone have a baby. And then I hear a scathing, snapping retort from an eleven-year-old boy born with the assistance of a sperm donor: "Yeah, right, what's so nice about the guy? He was just doing it for the money." Another "nice" man who donated his sperm to a lesbian couple showed up later like Rumpelstiltskin to claim his rights to his child, to see his "daughter" when he felt like it but pay no child support, and to deny the little girl's nonbiological mother the opportunity to become a legal parent through a co-parent adoption because, after all, he was the dad. If we are going to dispel myths and enable ourselves to think clearly, we must also have the courage to be realistic. We must be ready to take an honest look at the potential or presented downsides of donor and surrogacy births. Our story must embrace the good, the bad, and even the ugly. Only then can we understand the full experience, positive *and* negative, and work together to ensure the best health for the parents, for the children, for the donors and surrogates, and for all of us as a society.

MAKING PEACE BETWEEN OUR THINKING AND OUR FEELING

As those of you who have had children with a donor or surrogate know, it is not always a path without thorns. From the surrounding world you may confront not just people's uninformed prejudices and stereotypes, but also the high financial cost of assisted reproductive technology services, rejection by family members, lack of information about what to tell a child, and a lack of knowledgeable counseling services.

"Informed" social critics also step in your path. We have religious traditionalists who believe God's way, sexual intercourse, should be the only way to make a child. We have conservatives who believe only a man and woman *together* should have a child and that single-parent and gay or lesbian households represent the erosion of the family, if not all of society. We have philosophers, ethicists, and legal experts who worry that reproductive technology is a runaway train, going too fast for us to think through the pertinent moral, ethical, legal, and social concerns. We have political activists who object to all forms of genetic technology, including assisted reproductive techniques, viewing them as a threat to the health and well-being of our society.

If that is not enough to set you off course, these outside pressures get tangled up with a whole litany of inner stresses. You might encounter internalized guilt and anxiety about infertility. You might experience high levels of angst about viable pregnancies and healthy fetuses. You might not be able to shake off feelings of shame or failure induced by society's negative attitudes and behavior toward infertility, homosexuality, children born out of wedlock, or different kinds of families. You might feel insecure about forging a healthy bond with a child conceived by you and an outside party or by your partner and an outside party. You might feel confused and conflicted about telling your child about his or her conception. After all, you think, if the developmental experts have not been able to figure out this highly complicated issue, how can you be expected to? You might be worried about the prejudice, negativity, or rejection that could come your child's way from schoolmates, from schoolmates' parents, from teachers, from your friends, from your own extended family.

My story of children brought not by the stork but through assisted reproductive technology must therefore be an inside–outside story. It will have to weave together the external and the internal stressors and examine their effects on both parents and children. In that sense, it is not only a tapestry project but an excavation and illumination process. At times we will have to dig deep into our unconscious to pull up certain threads of the experience so they can be seen in the light of day and used to fill in the holes of our tapestry. Only then will we be able to see the full and rich spread of the fabric that will help us think about and think through the profound journey of family building with the aid of donors or surrogates.

I believe that harnessing our emotional, sometimes irrational fantasies to our more thoughtful, rational selves is the best insurance policy for a healthy and harmonious family life. The new ways of making babies create a rich breeding ground for imaginary stories and fictive fantasies. Here are just a few I have encountered. A couple who have a child conceived with a mix of the father's low-motility sperm and the sperm of an anonymous donor have decided never to tell their child about the circumstances of his conception. Over time both grow convinced that the husband is definitely the genetic father, even though the child has absolutely no resemblance to him and even though genetic testing is available to determine if he is or is not. A lesbian co-parent tells me that she actually conceived their child with her partner because she carried the baggie filled with sperm under her armpit to keep it warm on the way to the insemination. A man who donated sperm several times many years ago while a medical student denies having any connection at all to the children conceived with his sperm—he just lent his seed to science. All of these stories are myths, yet they also reveal deep *emotional* truths about our desires to be connected to the children we intend to bring into the world, or alternately, our desires to sever connections to the children we have helped create but have no intention of parenting.

These three tales also show how creating and raising children with the assistance of reproductive technology can generate immensely deep conflicts in all of us between our rational, conscious selves and our more primitive, unconscious selves. The time has come for parents, for donors and surrogates, for family members, for professionals, for friends, community, and policymakers all to work together so clear thinking and reflection are not thwarted by anxiety as we go forward into the fertile new world of assisted reproductive technology. This does not mean purging ourselves of our more primitive fantasies, but rather allowing them to come to the light of day and hitching them to our more rational thoughts.

Margolite loves her daughter, Stacey, more than life itself. She cannot believe she finally got the opportunity to become a mother with the help of the local sperm bank. But occasionally, when Stacey is driving her crazy with her demands, the thought runs through her mind, "I chose the wrong donor. This guy must have given her the screaming gene. I blew it. I wish I could trade her in." Then, horrified by these fleeting thoughts, she buries them deep in her unconscious and prepares for her speech at the local Parents Without Partners chapter, in which she will talk only of the great gift of donor insemination. And when she comes home, Margolite will grant

Stacey each and every one of her demands to compensate for any emotional harm she might have done in allowing her more negative feelings to surface. Perhaps we could say it is a ubiquitous wish among parents to distance themselves from the less endearing traits of their children, but in Margolite's case the wish collides head-on with her anxiety about a man she has never met but who perhaps has a strong (negative) influence on the child who is hers, but also comes from him. As a consequence, she is knocked off course, transforming herself into an overindulgent parent, good for neither herself nor her daughter.

To rid ourselves of any queasy feelings, we, like Margolite, may bend over backward to purge ourselves of any bad thoughts. Sometimes we do this by overemphasizing the virtues and denying the pitfalls of reproductive technology. For example, people talk about the "nice" man or woman who so generously donates sperm or eggs so someone can have a baby. Why can't the donor just be a person, neither nice nor nefarious? The experience of bringing a child into the world with the aid of a donor or surrogate is not either–or, not all bad or all good, but a mixed bag. It is a journey that criss-crosses unconscious stirrings and conscious intent, beliefs, and actions, in which positive, negative, and ambivalent feelings all swarm around each other. I would like to create a story that will help all of us negotiate the tensions between our unconscious stirrings and conscious strivings and between our irrational experiences and thoughtful reflections as we traverse the terrain of baby making with "you and someone else."

HOW IS THIS FAMILY DIFFERENT?

Let's return to the sentence "The experience is not either–or, neither all bad nor all good, but a mixed bag." If we step back for a moment, this statement captures the experience of *any* parent once he or she has decided to have a child. And if we zero back in on the parents who have turned to assisted reproductive technology, they are no different from any other parents who get up in the middle of the night to a crying infant, learn how to respond to a two-year-old's tantrums, play house with their preschooler, guide and follow their child's academic life, set curfews for their teenager, and launch their child into adulthood. Once a child is delivered to you, regardless of the delivery system, there is a uniform job description: develop a bond, protect, nurture, stay attuned, guide and support, set limits, love.

So, is that the end of the story? No, because there is another side to it. Families built with the help of a donor or surrogate live together and love each other (or not) like any other family. But they cannot avoid dealing with the reality that their family is not the same as other families—the daddy who raised you may not be the man who made you; or you grew in my tummy but from Auntie Doreen's egg; or you have two mommies, no daddy, and a man who gave us the seed so we could have you with Mommy Jean's egg; or you have one mommy, no daddy, and the man who gave us the seed so I could have you; or you have two daddies and the lady who gave us her egg and let you grow in her tummy with Daddy Joe's seed so we could have you; and so on.

Unique to assisted reproductive technology families is the presence of an outside party involved in the child's conception. Early in my research, while writing notes on surrogacy and gestational carriers, I noticed that I had mistakenly typed "birth other" instead of "birth mother." I laughed, realizing that my own unconscious may have been actively at work to develop more appropriate language for the woman who carries a child for someone else. Like parents who adopt, mothers and fathers using donated gametes or borrowed wombs to have a baby will inevitably parent with the presence of an outside party in their child's birth. Regardless of whether that outside party is an active member or merely a faint shadow in the family, he or she will always be there. That's true even if the parents choose never to disclose the "birth other's" existence to their child. As with adoption, there is no way to avoid the reality of the outsider. At the same time, there is no boilerplate, no one best way to include the birth other in the child's life, and each family must carve its own path for integrating that outsider's existence into their family experience. What they all share is that they do have to do this in one way or another.

Also unique to families using a birth other is the separation of sexual intercourse from reproduction. To qualify as such a family, parents have to plan to conceive a child but not have sex to do so. Some people experience this bifurcation between sex and reproduction as a minor detail of their child's origins. Others are haunted by it every day. A husband creates wild fantasies of his wife "doing it" with the sperm donor. A mother-to-be imagines her husband running off with the surrogate, who now has an intimate relationship with her husband via carrying his sperm within her body. With modern forms of birth control we have been able to take the reproduction out of sex, but with the fertile new world of reproductive technology, can we as successfully take the sex out of reproduction?

"Genetic asymmetry" is another feature unique to families using a birth other. In two-parent families, one parent will have a genetic link to the child and the other will not. The same is true, of course, in stepfamilies, except that those two parents come together later—one or both already have had children, either as a single parent or with someone else. A couple using a birth other to conceive has planned from the get-go to have that child together. They have full knowledge and anticipation that their child will have one genetic or biological parent and one social (nonbiological) parent, or one genetic and one biological parent in the case of egg-donor heterosexual couples or of lesbian couples when one mother is the egg donor and the other the gestational mother. In one-parent families, the asymmetry takes a different form. Two sets of genes came together to conceive the child, but only the bearer of one of those sets ever intended to raise that child. In some ways this is no different from the child conceived by a sexual union that was not intended to create a baby and in which the mother goes on to raise the child herself. Except that, unlike with the unintended pregnancies, no sex was involved and the one who will parent has planned for the baby before the sperm ever entered her body.[7]

You birth-other families share not only your uniqueness, but also your good fortune—the opportunity to become parents because of the revolutionary changes in reproductive technology. While you revel in your good fortune, your religious and social opponents may see folly instead. In the meantime, reproductive technology forges ahead, and your families are no longer a wave of the future but a strong surge of the present, caught up in rapidly expanding forms and waiting to be understood fully. The time has come for us to understand and facilitate, and that is what I'm inviting you to do with me.

TRUMPING ANXIETY WITH CLEAR THINKING

In *Adoption Nation*, Adam Pertman tells the story of a British gay couple who were unable to adopt or to hire a surrogate in England. They created embryos with a mix of their sperm and a California woman's eggs. The embryos were then implanted in another woman's womb. After giving birth, the surrogate signed over custody to the two fathers. This is the story of a transcontinental, homosexual, technological, expensive pseudo-adoption. Such new possibilities of family making create a fertile field for imaginary stories and fictive fantasies. They also offer the opportunity to stretch our thinking about families, about parent–child bonds, and about sex, love, and reproduction. The purpose of the journey I invite us to take together is to see if we can bring the thinking and feeling parts of ourselves together in creative tension in this groundbreaking terrain of baby making with a birth other.

I would like to guide our journey into the lives of birth-other families with three simple questions: Do we really know what we are doing here? What are we anxious about? What more do we need to think about to create a healthy environment for everyone affected?

Each of the following chapters will address one of the major life issues confronting men and women who choose egg donorship, donor insemination, or surrogacy as a way to make a family. First comes the pendulum swing between *power and powerlessness*: I am now granted the power to have a child and maybe even to preselect half his or her genes. But what if I don't conceive? What will it be like not to know totally from whence my child came? Why do I have to rely on all these doctors to do what should come naturally? This tension leads organically to the question of *ownership*: Whose child is this anyway? If I didn't make it, is it mine? If *I* made it, is it more mine? Closely following on ownership's heels is the problem of *collaboration*: What about that other person or all those other people involved—sperm donors, egg donors, surrogates, gestational carriers? How do they fit into my family? Inevitably, parents will also have to grapple with *belonging*: Before I decide whether to tell my child or not, what are my internal feelings about where my child comes from? Do I belong to her? Does she belong to me? To my partner, if I have one? What do I want other people to know or even want to face myself about her origins? The issue of belonging and *disclosure* go together like a horse and carriage: Fueled by our (my) own feelings about belonging, what exactly will we (I) tell our (my) child about her conception? What will we (I) tell the rest of the world? As a child grows, his or her own mental life comes into play, and now we must face the issue of the child's *fantasies* weighed against the realities of her parentage, family, genetic roots: What if my child converts the "nice man who donated his sperm" into the father of her dreams? How do I help her balance reality and fantasy while managing my own anxiety about her conception? Last, the issue of *resiliency and health* is ongoing throughout family life: How is my child doing? How do I help her with the challenges in her life, like the desire to find her donor or the worry that she will unwittingly marry her own brother or the teasing she might get at school or the secrets we may have to ask her to keep?

Every family grows in developmental stages. Any one of these key life issues may have primacy in a particular stage of family life. At the same time, all of the issues are interlaced throughout the family's experience, either as something to anticipate, something that is occurring in the present, or something that is now woven into the family history. Thus, each chapter will address one of the specific life issues—power and powerlessness, ownership, collaboration, belonging, disclosure, fantasies, or resilience and health—as it unfolds across the family lifespan.

In each chapter you will find a set of questions at the beginning to set yourself thinking about your own responses to the topic we are exploring. Then we will revisit the questions at the end of the chapter, so you can gauge how your thinking might have changed as we think together about the subject. Each time we do this, I hope we will bring ourselves closer to taming our anxieties, strengthening the clarity of our thinking, and most important, guiding us in what to *do* to raise healthy children in this fertile new world.

Let us now embark on our journey and tell the story, beginning at the beginning—when a child is first conceived.

The Power to Create, the Fear of Creation

> The irrevocable moment in becoming a parent is not the moment you conceive a child; it is the moment you conceive of her. . . . Maybe she looks partly like you and partly like your husband. Maybe she looks partly like you and partly like some handsome, genius sperm-bank stranger . . . whatever your idea of your child, once you have it, once you have thought of her as yours, nothing can stop you from wanting her.
>
> —Barbara Jones, a mother who couldn't conceive her own child[1]

Margot looks down at her swelling middle. She feels the baby kick. She's glowing. She cannot believe she's finally going to have a baby, after trying so long. Bill, her husband, is in the other room, getting her a snack. He's humming to himself, "Just Molly and me, and baby makes three," ecstatic about the baby he thought they'd never have. He's on top of the world, until a wave of panic hits him. "We don't even know who this guy is, the donor, and why should a baby made this funny way 'stick'?" The music stops.

To make a decision to have a child using a birth other is to chance a wild ride—a pendulum swing between power and powerlessness. The desire for a baby can be so strong, but there are questions to be thought about to steady oneself for the experience.

- How will it feel to have a child genetically related to only one parent?

- How will it be to have a child with genes from a total stranger or from a friend or from a partner's relative?
- What will it be like to undergo reproductive techniques that are not sensual acts of sexual union but instead "cold" laboratory or medical interventions?
- Is the baby going to suffer any harm from these scientific techniques?

DREAMING OF A CHILD IN THE FERTILE NEW WORLD

Children, especially girls but boys as well, grow up tucking their baby dolls, their stuffed animals, even their live pets into bed or maybe under their shirts. They imagine the time when they will bear a child of their own and be a real mommy or daddy. With a future of infinite possibilities, it never dawns on them that it could be otherwise. Many of those boys and girls go on to fulfill their dreams of parenthood. But well into adulthood a certain number find themselves up against a barrier—their bodies don't work right, or they don't have another body to work with to have their own biological baby.

Poets, psychologists, psychoanalysts, historians, anthropologists, and religious scholars have all tried to unravel the mystery of the desire to have a child. Yet nobody has really been able to explain why it happens. What we do know is that without the desire, we would not have survived as a species. Whether it's human nature or passed on to us through nurturing (or both), when that desire gets going, the surge of energy behind the wish for a baby becomes strong enough to be almost palpable.

Many look askance at people who seem madly driven to have their own genetically related children. With all the motherless and fatherless children all over the world in need of a family, why do people have to be so narcissistically invested that they are compelled to create a "bloodline" child? And with all the problems of overpopulation in the world, why not just take your infertility or lack of a breeding partner as a sign that you should be one who helps turn the tide and bring down the swelling numbers of people draining the earth's resources and challenging everyone's potential for survival? While these questions may be vital for us as a nation or as a species, they become cold and callous when put to any of you who are doing nothing more than wanting to experience the age-old, yet phenomenal, act of growing a child within your own body or making a baby from your own genes. Like your ancestors, you may long to carry on the intergenerational continuity of your mothers and fathers, grandmothers and grandfathers. Roots and bloodlines may have very special meaning. For lesbian and gay parents, a genetically related child may in fact be the *only* safe route to parenthood. Many states do not allow gay adoption at all. Even in those that do, the road to adoption may be very difficult, given homophobic biases of both public and private adoption agencies and the hesitancy of many birth parents in private adoptions to place their babies in gay or lesbian families.

When Dreams Don't Come True

Leslie was approaching forty when she finally met a man who looked like a "keeper." Some years earlier she had gotten pregnant after spending a weekend with a man she cared for but did not love, and she had decided to terminate the pregnancy. But now, with her biological clock ticking relentlessly and her new relationship quickly flourishing, the wish for a child pulsated within her with building force. She stopped using birth control and waited each month for the swelling in her breasts and the skipping of her period. But each month the blood flowed. She tried fertility drugs to no avail. The more she had to wait and the more she felt blocked in reaching her goal of becoming pregnant, the stronger the desire grew. Sometimes the tears flowed gently down her cheeks; sometimes she was racked with heavy sobs. But always the refrain was the same: "I want a baby of my own so badly; it's all I can think about." From initial hope and optimism she had slowly slipped into feelings of loss and despair.

Agnes Rossi, a novelist and short-story writer, wrote of her own battle between hope and loss as she tried to conceive:

> I talked about feeling defective, about the sadness I felt knowing I might live and die without ever feeling my baby's skin against my own, about finding out that something—someone—you'd always assumed would be a big part of your life and the best part, wasn't going to be at all. . . . The sorrow I felt when I confronted the possibility of never having a baby forced me to acknowledge how desperately I wanted one.[2]

Anyone who has gone through the pain of infertility will undoubtedly recognize these feelings. I was surprised to learn that many women confronted with infertility have the same levels of depression as women who have been diagnosed with heart disease or cancer or test HIV-positive. As expressed so poignantly by one woman who discovered she was infertile: "When you take away being able to have a child biologically, it is like having to face death—almost like having half of you die."[3] If you were born in the time of your ancestors, the only salve for such pain would have been to find someone or something else to nurture or to resolve the loss and move on to other life pursuits. But in this fertile new world of reproductive technology, hope follows quickly on the heels of despair. With each passing year comes a proliferation of new programs and clinics that promise a searching individual or couple a baby of their own, either through fertility drugs, birth technologies, or gamete donorship, surrogacy, or gestational carriers. If you're having trouble making a baby the "old-fashioned" way, the medical profession is here to save the day.

To Dream the Impossible Dream

Hope springs eternal as infertile couples or individuals enter the new terrain of using a little help to make a baby. Even if the odds are against them, with determination and courage they will sustain themselves through expensive and uncomfortable, even risky interventions. If those don't work, they may turn to donors or surrogates. As they pursue any of these assisted conceptions, they hold firm in their hope that they will beat the odds and have a child of their own.[4]

While these couples sit in the waiting room of the fertility clinic, caught up in their reveries of creating a baby against the odds, to their right or left may be some of their strange bedfellows—single, gay, and lesbian clients who have come to the clinic because they, too, have a strong desire to have a child and a brand new hope that a baby is within their reach.

Franny and Rachel met each other and fell in love when they were in their twenties. This was in the 1970s. They moved in together and became a couple. Both had a strong love of children. Franny chose to work with children in a preschool, and Rachel was the eldest of ten children, delighting in the experience of being a second mom to her brothers and sisters. Despite their strong maternal desires, they accepted that, as lesbians, they would never have children of their own, that this was the loss they had to accept in their love for each other. Until the revolution in reproduction hit. Living in the San Francisco Bay area, they heard about The Sperm Bank of California.

Run by women and opened in 1982, this revolutionary sperm bank welcomed all women—straight, lesbian, partnered, single. Franny and Rachel made an appointment. Then well into their thirties, they discovered that they were both still fertile. But because Franny was a few years older, they decided she would go first and Rachel would try to get pregnant a few years later, using the same donor. They chose a donor from the identity-release program, a man willing to have his identity revealed when the children turned eighteen, and after three attempts Franny got pregnant. Tears ran down both women's faces as they marveled at their good fortune. The loss they had resolutely accepted had transformed into an unexpected miraculous discovery—they could have a baby.

Carmen is yet another woman sitting in the waiting room of a clinic. Now in her early thirties, she had expected to start a family until she was diagnosed with cancer. As a result of her treatment, which involved hysterectomy, chemotherapy, and radiation, she can no longer bear a child. Sitting next to her is her husband, Danny. On her other side sits Pamela, Carmen's sister. Prior to Carmen's cancer treatment, she and Danny decided to harvest her eggs, fertilize them with Danny's sperm in an in vitro procedure, and freeze the embryos. Carmen has faced her own mortality and survived her cancer. A child born of her own eggs now becomes a critical part of her recovery, providing an affirmation of the genetic continuity of her life. Her sister, Pamela, has offered to be the gestational carrier who will bring their baby to term so that Carmen and Danny can have the child of their dreams and Carmen can fully embrace life again.

With all the possibilities of assisted conception, either hope springs eternal or a pipeline of hope is newly laid. But almost inevitably, the excited hope is accompanied by opposite feelings—queasiness about "defying Mother Nature," the lack of any guidance in the decision-making process, and the turbulence of "shopping" for the right child. Tension between the power to create and the fear of creation is built into the decision to have a baby with a birth other.

SOARING FANTASIES OF BABY MAKING

Anybody turning to assisted conception is committing an act of defiance—either defying the odds or defying Mother Nature. This is an extremely powerful position. Mother Nature has taught us that the way to make a baby is for a male and a female to get together and create a union of their gametes, which will turn into an embryo that will turn into a new member of the species. We mammals do this through an act of sexual intercourse. But science has transcended nature by divorcing the sexual from the reproductive act, and, as the little children teach us, now you can even do it in a dish. A turkey baster or syringe containing sperm can be placed in a woman's vagina, an egg can be extracted from a woman's ovary and joined with a sperm outside of her body, a single sperm can be injected directly into an egg, an embryo can be implanted into a uterus that has no genetic relationship to the embryo. . . .

These are acts of defiance that bring with them amazing fantasies of possibility. Dr. Shana Millstein, who is conducting a study at the University of California San Francisco on decision making among infertile couples, mentioned in conversation that infertile couples are so driven by their desire to have a baby that in the end nothing will stop them—not the great odds against them, not the possible medical risks, not the exorbitant cost, not even bad news about the possible developmental anomalies that may come the way of their child (small risks of some of the new reproductive techniques). Instead, if couples don't like what the doctor has to say, they move on to another specialist.[5] What's happening here? I think Dr. Millstein is witnessing the expectant parents' soaring fantasies about the baby who will be born to them—somehow.

Gigi was thirty-nine. She had been married to Marty for three years. Although she dearly loved Marty's two children from his first marriage, she began to long for a child of her own. Many years ago, in her twenties, she had gotten pregnant accidentally and had an abortion. Fifteen years later, she was in the same doctor's office, but this time to help her have a baby. Upon examination, he told her she had significant scar tissue blocking her fallopian tubes. She underwent surgery to have it removed. She and Marty then tried and tried, for six months, for twelve months, with no luck. So back to the doctor's office. This time the doctor told Gigi that her hormones were off and her eggs not that good. So she began a regimen of hormone therapy. Twelve months later, no baby. Now came a visit to a fertility expert. Marty's sperm was tested. It was fine. But Gigi wasn't producing very many eggs. So began a regimen of fertility treatments with pills and painful shots. Twelve months later, no results. After a new work-up, the fertility doctor finally delivered the news no woman wants to hear—there was almost zero chance she could have a baby of her own. Gigi wasn't convinced, so she visited a Chinese doctor, who gave her herbal jaw-breakers to swallow every day, accompanied by weekly acupuncture. No results.

With a look of fierce determination, Gigi sat across the restaurant table from me with her bag of herbal remedies by her plate. "I guess you think I'm crazy, Diane," she said, "but I *know* that this baby I've dreamed about every night for years now is going to happen. I can do it. I know I can. If Sarah could do it in the Bible, so can I."

So what about Sarah? Carl Jung introduced the concept of the collective unconscious—dreams, notions, and fantasies that a whole culture shares. In Western culture, we share phantasmagoric stories about children born through fantastic means, stories that we carry deep in our bones. Assisted reproductive technology may have ushered in a fertile new world, but our fascination with children born other than the traditional way is age-old, going way back in written history and mythology. First there was Athena, believed to be born not from a mother but from her father, Zeus, and not through a birth canal but from his head. Then came the Old Testament story of Abraham, Sarah, and Hagar. Hagar had a child, Ishmael, for the elderly Abraham and barren Sarah, and then Sarah, at the ripe age of ninety, gave birth to their second child, Isaac, with help from God. We could say that Jesus is the archetype of the sperm-donor baby, conceived not from a sexual union between Mary and her husband, Joseph, but from a spiritual union between Mary and God.[6]

If you turn to assisted reproductive technology, you will find yourself in the company of the original fathers and mothers of Judaism and Christianity and the grandest heroes and heroines of antiquity. Buoyed by fantastic birth stories embedded deep in our collective unconscious, you can envision moving mountains and challenging the heavens to overcome what nature said could never happen.

Bob Shacochis, a writer, shared his wife's pain that she could not conceive a child of her own. He and his wife then discovered they could transcend Mother Nature by using his sperm and an egg donor and implanting the embryo in his wife's womb. The result? His wife gave birth to a healthy baby. The way in which their baby was made was fact, not fancy. But we could say that the "magic" of science created what felt like a miracle to Bob and his wife, a miracle once found only in biblical accounts, ancient myths, and folktales.[7]

For any of you who have come of age in the second half of the twentieth century, this magic of science may correspond perfectly with your sensibilities about life. You may be among those who put off motherhood or fatherhood, setting your career in motion or sowing your wild oats well into your thirties, maybe even your forties, before finding a parenting partner and being ready to settle down and contemplate the responsibilities and demands of parenthood. All this time you may have felt totally on top of your own destiny, until you bumped up against the one thing not in your control—the ability to conceive or bear a child. Now you are both the gleeful recipients of and the movers and shakers in the explosion of new alternatives to the stork. Among you are the pioneers and driving force behind the ever-expanding scientific discoveries in the field of reproductive technology, advances that ostensibly put people back in control of their lives and reinfuse them with the hope that the world is their oyster that will now produce new little pearls.

THE AWE AND FEAR OF CREATION

Regrettably, the soaring fantasies and reinfused hope are punctured by poignant pricks of anxiety. We're all excited by magicians' tricks, but they also make us nervous. What if the pretty young woman in the trunk is really cut in two? What if the young volunteer never gets released from the handcuffs? We seem to feel the same furtiveness about the magic of donated gametes and borrowed wombs. We are caught between the gratifying surge of power and the tremors that shake our foundations when the impossible becomes a reality and Mother Nature is defied. A barren woman can bear a child, a virgin can become pregnant, a man can have a baby with his infertile wife or gay partner, and so on. We all know what happened when Daedalus built wax wings for himself and his son, Icarus: Icarus was so taken by gaining the power of flight that he flew too close to the sun, against his father's admonitions, his wings melted, and he plummeted back to earth. For defying nature, Daedalus was punished with the death of his beloved son. Consciously or unconsciously, we feel the same anxieties about "defying the gods" when we tamper with Mother Nature's way of bringing babies into the world.

Recently I was having dinner with a female colleague and both our husbands. We were discussing my writing and thoughts on reproductive technology. My colleague's husband asked whether I would be taking a stand on the ethics of reproductive technology in the book. No, I responded. My intent was to make sense of the parents' experiences and think through the difficult questions confronting families using assisted reproductive technology so their children can grow well. I wasn't planning to condemn or condone assisted conception. But he continued to pursue the question, touching a tender feminist nerve: "Do you think it's ethical for postmenopausal women to get pregnant when they might very well not be alive to see their children reach adulthood?" "Let's see," I answered. "I'll consider the question only if we apply it to men as well: Do you think it's ethical for older men, like Picasso, to sire children when they might very well not be alive to see their children reach adulthood?" Truthfully, as a trained psychotherapist, I was more interested in the question than in the answer. What angst gets stirred up in us now that we have replaced biblical stories with scientific evidence of a woman as old as sixty-six who gave birth to a baby girl conceived through in vitro fertilization using sperm and egg from anonymous donors and a sixty-three-year-old woman who has given birth to a healthy child with the aid of an egg donor and an in vitro insemination with her husband's sperm?[8] What Pandora's box do we fear opening?

Playing God Is Not the Same as Playing House

When we are little, we push doll carriages, feed our baby dolls pretend mush, and give little thought to how they got to be ours. But if you have grown up to discover that real babies are much harder to come by, and you are thinking about getting some extra help to have one, this might be a good time to pay attention to anxieties about "playing God" that might intrude on your excitement over having a baby.

Think about your own Pandora's box. On the surface, we may all marvel at the expansive capacities to create life afforded by the new reproductive technologies. But we may also be haunted by some memories of an earlier time in our life, a time when we depended on our mothers, fathers, and teachers to rein us in so our fantasies wouldn't get out of control. I am specifically speaking of fantasies about babies—where they come from, how we get them, who we want to have them with.

When people, like my colleague's husband, object to older women bearing children, their concern is usually couched in the best interests of the child. They say it is not fair knowingly to deny the child access to a vital and functioning mother throughout childhood. They say having the child is an act of sheer narcissism on the part of the older mother, who denies and defies the aging process in a selfish quest to satisfy her own hungry desire for a baby. Yes, it is important to have a mother, but, I think to myself, no one seems to be objecting so adamantly to the swelling number of grandmothers who are raising their grandchildren. And no one a hundred years ago counseled women not to bear children because they might die in childbirth or of natural causes well before their children reached adulthood, even though there was a strong possibility that this would happen.

Sarah may have been ninety years old when she walked the earth pregnant in the book of Genesis, but many of us grow queasy—"It just isn't natural"—when we imagine a gray-haired woman with wrinkles and a swelling belly walking the earth today. And that reaction isn't limited to old ladies having babies. Having a baby using your mom's womb or your daughter's eggs may stir up fantasies from your early childhood that you thought you had put to rest as you moved along to become a healthy grown-up.

Let me explain.

A little boy named Ramsey wrote a note to his mother: "Dear Mom, I love you and I think you are the best mom in the whole world, but if you see this, why do you still love Dad?"[9] Ramsey entertained fantasies that he could hook up with his mom in a romantic tryst, if only his mother would ditch his father. Ramsey is having what we in the field call an "Oedipal fantasy." In this drama, little boys or girls can marry their mothers or fathers, just like Oedipus unwittingly did after killing his father and falling in love with his mother. When my own daughter was three, and I was pregnant with our second child, she announced to my husband, "Daddy, let's go move to Ho Chi Minh Park. And Mommy can visit us—once in a while." An amazing statement from a little girl who from infancy on was nearly glued to my hip. But she too was having her Oedipal, or more accurately, her Electra, fantasy of marrying her daddy. When my son was just a little bit older than that, he was struggling to wrap my Mother's Day present. My husband offered to help him, but he refused: "No, only Mommy can do it. She wraps better, and she smells better." And then I'm reminded of the poem my mother remembers to this day from her elocution lessons as a very young child: "If Daddy hadn't married Mommy, he would have married me." An Oedipal fantasy transformed into a little ditty, in which daddy is quite an old husband for the little girl, and the little girl will be quite a young wife. And then what?

Well, then comes baby. Many of these Oedipal or Electra fantasies are replete with future plans for little babies, with mommy or daddy as the chosen other parent. And in these preschool tales babies show up in the funniest of ways—pooped into toilets, dropped out of shirts, and so forth.

By the time children are six or seven, these fantasies go by the wayside, replaced by a wish to find one's own partner some day and a scientific under-standing of how babies are really made. But these fantasies don't necessarily disappear. Instead, they are put in cold storage deep in our psyches. Then along come all the new reproductive possibilities, and out trot these early fantasies that we thought we had foreclosed and repressed. If you are con-templating some form of assisted reproductive technology, you may be sur-prised to find that some of the wild and fantastic images of pregnancy and birth that we so reveled in as young children are not just silly dreams but can actually come true. You may be catapulted back to an earlier developmental period of tumultuous psychic drama where anything goes and everything explodes—little girls can marry their daddies, daddies can have babies, little girls can steal babies from their mommies, mommies can steal their little girls' babies—swirling tales of "In the Night Bedroom" far more outlandish than the escapades in Maurice Sendak's famous children's book, *In the Night Kitchen*.

Myra was pregnant with her first child. She had tried for years to get pregnant, and finally, with the help of an egg donated by her older sister, she was carrying a child. She thought she would be ecstatic and was taken aback when every night she had a recurring dream of her sister running inside her belly and then popping out of her mouth. Then she started having a different dream—her sister was actually her mother, married to their father, and the baby being born was Myra. She was troubled by these dreams, worried that they were a harbinger of bad things to come from her choice to be an egg-donor mom. But then she began to remember how she used to think that ba-bies came from eating marshmallow chicks that hopped around your belly until they were ready to jump out of your mouth again. And she remembered that it wasn't her sister, but she herself who she had envisioned marrying her father. After she made these links, the dreams became less disquieting. She could even laugh about them. Although Myra couldn't know for sure, she wondered whether using her sister's eggs in this fantastic new way of having babies made her dreams different than if she'd gotten pregnant the old-fashioned way, calling forth more poignantly some long-buried childhood nar-ratives of "sex with the improper parent" and absurd theories of procreation.

The Earth Moving under My Feet Makes Me Queasy

Stephen Byrnes, who is gay, writes about his and his partner's journey into parenthood using his sperm and a surrogate mother:

It took a lot of inner work for me to say I was ready to be a father. Work that most straight people don't generally have to go through, because for them it's usually a less self-conscious act. Few heterosexuals ask: Am I worthy to be a parent? For me, and I suspect most of my gay brethren who have taken the leap, finding myself worthy to be a parent has been the ultimate act of self-acceptance. It is also probably the most important and profound political act that I will ever make. Once I found myself worthy, nothing could hold me back.[10]

I wondered about another piece of unspoken inner work for Stephen Byrnes, beyond establishing his self-worth as a gay father. He and his partner were not going to have a baby like the books told him when he was a child. He was not only defying social norms by becoming a gay dad to his own biological child, but also defying the traditional story of sex, reproduction, and birth. With no sexual union, he was implanting his seed in a woman's body, a woman who had before that been a total stranger to him, a woman who was married to another man. His child was growing in the same womb that had housed this couple's two children. He was waiting for his baby to be birthed by this other woman and then delivered to him and his partner as *their* child. How different is that?

If you start out on the journey to have a child using new alternative reproductive techniques, you may find the earth moving under your feet while an uneasy still, small voice cries out from inside, "What are you doing? This is not how it is meant to be." I often imagine that a hundred years from now people will read of our squeamishness and fears about assisted conception and scratch their heads. How primitive and provincial we were in our thinking and feelings about making babies, they'll say.[11] But for now we live at the edge of a horizon that still feels new-fangled and unnatural as we conjure up images of babies in test tubes or petri dishes, babies conceived with no sexual union, fetuses with no genetic relationship to the womb in which they grow, adulterous liaisons, married people "doing it" with someone else, virgin mothers, even babies that can be their own grandparents.

Edward and Robby have been a couple for five years. Robby has gotten the "baby bug"—it feels like it is all he can think about. Edward is not so sure. A friend of theirs told Robby about a place called Growing Generations, a surrogacy service catering only to gay men. Lots of men go there and find one woman to be an egg donor and another to be the surrogate. Robby is excited and even has the idea that he and Edward could mix their sperm so that each would have a chance of being the genetic dad. Unfortunately, Edward does not share Robby's excitement. Edward grew up in an Orthodox Jewish home. Coming out was enough of a challenge to the religious beliefs he was raised with. The idea of mixing up two men's sperm and then putting the mixture in a petri dish with some woman's eggs and then injecting the tiny baby-to-be into another stranger's uterus was more than he could get his head around. Edward lost sleep for several nights, and the tension between him and Robby mounted until one day they went to see a movie. It was Johnny Symons's documentary *Daddy and Papa*, a film documenting the experiences of gay fathers. One of the families in the film included a woman who had had a baby for a gay couple. Edward was so moved by the pleasure and happiness he saw in the fathers' faces and in their interactions with their daughter that something cracked wide open for him. His squeamishness never entirely vanished, but it was overshadowed by the realization that he and Robby could actually have a child of their own in a happy, healthy family.

Squeamishness like Edward's is not limited to the men and women who embark on the journey into parenthood using assisted reproductive technology. "Icky" feelings reverberate loudly and clearly from people all around, in fact even more so because these folks have no investment in getting over their anxiety as they're not the ones who are hoping for a baby.

Jerry and Paula had been married for five years. Jerry had been adopted at birth in a closed adoption and knew nothing of his birth parents. Just as they were about to begin planning a family, Jerry was diagnosed with a serious genetic disease, one that had a very, very strong likelihood of being passed on to his offspring. He and Paula agonized together and made a hard choice—Jerry would not be a biological father to their children. They would have a baby using donor insemination, with an anonymous donor from a local sperm bank. Once resolved in their decision, they approached their parents to tell them. They wanted no family secrets. Jerry's parents handled it well. They themselves had grappled with infertility and ultimately turned to adoption. They knew that parent–child bonds were forged not from blood but from love and emotional connection. Paula's parents were another story. Practicing Catholics, they condemned any form of procreation that challenged "God's way." They railed at Jerry and Paula for not taking their chances at having their own biological child. As far as they were concerned, whether the child would inherit the illness should be left to God's will. If Jerry could deal with his disease, so could his child if it was passed on.

Paula's parents accused Jerry and Paula of making it one hundred percent sure that their child would be a freak, unaccepted by his family and spurned by his peers as an unnatural being. Ironically, they had just read a story about a child in their community who was teased on the playground for being a test-tube baby and an alien, and they used this account as ammunition in their plea to Paula and Jerry to dispense with their unconscionable plan.

Paula and Jerry were crushed and began to wonder if they had made the right decision. No movie like *Daddy and Papa* was there to raise their spirits—only their commitment to each other and their conviction that their child would be a treasure, not a freak. Still, they decided to consult with their family doctor about the decision they had made to have a baby with a sperm donor—was it against nature, and would they be doing something harmful to a child so born? Fortunately, their doctor was a progressive man who assured them that the desire to have a child and the willingness to sacrifice Jerry's blood ties to ensure their child's health was not an act of blasphemy but a gift of caring. Despite Paula's parents' unrelenting pressure, they went on to have the donor child of their dreams.

The earth not only moves under your feet; an earthquake rumbles as the pressure from friends, family, and countrymen collides with a parent's inner doubts or questions. The turbulence can run very deep, straight to the core of one's religious or moral beliefs. Jeanette and Donald decided to have a baby using a donor egg after they discovered Jeanette had no viable eggs of her own. They were ecstatic when Jeanette became pregnant, until she miscarried at eleven weeks. They grieved the loss of the baby they had thought would be. But Jeanette also grew increasingly agitated—she believed that God was punishing her for defying the doctrines of her church, which prohibited anything but sexual intercourse as a way to have a child. Maybe her miscarriage was confirmation that no good could come from tampering with nature. She began to wonder if someone was sending her a message that she shouldn't be a parent at all, that she was bad for wanting to be one. She located a Unitarian minister in her community. The minister reminded her that we are all God's creatures and that our mission is to embrace all children on earth, no matter how they come to us. Jeanette went on to become pregnant again using a donor egg, this time carrying a healthy baby to term—but only after she had done some "earthquake proofing."

I am sure many of you who have decided to have a child with a birth other will have your own stories to tell—accounts of raised eyebrows, worried looks, nervous laughter, rude questions, harsh judgments, and your own inner rumblings. You are swimming against the current, stroking hard to maintain your hope and optimism against the flow of cultural aspersion and internal misgivings. You need supports to stay afloat. It behooves every one of us—family members, professionals, or concerned "villagers"—to provide "water wings," educating ourselves so we can replace knee-jerk reactions with informed responses and substitute compassion for condemnation. We will need some help from the experts to do this.

WHERE IS THE PROFESSIONAL HELP?

Colleen sat in my office sobbing. Her life with her thirteen-month-old daughter, Olivia, felt ruined. She and her partner, Suzanne, had decided to have a baby together. They asked a friend of Colleen's to be the sperm donor. At the time, they thought it would be neat to put his name on the birth certificate, just so their baby could always know she had a genetic father. She and Suzanne would go on to live their lives as Olivia's two mommies. No one counseled them that by putting the donor's name on the birth certificate they would be granting him legal rights as a father, which he indeed went on to claim in Olivia's second six months of life, totally disrupting the harmonious threesome of Colleen, Suzanne, and Olivia. Now they had to make room for a third parent, a person they never intended to include in their family life. Colleen and Suzanne may have been naive in signing away paternal rights to this man they meant only to be a donor. Still, so much of this turmoil could have been avoided if, in their intense desire to have a child of their own, someone had sat down with them before the fact to walk them through the process and help them think through all the feelings and thoughts they had about having a baby with a donor. Why didn't this happen?

The Professional Blind Spots

As parents struggle with the tension between the desire to create a child and their confusion or fears about the creation, no net of professionals is there to catch them if they fall or to keep them from falling. I have been pleased to learn that more and more fertility clinics are offering counseling services in conjunction with their medical procedures, particularly when surrogacy is involved, but until recently, the medical services of assisted reproductive technology have been virtually divorced from mental health services that could help parents negotiate the experience emotionally.

The power of discovering new ways to conceive babies has been exciting not only to prospective parents, but to the medical experts who are at the cutting edge of this exploding field of research and clinical practice. In the exhilaration of making the baby, the medical professionals, along with the parents, are often so focused on the "miracle" of creating a baby prior to the birth that they are ill prepared for potential problems later. Our country has yet to establish federal guidelines for assisted reproductive technologies. For example, other countries limit the number of embryos that can be implanted in a woman to protect both mother and babies, as multiple births have a higher level of complications for the pregnant mother and greater risks of developmental problems for the babies. But fewer embryos mean fewer chances of getting a baby, so in our country many doctors still implant multiple embryos in the womb to elevate the success rates of baby making. They do this regardless of the distress for parents if they have to make a decision about fetal reduction (aborting one or more of multiple fetuses) or struggle with medical complications for mother and baby(ies) or deal for the rest of their lives with the financial and emotional burdens of raising triplets, quadruplets, or even greater numbers of multiples, any of whom may have special needs.

A colleague called me recently, wanting to talk to me about something: "Maybe it's just a fluke, but I've been wondering. All three children I see who are egg-donor or sperm-donor babies have a neurological problem. Do you think there's something going on here?" She's not the first to ask or notice. Many of us who work as developmental child clinicians have observed developmental anomalies or learning disabilities in a fair number of children born with the aid of reproductive technology. We have wondered together whether later parenthood, the effects on the fetus of manipulation of eggs and sperm in new ways, or the general increase in such problems in the culture at large could account for the children's problems. We recognize that these are just collective clinical speculations, but, as we will discuss later, recent research studies have begun to corroborate our impressions about increased risks for the children. Yet typically fertility experts do not appear to be focusing on these risks as they offer the promise of babies to hopeful parents. It seems that the left hand does not know what the right hand is doing when it comes to the medical experts doing their work *before* birth and the parents and professionals who care for the children *after* birth.

Lack of coordination between medical and mental health experts is an old story. But the stakes are quite high when the medical experts on one side have only one goal in sight, to make a baby for an individual or couple who strongly wants one, without keeping in mind the neurological or psychological effects on that baby (who will go through life having been made in this new way) or without paying attention to the emotional effects on the parents who will raise the baby. All of you parents will benefit enormously if we professionals can get our act together and build a bridge between the "before the baby" and "after the baby" folks.

We have yet another professional blind spot—information from the adoption field that *could* but continues *not* to inform us as we strive to understand the needs of children conceived with a birth other. Two generations ago it was standard fare for adopted children to be shielded from the knowledge of their origins. Decades of research and clinical experience have contributed to a complete reversal in that position. Now adopted children should be told of their origins and given the opportunity to search for their birth parents or have contact with them throughout their childhood. The Fall/Winter 2003–2004 *Adoption Book Catalog* from Tapestry Books included no fewer than forty titles on the subject. Yet in reviewing the professional literature on disclosure of donorship or surrogacy to a child, amazingly little reference is made to the knowledge that could be gleaned from the adoption field. And, although the terrain is quickly shifting toward advocating disclosure, many experts still advise parents never to tell their children about their conception using a birth other, believing that family harmony is more important than family honesty.

Of course, a baby conceived through a sexual union between two people and later placed for adoption is no doubt different from a baby planned for by a parent or parents who used an outside party to have their baby. Yet the two forms of birth have something very important in common—in each case a child has a birth history that involves "someone else" besides the parent or parents who raise the child. Interesting, then, that so many of the experts in reproductive technology (and, I think, many parents as well) ignore the more recent findings from the adoption field that children do better when they are honestly informed about their roots. There has often been a stigma around adoption. In the excitement about the new scientific miracles of reproductive technology, it is understandable that we would all divorce ourselves from the "darkness" of adoption. But it doesn't make sense. It's not just our excitement, but our anxieties about making babies using donated gametes or borrowed wombs that blind us to the wisdom from the adoption field as we sort through the long-term effects of concealing versus disclosing donorship or surrogacy to a child and to the rest of the family. Here again, the tension between the power to create and the fear of creation compromises our ability to think clearly, which in this case would involve extracting the wisdom from the adoption field as we reflect on whether to tell a child about his or her conception with a birth other.

Is There a Counselor in the House?

So what help can a parent expect in sorting out the decision to have a baby using a birth other? Regrettably, to date, our mental health community offers you nothing systematic. The adoption community has established comprehensive counseling services both to screen prospective adoptive parents and to guide them through the emotional throes of deciding to adopt, looking for, and then adopting a child. You will find no consistent carryover of these services into the field of assisted reproductive technology. Although some clinics now provide it, you cannot automatically expect to find a trained social worker or psychologist waiting to help you sort through all your hopes, fears, anxieties, and hesitancies as you face one of the most important decisions in your life. In the fervent efforts to promise people the children they never thought they could have, often with the biological clock ticking away, the revolutionary zeal of doctors potentially precludes incorporating mental health services into their protocols. If only doctors weren't compromised in their thinking by this zeal, parents could receive support services that would help them stop and take a look, asking the questions I posed at the beginning of the chapter and others as well: How will you feel having a child with a birth other? How is it going to feel conceiving through a scientific procedure? How will it be having a child who is not genetically related to you or genetically related only to your partner? What do you want to know about the donor or surrogate? What are you thinking you might want to tell your child? What will you tell your parents? Your friends? Is your baby going to be okay?

For so many parents, there is no turning back; nothing will stop their burning desire to have a child. So what would be the benefit of a counseling program? And why should parents using assisted reproductive technology have to examine their decision any more than parents choosing to have babies the old-fashioned way? Because the tension between the power to create and the fear of creation in assisted conception can cause a great deal of anxiety. Complications can arise in figuring out how to weave into your family tapestry the fact that your baby was born with the aid of a birth other. Mourning the loss of the opportunity to have a genetically related child may come up, along with facing the internal discomforts or external pressures that may make you question whether this is really a good thing to do. Nowhere else could the Boy Scouts' motto, "Be Prepared," be more pertinent. You don't necessarily need answers. Just thinking about all the questions and untangling potential emotional knots early on will pave the way for maneuvering around the inevitable bumps and potholes along the way.

So why haven't we mental health professionals pushed to make sure that counseling is available to all prospective parents turning to assisted reproductive technology? The original assisted reproductive procedures, specifically donor insemination for infertile men, were often cloaked in a veil of secrecy and shame. Donor insemination was seen as a way to provide an infertile couple with a child without anyone else ever having to know. No one wanted to stigmatize the men who couldn't sire their own children. This shroud of secrecy and protection laid the groundwork for keeping all assisted conception a confidential medical procedure, shared only between physician and patient. This means that up until recently little attention has been given to the emotional meaning of having a child in this way. Feelings of would-be parents using assisted reproductive technology are even pushed away as irrelevant to the process.

Fortunately, times are changing. The shame surrounding male infertility is subsiding, and not just infertile men, but women, both fertile and infertile, and fertile men, both gay and straight, are the new clientele of assisted conception services. As everyone gets more seasoned, medical and mental health experts alike are recognizing the need to work together and pay attention to the psychological components of the experience. If psychological services are not built into a fertility clinic's structure, there are enough sensitized mental health professionals in the community that I would encourage all parents to seek out services for themselves if they aren't automatically provided. But in the meantime, the emotional complexities are still often overlooked. Instead, a prospective parent may find a professional offering the glib assurance "Once the baby's conceived, you won't even remember how it all began. You'll just go on to be a parent like any other parent."

Oh, By the Way

If you have chosen assisted conception, you *will* go on to be a parent like any other parent, getting up at night, changing diapers, marveling over first steps and first words, and so on. But my clinical experience tells me that if you do not remember how your baby's conception all began, it is only because you have pushed the memory aside. Actually, I've yet to meet a parent who has successfully done this. Instead, the information often comes across as a seeming afterthought. Parents come to me to consult about something that is troubling them about their child. We begin to think about it together. I may even have started meeting with the child when one day, in a session, a parent will say to me, "By the way, there's something you might want to know. I didn't think it was really important, but our child is a sperm-donor baby (or egg-donor baby or surrogate baby)." Inevitably, this fact turns out to be profoundly important in one way or another, both for the parents and the child and for the family as a whole.

The first time I encountered the "By the way" scenario, I was somewhat taken aback. How could parents overlook giving me this critical piece of information about their child from the get-go? But then it started happening over and over again. In looking back at my experiences working with parents and children, I realized that when a lesbian or gay family came in to consult with me, it was obvious and self-evident that I would ask how their child was conceived or how their child came to them. The same was true when I met with a single parent, gay or straight. Yet, as a standard practice, I never posed the same question to heterosexual couples. I have now learned to ask all parents to tell me how their child was conceived, and I no longer take it for granted that the child was born the old-fashioned way.

Posing the question about conception as standard practice is one way we health and mental health professionals can be better caretakers, helping parents with the hesitancy to bring up their child's assisted-conception birth or with the resistance to seeing it as important in their child's development. Plus, it educates all of us to stop assuming that all babies are the product of sexual intercourse between a man and a woman. But we should not forget that our oversight in leaving this question out when taking a developmental history, along with parents' failure to tell us, goes back to the lack of coordination between medical and mental health professionals. We have failed to set a self-reflective process in motion for the men and women who are building families with donors or surrogates. If you're thinking of having a baby using assisted conception, you should have access to that kind of support system far earlier than birth or even gestation. At the same time, it is never too late to begin this process. This I have learned from many moving experiences sitting with mothers and fathers in my consulting room as they sort through the feelings they have had throughout their own wild ride in the pendulum swing between the power to create and the fear of creation. Subsumed in each of their stories is a wish that someone had helped them with this sooner.

SHOPPING FOR PERFECTION

Returning to swimming against the current, we now know that its force is swelled by parents' misgivings, the potential disapproval or discomfort of the people around them, and the lack of supportive guidance. Still, as parents swim, they will notice a lot of other people in the water. In a previous book, *Spoiling Childhood*, I identified a new diagnosis of the millennium: chronic parental anxiety. Modern parents are confronted with the professionalization of parenthood and increased emphasis on crafting the perfect child as perfect parents just at a time when there is less and less time to parent and more and more felt threats to a child's well-being. As a result, mothers and fathers are reeling from the pressures of raising a healthy, happy child with a dearth of time and social supports. The medical profession alerts us to all the things that could go wrong with our child, abnormalities that can show up on a sonogram screen before the baby is even born, and experts itemize all the precautions we should take to avoid harm and ensure our child's well-being. These are the social–medical waters in which *all* parents must swim. But when we factor in the elements of infertility, financial investment in expensive technologies and procedures, newfound hope that a baby so badly wanted is now within reach, and the cliffhanging angst that it still might not ever happen, we can only begin to imagine the skyrocketing of this chronic parental anxiety and the strength of the cross-currents when you make a baby using assisted reproductive technology.

So What's to Worry About?

If a prospective parent pays attention to the information just beginning to unfold about the potential risks to both parent and child from the use of fertility drugs and alternative birth technologies, the alarm sirens can begin to wail quite loudly. Oncologists, gynecologists, and endocrinologists worry about the effects of massive doses of fertility drugs on women's reproductive and general health. There is some anecdotal evidence that hormones used to promote egg receptivity may have lasting effects on the women receiving them. Some women just do not return to their normal functioning. There may even be an increased risk for certain kinds of cancer, particularly ovarian. Epidemiologists, neurologists, neonatal and pediatric medical experts, and developmental and clinical specialists have all expressed concerns that infants conceived with the use of assisted reproductive technology might have an increased risk of birth defects or developmental anomalies because of the tampering with sperm and eggs outside the body, the effects of fertility drugs or the medical procedures for impregnation, the advanced age of the eggs, sperm, and uterus, or the crowding of the womb with multiple fetuses.

A study conducted in Australia found that infants conceived with either in vitro fertilization or intracytoplasmic sperm injection procedures were significantly more likely to be delivered by cesarean section, to have low birth weight, and to be born before term. Further, they found that those conceived with such procedures were more than twice as likely as naturally conceived infants to have a major birth defect diagnosed by one year of age, particularly cardiovascular, urogenital, chromosomal, or musculoskeletal defects. A U.S. study found a significantly higher risk of low birth weight in babies born with assisted reproductive technology. A Swedish study found a higher rate of neurological complications and developmental delays in children conceived through in vitro fertilization, but some of this effect was attributed to the high incidence of multiple births among these children.[12] It should be pointed out that the absolute risks are still very low and that the majority of children so born, over ninety percent, will be just fine, at least as evidenced in their first year of life. These small risks may be quite inconsequential in any individual's or couple's decision to have a child through these procedures. Nonetheless, the risks are there. As such studies become more publicly disseminated, we'll have to add worry about developmental disaster to queasiness about unnatural means of conception in itemizing the fears of creation.

No parent can ever be fully prepared for the announcement that his or her child is afflicted with a physical or developmental anomaly. Not just parents creating babies with a birth other, but more and more parents of every variety—biological, assisted conception, adoptive, step-, foster—are alerted to the possibility of bad things happening and worry about it. To assuage angst, you can engage in a psychological ploy: turn up the amp of perfection to drown out the wailing siren of developmental disaster. If you eat the right foods during pregnancy, play the right music to your fetus, buy the appropriate cognitively stimulating toys for your infant, enroll your children in the right preschool, and find the best enrichment programs, your child will be resilient and successful and inoculated against developmental disablers. Many people accuse contemporary middle-class parents of having gone hog-wild—narcissistically overinvesting in their children's accomplishments, pampering and pressuring their children toward successes that will reflect well on themselves. While there are certainly some parents like that, the vast majority are not. They are just trying to manage their chronic parental anxiety by tempering it with ever-present evidence that their children are doing well—or maybe even perfectly.

The wails may reverberate even louder if you are a parent using assisted conception: Will you ever have your own baby? Will that baby be at higher risk for developmental anomalies? Will your baby be unnatural? Will other people see it that way? Will you be able to bond to a baby who is yours and someone else's?

Stop Your Worries, Go Shopping

To assuage your worries, you may find yourself engaged in a unique psychological defense against calamity. It is an opportunity not afforded to your contemporaries having babies the old-fashioned way but just as worried as you about their child being okay. You can go out "genetic shopping." You can embark on a quest for just the right donor or just the right surrogate. These days, old-fashioned parents-to-be can rely only on the primitive, gestational forms of genetic engineering to get them by, but you can actually shop. You can even go on the Internet in search of just the right person to be the birth other of your child. Customers looking for donor sperm can browse sperm banks' Web sites for basic information free of charge. With credit card in hand, they can then download potential donors' baby pictures, audiotapes, and personal essays.[13] Sophie Cabot Black, a mother in a lesbian couple, couldn't have said it better: "Once we made the leap into looking at sperm banks, it became a lot like shopping. Asking around, browsing catalogues, comparing prices."[14] Suddenly, you can feel like you have the whole world in your hands again as you discover the power to craft the child that will be yours.

The shopping expedition is not just an antidote to chronic parental anxiety. If you have confronted infertility, the sense of control taken away upon discovering you could not conceive your own child is restored with a compensatory form of power. You can carefully select half or all of the gametes of your child. If you are a single parent or gay or lesbian, your control is taken away by the absence of an intimate other who can make a baby with you, but you can regain control in the power given to you to shop for a donor or surrogate. For any of you who are part of a couple, the shopping expedition provides the opportunity for the nongenetic parent to play an active role in making your baby by participating in the shopping expedition. In the genetic shopping spree, we watch the pendulum of fear and hope reverse directions: The doubts about creating lead to an emboldened power over creation. Parents can become informed consumers searching for the best baby. Lynn Macklin, administrator of the Center for Surrogate Parenting and Egg Donation in Beverly Hills, tells it this way: "It's like shopping. If you have the option between a Volkswagen and Mercedes, you'll select the Mercedes."[15]

In 1999, an infertile couple made front-page news and all the tabloids when they advertised in Ivy League newspapers for an intelligent, athletic egg donor who was at least five feet ten inches tall and had an SAT score of 1400 or higher. They were willing to pay $50,000 for one cycle's worth of viable eggs.[16] People were horrified that someone could shop for a child like purchasing a fancy car, or invest in ova as if they were a good stock option. Widely publicized ads like this couple's have given a bad name to the vast majority of infertile couples or single or gay or lesbian parents who are not shopping for a Mercedes of a child but just trying to make a baby happen. Nonetheless, we cannot get around the fact that the opportunity to choose half or all of your child's genes in advance can lend itself to a sense of omnipotence and grandiosity.

Playing God to Your Majesty, the Baby

Being able to shop for your child's features among potential donors or search for a surrogate with the healthiest available womb only fuels the excitement and the power to craft a perfect child that is the overall ambiance of parenting today. The genetic shopping spree happens in the midst of a frenzied atmosphere in which childhood has become glorified and babies have become precious commodities for all parents. Newborns are no longer just little bundles that are delivered to your doorstep. They have been elevated to the status of "your majesty, the baby" and often maintain their place on the throne through their entire childhoods.[17] This cult of glorifying the baby affects most parents today. It only gets magnified when you've spent months, even years of your life searching for a donor or surrogate, drained your financial resources paying for high-priced procedures, or put your body through hell. By the time the baby arrives, it is like the coming of the Messiah, the miraculous baby who will bring power and glory to the waiting parents.

The exertion of power is at its height when a couple advertises a $50,000 payment to a tall, smart college co-ed so they can harvest her eggs to have the baby of their dreams. It is also at its height when the medical profession promises a customized baby. A clinic at Columbia–Presbyterian Medical Center will tailor-make an embryo for prospective parents by choosing both an egg donor and a sperm donor to match their desires. In southern California, Robert Klark Graham established the Repository for Germinal Choice. He collects the sperm of Nobel-prize-winning scientists and geniuses and then offers them only to highly intelligent women. The women must be members of Mensa, an international society of people tested to be the brightest two percent of the population. Victoria Kowalski was the first child born using Graham's sperm bank. Soon after Victoria's birth, her mother announced to the press, "The odds are very good that our little girl will be a genius. I imagine her as a child studying college textbooks." Victoria's father shared those sentiments: "We'll begin training Victoria on computers when she's three, and we'll teach her words and numbers before she can walk."

Every parent is entitled to engage in soaring fantasies of the endless possibilities for their newborn child. It is what I refer to as "expectable parental narcissism." It is the birthright of mothers and fathers as they forge a love bond with their new little being.[18] But I shudder over Victoria's parents' sense of engineering and control over a child who will lose her own identity as it is replaced by her parents' preprogrammed expectations. Such self-involved investment can be profoundly dangerous to a child's well-being. Where is the room for Victoria to unfold and become her own person, rather than the object of her parents' desires?

Control over perfection is at best only approximate, if not totally illusory. After all, just because you're tall doesn't mean your child will be. Just because you're a genius doesn't mean your child will follow suit. The reverse is also true. Parents of average intelligence have produced geniuses, and short parents have given birth to children who grow very tall. With that said, imagine the pressure on the child and the parents' deflation when all their careful efforts do not produce the child of their dreams. In our present era of consumerism and child perfectibility, the urge to play God in crafting a perfect child in a shopping expedition for the highest-quality gametes or wombs is compellingly seductive for any parent turning to assisted conception. After all, asks one couple who conceived a child with high-IQ sperm, "Why is it okay for people to choose the best house, the best schools, the best surgeon, the best car, but not try to have the best baby possible?"[19]

Perhaps because the quest is infused with a dangerous level of hubris, a false belief in one's ultimate control over nature by molding a child to precise specifications and an unwillingness simply to receive the child who comes to you. Remember, we are talking about a generation, now two generations, born in an era in which "having it all" and "taking control" have been people's mantra. This silver-spoon-in-your-mouth sensibility doesn't prepare people well for the realities of a life not always lined with silk. This leaves those among you who have chosen assisted conception susceptible to a particular form of this illusory control. If you search for perfect genes and believe you can craft a perfect child, you are fueled by and simultaneously fuel a soaring hope—you thought you could *not* but then discovered that you *could* have your own baby. The shopping expedition proves it's true.

The illusion of consumer control and perfectibility is also alluring for anyone who has struggled with infertility. What is on the other side of the pain of trying, again and again, of having gone through the psychological wringer, subjecting your body or witnessing your partner's body being subjected to repeated medical interventions, even breaking the bank in the process? The staunch feeling that this whole effort to make a baby has got to be worth the trouble. People often turn up the amp on the virtues of both the shopping expedition and the quest for perfectibility to drown out the deeper static of despair about getting a baby at all—I'll never have a baby, stop dreaming the impossible dream, it'll never really work, and it's definitely not worth the effort given the cost to my body, my psyche, my pocketbook, and/or even my relationship with my significant other. So why wouldn't any prospective parent embrace the shopping spree to hold on to a sense of power, optimism, and control in the face of these deeper anxieties about fertility and reproduction?

STILLING THE PENDULUM SWING
BETWEEN POWER AND FEAR

Unfortunately, the surge of power, optimism, and control is subject to blow-outs. It is hard for a parent to shake the gnawing realities of medical interventions, fertility drugs, bought gametes, or borrowed wombs, constant reminders of possible lurking disasters. In the case of egg- and sperm-donor babies, whose genes are these really, anyway? What if they are damaged, or not as good as the ones my partner or I could not provide? In the case of surrogacy, what if the surrogate has a festering womb, negligent pregnancy, or botched birth experience? How will I control that? What if the donor or surrogate comes in search of my child? What if the studies suggesting babies born with assisted reproductive technology are at higher risk for medical complications apply to *my* baby?

Worst of all, what about the human failures in these new technological interventions? Even though they may be playing God in these new miracle births, the medical personnel are, after all, only people. And people make mistakes. The most dramatic "gulp" in response to assisted reproductive technology is when there are baby mix-ups. In 1999, Donna Fasano, using in vitro fertilization with her eggs and her husband's sperm, gave birth to twins. The problem was that one was black. Neither she nor her husband is. It appears that the embryologist knew from the beginning that he had made an error in switching embryos, but he did not disclose or take responsibility for it. In a heart-wrenching decision, the Fasanos gave the black baby back to his genetic parents, even though they had grown to love him in the three months since his birth. They only hoped that the two babies, who had shared a womb inside Ms. Fasano, would remain in contact throughout their lives.[20] That is not the only time a mix-up has occurred. Race is an obvious giveaway that a mistake has been made, but parents can only begin to wonder about all the other potential hidden mistakes wrought by the new kind of baby making controlled not by heaven or their own actions but by overworked or careless medical experts and technicians susceptible to human error. Fantasies about such nightmarish fallibility are enough to take the wind out of anyone's sails.

Typically, parents like to feel at least partially in control of their children's destiny, even if this is a delusional belief. It is a protective coating, but one that is especially vulnerable to punctures when half of the child's very flesh and blood comes from an outsider, when the scientific community is beginning to suggest that the children so born are at risk for medical problems, and when the baby is conceived not by an act of love in bed but by medical personnel who could make a big mistake.

When your emotions are swinging like a pendulum, it is hard to think clearly. This is exactly what happens when parents using a birth other vacillate wildly between the sense of power in creation and the fear of damage to their creation. I am going to fast-forward to the story of Katy, the girl from Chapter 1 who Sylvie thought had a father *somewhere* out there. Katy's mother, Edie, a single woman who was over forty when she conceived, did all the right homework to choose an anonymous donor with strong intellectual and athletic abilities, a stable professional identity, and a similar ethnic background to her own. She reveled in her good choice, until her child showed some mild learning difficulties. Then the wall of good fortune came tumbling down, as she scrambled from specialist to specialist, trying to find the perfect cure and wailing that it was too late, she had chosen the wrong donor, and her child now faced a horrible future, a child who, in Edie's anxiety-distorted vision, was transformed into a mentally retarded daughter.

To attend better to Katy's learning needs, Edie had to release herself from the tensions between power and powerlessness so she could see and think more clearly, freed from the tyranny of her irrational fears. Because Edie herself had been quite outstanding in her academic career, the jolt of having a child who carried foreign, defective genes was almost more than she could bear. Her task was to step back and let Katy be a regular child with some minor problems just like any other child might have. It was not an all-or-nothing phenomenon. She had to face the delusional sense of power that had fueled her entry into parenthood and dispel the fantasy that the opportunity to shop for a donor was an insurance policy accompanied by a guarantee of child perfection. Simultaneously, Edie had to dig deep within herself and uncover the anxieties that were there from the beginning—that relying on a doctor, a syringe, fertility drugs, and the genetic material of a medical student young enough to be her son was risky and strange business. With the help of her therapist and her brother, who repeatedly nudged her to lighten up on both herself and Katy, Edie did this personal excavation and resolved that she neither controlled her child's destiny nor had caused her any harm by having her with an anonymous sperm donor.

The story of Katy and Edie is a lesson for all of us. It reveals the tension between the power to create and the fear of creation that can permeate the experience of parents who use assisted conception. The pulls between omnipotence and disillusionment or fear are in full gear before the baby is even conceived. And they never go away. Katy was nine years old, and her mother was still ruminating, even agonizing, about the shopping expedition gone awry—with all her careful perusal of a donor's characteristics, she still ended up with "damaged goods." Edie's main work was to drag to the surface deeply embedded thoughts and fantasies, some of which were buried in her unconscious. This allowed her to find her footing and stay on course.

It is both scary and exciting to have a baby using a donor or surrogate. Anxiety is an almost inevitable ingredient of this experience. The best way to manage that anxiety is to confront it head-on, rather than bury it. If you don't, not only might your anxiety keep growing, you might also build up a wall of defenses to protect yourself against its onslaught. When this happens, you're rendered far less effective in your mindfulness as a parent and in your responses to your child. Dealing with fears of creation head-on will counteract the tendency toward grandiose compensatory fantasies of playing God. How do you do this? Go back to the questions at the beginning of the chapter: How do you feel about the procedures, the use of someone else's gametes or womb, the effects on your child? How would you answer the questions now? Is there room for both positive and negative responses? Being able to answer the questions is not as important as the freedom to think fully about them—taking in the good, the bad, and the ugly and weaving them together. To do this is to facilitate a much smoother journey, beginning with the strong desire to have a child and ending with the actual existence of the child.

Katy and Edie's story also reminds us of another key player—the birth other. You will notice that in the preceding discussion of the power to create and the fear of creation one critical ingredient was left out: the presence of an outside person in the process, the donor or the surrogate. D. W. Winnicott once said that there is no infant without a mother, meaning that a child cannot survive in isolation and can be understood only in context of his or her relationship with his or her mother (to which I would add father). In the case of alternative-to-the-stork families, there is no infant without a mother or mothers, father or fathers, and birth others who participated in that child's conception. It is to that phenomenon, procreation with the proper stranger, that we will now turn.

Procreation with the Proper Stranger

> We have conceived a child without sex. . . . This was an extra-marital pregnancy. Our anti-adultery instincts certainly get alerted by that.
>
> —Mary Ann Thompson, a surrogate for her two close friends[1]

"No sperm, we get sperm. No egg, we get eggs. No uterus, we rent a uterus." These are the actual words of a reproductive endocrinologist barking his wares to any individual or couple trying to have a baby and willing to buy his services. How lucky for prospective parents in need of such ingredients—discovering they are now available for sale, culminating in the baby so badly wanted and finally within reach. Our kind doctor has overlooked one important fact—the sperm, the eggs, the uteruses do not come off the supermarket shelf. They come from whole people with minds and feelings, people who through the donation of their eggs or sperm or use of their wombs will inevitably become human participants, the birth others in these families.

The narrative of the birth other who helps make the dream of a baby come true is a very long story that weaves in and out of the entire lifespan of any family formed with assisted conception. Who will you choose to be the birth other? Will you want that person to be someone close to you? Will you even want to know who that person is? Will that person want to make him- or herself known or even claim some rights to your child? Will that person be part of your family's life? It is an endless stream of questions extending across many, many years, but for right now I want to stay focused on the beginning stage: making a baby with a someone else.

As we think through this process, here are some very specific questions for parents to ask:

- When I think about the donor or surrogate, what images come to mind?
- Are any of these feelings uncomfortable?
- Do any of them have to do with sex or erotic fantasies?
- Am I jealous, envious, or threatened by the birth other's participation in my child's birth?
- How does my thinking change if I think about an egg or a sperm or a womb versus thinking about the donor or the surrogate?

AND BABY MAKES TWO—OR THREE, OR FOUR, OR MORE

A few years ago, I attended a meeting bringing together gay men adopting children through foster care and clinicians working in a foster care project. One of the fathers told the story of a five-year-old boy adopted by a gay couple in an open adoption. One day, a little girl in his class at school got right in his face—"Wait a minute. How did you get born? You need an egg and a sperm to get born, and your house is all sperm. You need an egg." The little boy did not miss a beat. He glared right at her and snapped back, "I do too have an egg. She just doesn't live with us."

In the fertile new world of baby making, an egg has an address while a person is reduced to reproductive material in a dish. "Doing it"—creating a baby from a sexual union of love or a night in the hay—is now only one of several ways of "getting knocked up." In January 2003, a news report highlighted the number of men in the American military who were flocking to banks before being shipped off to Iraq—sperm banks. In the event of chemical warfare that might render them infertile, they wanted back-up sperm. Men both single and married were depositing their sperm in the bank. I believe this is the first time soldiers have gone off to war leaving their frozen sperm behind. In the past they just left their wives and girlfriends. Born in

1946, I was in the first cohort of the post-World War II baby boomers, children born nine months after their fathers returned from the warfront to the sexual intimacy of their marriages. Now the new return from war may be not to the bedroom but to a sperm bank and doctor's office.

We're not just talking about frozen sperm. Add a whole other cast of characters to "Just Molly and me" in the new birth stories. Imagine receiving an invitation like the one sent by two couples, the wife of one serving as the surrogate for the other: "Come and talk to four people who made a baby."[2] Four today. How many tomorrow?

A few years ago, I was reading an article about erotic feelings that surface in psychotherapy. I came to a halt when I read the following sentence: "Each of us is conceived out of the desire of two significant others."[3] Maybe some of us, but not all of us. Not anymore. Let's leave for the moment age-old situations of rape or sexual unions borne of violence or treachery leading to unwanted pregnancies far removed from desire. In our fertile new world, the quote that brought me to a standstill would need to be amended to read, "Each of us is conceived out of the desire of one or two people and possibly the help of one or more other people who participate in our conception not out of sexual desire but as a result of lending their bodies or their gametes so a baby could be made." If we take "the desire" to mean *sexual* desire, rather than desire to have a child, then sexual desire may be far removed from the laboratory procedure that led to a baby. Sexual desire is no longer a requisite for conception. Nor are two sexual partners. Indeed, science has allowed us to totally remove sexuality from reproduction, just as it previously allowed us to remove reproduction from sexuality after the discovery of effective birth control methods. Or has it?

YOU CAN TAKE THE REPRODUCTION OUT OF SEX . . .

"Couples who ultimately choose this alternative means of family building must be able to separate the act of lovemaking from the act of procreation."[4] This is the advice of Susan L. Cooper and Ellen Glazer in their book *Beyond Infertility.* My response: Easier said than done. It is my strong belief that we can take the reproduction out of sex, but we cannot so easily take the sex out of reproduction. At least not yet. Once having learned the story of sexual intercourse and baby making, we are hard pressed to rid ourselves of the scenario of man, woman, sex, and pregnancy. Fantasies of illicit sex, adultery, and a ménage à trois dance in our heads as soon as someone talks about making a baby in these revolutionary ways.

Maureen and Craig very much wanted a baby but discovered that Craig's sperm count was so low that it was impossible to conceive. They decided, while living abroad, that they would turn to donor insemination as a means of conceiving a child. They found an anonymous donor from southern France. All they knew about him was that he was a blond heart surgeon. Years later, they sat in my office talking about their decision to withhold the information from their son, Eli, that Craig was not his biological father. With long dark hair and sparkling brown eyes, Maureen was an intense, vibrant woman who looked far younger than her forty-some years. Craig, in his jeans and work shirt, was much older and had a softer, well-worn look about him, with an ethereally handsome face. Maureen let me know that she was clear in her conviction that withholding the information about insemination from Eli was the right thing to do, that it would be much better if Eli did not know, not now, not ever. Craig, on the other hand, had his doubts about concealing this information from him, worried about being dishonest with his son. He wanted to tell him now, when he was seven and old enough to understand, and not wait until he grew up and ended up feeling duped by a lie about his origins. The tension between Maureen and Craig—to disclose or not to disclose—piqued my curiosity, as it is typically the nonbiological, not the biological, parent who is more squeamish about telling their child that he or she is not the genetic parent. Why was Maureen so insistent about secrecy in the face of Craig's uneasiness about nondisclosure?

What surfaced was Maureen's tremendous discomfort when she contemplated communicating to their son her and Craig's personal history with sex, infertility, and reproduction. That's a really hard thing for any parent to do. Maureen also worried that if they decided to tell their son, Eli would quickly move the insemination information into a sexual scenario: "You mean you did it with someone else, Mommy?" Having had the opportunity to meet Eli, I was able to offer Maureen reassurance that their seven-year-old was more interested in his superhero figures than in the sexual activities of his mom and dad. I grew to understand that Maureen's worries about telling Eli had more to do with her own disquieting sexual thoughts than with any harm she might do to Eli. Maureen was a very attractive woman and herself daydreamed about sex and romance quite a bit. In one of our sessions she began to tell me about the circumstances of Eli's birth, which, as I mentioned, took place while they were living abroad. When it came to reporting the situation with the sperm donor, her whole demeanor changed—her voice lowered, and her face took on a dreamy look as she reported with obvious pride that Eli's donor was a blond heart surgeon from southern France. It was as if she were describing the most erotic of intimate rendezvous, rather than a medical procedure. Indeed, in her deepest private fantasies maybe she did "do it" with someone else, a French doctor to be exact.

It was hard for Craig to tolerate this, or leave room for Maureen to talk about her fears. Instead, as she told her story, Craig sat across the room from her—vacillating between anger and total deflation. Maureen and Craig were unable to resolve their differences and eventually separated. Several years later Maureen remarried—an American surgeon who became Eli's stepdad.

Maureen had anxieties about her illicit sexual fantasies. Craig could not tolerate hearing them. He was absorbed in remorse about his infertility and his need to overcome the shame of it by coming clean with his son. This prevented both of them from being able to think together about Eli's best interests.

You may have faced shame and remorse about infertility. You may have found yourself feeling squirmy because you felt like you were "doing it" with someone else, cheating on your partner. You may feel crazy anger because you find yourself feeling your partner was cheating on you, "hooking up" with a relative, friend, or stranger. You may feel disappointed because you don't have an intimate partner to "do it" with. These are all ingredients for anxiety trumping clear thinking as you fervently try to take the sex out of reproduction in your assisted conception. The anxiety can send you running in opposite directions. Sometimes you may put all your efforts into reducing the birth other to a thing or a part. It's far less likely you'll have sexual feelings toward an egg, a sperm, or a womb than toward a person. Other times you may find yourself creating a whole person in your fantasies when all you know about is a vial of sperm, a transferred egg, or a borrowed womb. And these fantasies can get pretty racy. Whether you find your psyche rendering wholes into parts or parts into wholes, both techniques are ways to negotiate the sexualized feelings that can get stirred up in procreation with the proper stranger. Typically, these are very unnerving feelings that no one wants to talk about, but it is far better to admit to and negotiate them than get tied up and contorted by them.

X-Rated Conception

Assisted conception has the potential to transform itself into a drama of illicit sex, adultery, and ménage à trois. The sperm donor, egg donor, or surrogate is not only a nice man or woman (if that), he or she may be another person who enters the sexual arena of man and woman, woman or man alone, two women, or two men, an interloper who treads on the erotic terrain where babies are made.

Scientifically, sex is separated from reproduction in the new forms of assisted reproductive technology. Any of you who have gone through high-tech reproductive procedures may have experienced the sterility and anti-sexuality of the experience. Hear the pain in this mother's words, a woman who used in vitro fertilization to conceive a baby:

> The substitution of aluminum probes and fluorescent lighting and lab attendants chatting about their weekends for copulation, flesh into flesh, grunting and groaning, had to be bad, had to cast a shadow, set a tone. I wanted my baby to begin life in the dark and bloody interiors of my body, not in a cold and sterile Pyrex dish. . . . I didn't want to believe that I was handicapped to the extent that I needed drugs, doctors, an operating room, and a laboratory to do what I should have been able to do simply by having sex with Dan.[5]

How could it not take the romance out of procreation when it happens in a cold sterile lab or between you and a turkey baster, or in an exquisitely timed choreography between an egg donor and recipient, or after an ejaculation into a jar that will be shipped off to the surrogate by special delivery? Surprisingly, it doesn't. Even with this strange phenomenon of sexless conception in the afternoon (or early, early in the morning, as many medical facilities would have it), sexual feelings don't just go away. Our psyches, because of genetic preprogramming and/or deeply rooted social conditioning, don't easily allow for the total expulsion of sex from the garden of baby making. With a sleight of the psyche's hand, sterilized conception is transformed into sexualized procreation—in the form of dreams, fantasies, and anxious musings.

"I've never told anyone this, but my husband is the only man I have ever had sex with. I'm afraid that having another man's sperm inside me would make me feel like I was sleeping with someone else."[6] A mother contemplating using donor sperm grows squeamish when the thought of the insemination stirs up fantasies of illicit sex with another man. Up pops another form of strange bedfellow—the birth other, actually in bed with you, albeit in fantasy.

Alexis, a single woman in her early forties, decided that she no longer wanted to wait to have a child—her biological clock was ticking with alarming volume. She decided to look for a known donor, someone who might also be interested in co-parenting a child with her. She found just the right man through her contacts in the gay community. She and James met and decided to go forward with an insemination procedure. During the period when the inseminations were taking place, Alexis shared with me romantic and sexual fantasies she was having about James. Even though he was gay, she began to wish they could get together and "do it." She daydreamed about how his body would look and how it would feel to be with him in bed. These thoughts brought her great pleasure, but also disappointment, because she knew it would never come to pass.

Mary Ann Thompson, who became a surrogate for her close friends, had her own erotic encounters with Mandel, the father of the child she was carrying: "Mandel and I glanced at each other—I felt shy and excited observing him with completely new eyes…Mandel is a wonderful man, but to be having such intimacy with the husband of a friend was anomalous."[7] All throughout her pregnancy such "anomalous" thoughts reverberated through her head. In her fantasies, Mandel had crept into her bed.

Charlie and Jo were now divorced. But many years before, when Charlie discovered that he could not reverse his vasectomy, he and Jo decided to have a baby using an anonymous donor. Rather than using a sperm bank, they solicited the donor through their community networks. The donor was supposed to remain anonymous, but both Jo and Charlie, through a sequence of coincidences and leaks, figured out who he was. Actually, he was no stranger, but someone who had been part of their social life in the past. Although he was now married with children of his own, Jo rekindled their friendship, visiting his family and making repeated references to him in Charlie's presence. Like Maureen talking about the French doctor, Jo's whole self seemed to soften and even undulate as she spoke of this attractive man whom she believed to be the genetic father of her child. This drove Charlie up a wall, and what surfaced, in addition to the threats to his legitimacy as their child's father, was his raw jealousy, envy, and rage in the face of the erotic connotations of Jo's renewed connections with this man. No longer was the donor a generous man who selflessly gave his sperm so Jo and Charlie could have a child. To Charlie he was a sexual threat and competitor, even several years after he had divorced Jo. And for Jo he temporarily became the object of her erotic fantasies. Charlie and Jo were unable to talk to each other about these feelings. However, as the heat died down for Jo and as she was able to offer Charlie assurance that her primary interest in the donor was to secure for Caroline knowledge of her genetic roots, the sexual drama faded into the background.

A lesbian mother in a couple had her own creative response to this potential sexual competitor, the donor. The couple's child had been conceived by her partner and a known sperm donor. She accompanied her partner to the insemination, tucking the bag of fresh sperm under her armpit to keep it warm on the way to the doctor's office. She developed a new narrative to the birth story—she and her partner, rather than her partner and the donor, had conceived a child together, because, after all, she had hand-delivered the sperm that made the baby. Her tale is emblematic of creative birth concepts evolving from assisted reproductive technology, concepts that I have come to think of as "immaculate deception." Immaculate deception allows this mother to delete the donor from the conception process. Simultaneously, she could reinvent herself as the only partner in this sexy conception. She drew pleasure from the erotic imagery of the warm sperm so close to her body, of her own physical closeness to her partner as the sperm that was kept alive only because of the heat of her own body went up her lover's vagina. From that intimate, erotic closeness a baby was made.

Which Is Sexier—Sperm or Eggs?

All of these stories are about people who injected sexual fantasies into the medical procedures of assisted reproductive technology. And in each of these situations the fantasies or anxieties emanated from the act of procreating with *another* man's or *any* man's sperm. If you have chosen donor insemination as the way to have a child, you may be especially vulnerable to sexualized images. In our culture, sperm have been inextricably linked with sexuality, in a way ova never are. Eggs symbolize birth, purity, even housing for the young. We eat eggs for our nourishment. We have an Easter egg, but no comparable Easter sperm. We have Humpty Dumpty—the anthropomorphized egg who had a great fall—but no comparable Spermy Wormy in our cache of children's nursery rhymes. Instead, sperm symbolize sexual passion, male virility, even male dominance, more likely showing up in dirty jokes and pornography than in children's toys or tales.

I believe this sensibility regarding sex and sperm is deeply embedded in our unconscious, despite our conscious awareness of sperm as merely the male seed that connects with the female egg. Indeed, sex is what made one mother decide not to use her infertile husband's father or brother as a sperm donor: "Lou's father and brother both offered to donate sperm, but Felicia was repulsed by the 'incestuous' aspect of using either man's sperm. However, Felicia said that if she had been infertile, she would not have had a problem using her sister's eggs because they bore none of the sexual connotations that sperm do."[8]

But is it true that egg donation will totally quash any sexy thoughts? If you are a woman, probably yes. When you borrow someone else's eggs in order to conceive, you are placing something in your body that your own body would normally produce, rather than borrowed semen from a man. It is a woman-to-woman phenomenon. Implanting eggs has connotations of fecundity, pregnancy, and motherhood, rather than being associated with sexuality and lovemaking, as sperm are.

If you are a man in an egg-donor family, your sexual thoughts might not be so easily quashed. The connections to fecundity, pregnancy, and motherhood may not stop you from fantasizing about the woman whose egg joined with your sperm to create the baby who is growing inside your wife or partner. Bob Shacochis recalls his experience reading the questionnaire filled out by the anonymous twenty-three-year-old woman who was his and his wife's egg donor and with whom "two days previously, I had had test-tube sex." The night before, he had a dream: ". . . I had dreamed about this young woman I will never meet, we sat in a room together and talked, although I could not remember what we said."[9] He reported this dream to his wife. She wondered what the young woman looked like. She hoped that his dream image might provide a forecasting of her own child's looks, half of which would come from this dreamed-about woman.

Given Bob's allusions to test-tube sex, we can wonder whether the room and the talking in the dream were as innocent as that. Under any other circumstance, I can imagine a wife becoming understandably unsettled if her husband tells her a dream about a private tête-à-tête with another, younger woman. Yet Bob's wife's curiosity was piqued only by her associations with their own child-to-be. In his account of the dream neither Bob nor his wife was attending to the possible sexual connotations of his fantasies about this young woman with viable eggs to give, the young woman with whom he had had, by his own account, "test-tube sex." When it came to the sexual innuendos surrounding the egg donor, he only alluded to it and his wife deftly avoided it.

The "Affair"

We cannot get around it. There is sex in the air when sperm donors, egg donors, and surrogates enter the scene. This creates angst. Sometimes the anxiety is transferred into worries about the children. It is almost standard fare in a discussion of assisted reproductive technology to have someone bring up the hair-raising question "But what if a sister unwittingly marries her brother?" The likelihood of half-siblings of the same anonymous donor meeting up with each other and falling in love is small, but the concern, of course, is real, given the taboo on incest and our scientific understanding of the potential physical damage to offspring conceived from a union of close blood relatives. I also think the question of unwitting incest so readily pops to mind because of the disquieting undercurrent of eroticism that gets activated when men and women turn to an outside party to make a baby.

Eroticism permeates the conception experience. For both single and coupled parents, no holds are barred for fantasies of illicit sex, adultery, or even sex across boundaries of sexual orientation. For mothers and fathers who are in couples, whether same sex or opposite sex, the presence of a birth other is especially ripe for ménage à trois dramas.

"I felt like the odd woman out in the donor egg process, as my old friend from college was my donor, but this meant that her eggs would be fertilized by *my* husband's sperm. They are making the embryo/baby while I wait, then I'll carry *their* embryo that I didn't contribute to making."[10] If we boil her feelings down to their essence, this mother feels she's been put in the position of watching her husband get together with another woman while she sits on the sidelines and even participates in their lovemaking by carrying *their* child. And what she may be reexperiencing is a very old feeling from her childhood. The position of this mother as "the odd woman out" was labeled many years ago by Sigmund Freud as the primal scene, the early and upsetting knowledge that your mother and father are engaging in a sexual act together, an act that excludes you.

Beginning with Freud, psychoanalysts have argued that the primal scene is part of the universal human condition, while others have called it a social concoction. However, most agree that within Western culture children are intrigued by what goes on behind the bedroom door, particularly their parents' bedroom door. In this scenario children grow simultaneously excited and disquieted by the entry of a third person, whether it be themselves or someone else, into the intimate scene behind their parents' closed door. Over time this disquiet dissipates, but it never disappears. We can locate the residues of the drama in our intimate adult relationships. There is nothing more intense than the rage and distress that arises upon discovering a spouse or partner's love affair with someone else. And, sure enough, the drama also finds its way into assisted conception.

Bringing an egg or sperm donor or a surrogate into baby making can stir up these archaic bedroom scenarios, stimulating fantasies of illicit extramarital sex or ménages à trois. The fantasies spill out in all directions, and they dance in other people's heads, not just the parents'. For example, if you are a husband of a surrogate, you may need support in the face of friends' or family's questions about how you could let your wife get pregnant by another man. Not only are the queries judgmental, they are also laden with sexual innuendo about the husband's wife "doing it" with another man right under the husband's nose.[11] Recipients, donors, surrogates, significant others—it will help if you all prepare yourselves for the eroticized connotations of procreation in the afternoon. And it will help if all of us around you sensitize ourselves to our own infusion of sexuality into the process of assisted conception lest we unwittingly "lay a trip" on the mothers and fathers who are building their families in these fertile new ways.

At a deeply unconscious level we all fight against the resurfacing of these sexualized images, as they make us uneasy, even queasy. And at a conscious level we assuage our anxieties by reducing the threatening birth others to sperm, eggs, or uteruses. Alternatively, we may transform them into nice, generous men or women who dispassionately dispense their sperm or eggs or offer their wombs as selfless and sexless gifts to the childless. A better solution is simply to acknowledge the erotic feelings and accept them, at least at this moment in history, as coming with the territory of assisted conception. Rather than fight against them, you can pay attention to and talk about them and be ready to acknowledge your intimate other's feelings as well, so they don't fester as shameful or hidden secrets. In the end, these feelings are just part of doing what comes scientifically.

INFERTILITY, *MACHISMO*, AND *FEMINISMA*

Sex can also creep into reproduction through two other back doors. The first is infertility, and the second, which goes hand in hand with infertility, is *machismo* for men, *feminisma* for women. The pain of infertility is an age-old story, going back to the woes of Sarah in her failure to produce a child for Abraham. If you are heterosexual and have chosen assisted conception, your choice is typically a second choice. The first choice, particularly if you are in a couple, would have been to conceive a baby through sexual intercourse with an intimate other. If it was infertility or disease that thwarted your first choice, you may have to mourn the loss of the possibility of making a child of your own.[12] Those of you who have left your first choice to turn to assisted conception to have a baby may then find yourself facing yet another affront to your sense of self—your manhood, your womanhood. Who is challenging your self-concept as a "whole" man or "whole" woman? The birth other, the fertile man or woman who will take your place in the scenario of procreation with the proper stranger, the person who may make you feel like a "birth nobody."

No Mother Wants to Be a Birth Nobody

Agnes Rossi coined the term *feminisma*, saying "the essence of feminisma is the ability to create a living, breathing human being in the space between one's hipbones."[13] I would not go so far as to say every woman carries or breathes that essence. Yet when it does infiltrate your being and you find yourself deprived of the opportunity to make and carry that little being within you, you may be left with the sad feeling that you've lost your womanhood. You grew up imagining that the doll in your carriage was your own, and now you discover it never will be, at least not one made by your own eggs. Often there is no time to mourn this loss, because time is of the essence and deep maternal desire can drive you forward at a rapid speed. So think about it this way: You may be someone who is still reeling from the experience that you will never conceive or bear a child, and now, if you turn to an egg donor or surrogate to have a child, you will be letting in your life another woman who faces no challenge to her *feminisma*.[15] You'll be joining with another woman who can produce viable eggs by the thousands or bring healthy fetuses to term between her hipbones, not only for herself but for others as well. To add insult to injury, if you are an egg-donor mother or if your child was born to a surrogate, you may also find yourself collaborating with a woman much younger (maybe even more beautiful) than you or with a sister, relative, or close friend who can do so easily what you haven't been able to. Even if you never meet this woman, she still exists in fantasy.

Seven years after her son's birth, Natalie sat in my office fretting over the one thing she hadn't taken care of—she had never gotten around to sending a letter to the egg donor thanking her for the wonderful child that she had helped Natalie have. Like Natalie, many mothers often express deep gratitude toward the egg donors or surrogates who have generously given of themselves so that the mothers can become mothers. Yet what often bites these mothers from behind is the sensation of unexpected but intense envy. And, as rumor has it, there is a long history and no bounds to a woman's envy. Way back in the Old Testament, Sarah banned Hagar from her land because Sarah could not tolerate her own jealousy toward this handmaiden who had borne a child for her.[16] You may not just be jealous of the other woman who, in fantasy, "did it" with your partner. You may also deeply envy what that other woman has—the ability to get pregnant or bear a child. It may be so much what you wanted for yourself, and the frustration of not having it can become a constant and sometimes consuming source of pain in collaborating with an egg donor or surrogate who does have the ability.

Melanie Klein, in her psychoanalytic theory of development, defined basic envy as an attack on what is perceived as good—most specifically, the mother. The frustration of not having what the mother has or not getting what the mother has to offer can sometimes lead the infant to want to spoil things, to get inside and attack the good mother, according to this theory. With time, the infant develops the capacity for gratitude for all that the mother gives, and that sense of gratitude calms the tides of envy so that the child can go on to live a productive and healthy life. But that earliest of feelings, intense envy toward someone good, can resurface at any time in life under the proper circumstances. When you are a mother-to-be who must make use of another woman's body to have a baby, you may encounter just such a circumstance.

To be prepared to negotiate the full experience of procreation with a birth other is to recognize that the flip side of the feelings of gratitude toward the birth other is a darker side—a strong sense of envy, even hostility or hatred. Veronique was shocked to find herself tearfully tearing up the photograph of Martine with her swelling belly. Veronique had discovered that endometriosis and fibroid tumors prevented her from ever having a child of her own. Martine, Veronique's cousin, agreed to be a surrogate for Veronique and her husband. Martine lived several states away. She had made an arrangement to send Veronique a picture every month so Veronique could see her baby growing. Every month Veronique waited eagerly for the picture and reveled at the quick pace of her baby's growth inside Martine's womb. Until that one afternoon when something snapped. Veronique remembered all the ways she always felt inferior to Martine. She tore the picture of pregnant Martine into shreds and then collapsed in a heap. She thought she was going nuts and became scared that she had made the biggest mistake in her life, doing this surrogate thing.

Rather than being frightened by her rageful feelings, it helped Veronique to discover that her feelings were merely an outgrowth of the challenge to her *feminisma* as she faced both the failures of her body and the need to turn to her cousin with a body in working order to have the baby of her dreams. She did this by going on-line, contacting other mothers who had used surrogates through a chat line, describing what had happened to her and asking if any other mothers had had similar experiences. She received an outpouring of responses, all with variations on the theme of her own "green with envy" destructive moment.

A woman's experience of collaborating with a donor or surrogate to have a child may evoke the very earliest feelings of dependency on another female body that had everything the mother did not. Even when we replace the concept of infertility with the notion of alternative conceptions, we cannot totally soothe the pain if your own body didn't work as you had planned, and, hard as you tried, the only thing you could do to have a child of your own was to turn to another woman's body.

Mary Ann Thompson, the surrogate, was struggling with the erotic rumblings in her interactions with Mandel, the husband of her friend for whom she was being a surrogate. But she wasn't the only one struggling. Alycia, the mother-to-be, couldn't even bear to be around Mary Ann during a good part of Mary Ann's pregnancy. Alycia resisted watching her friend's belly grow with the child conceived by Mary Ann and Alycia's husband. Mary Ann describes Alycia's experience as seen through her eyes:

> The iron bar of her [Alycia's] self was heated from the inside. It began to heat from the hurt, the anger, the frustration of her infertility, of all the emotions of our pregnancy and our broken relationship, from the cultural expectations, from factors she could not even identify. . . . Those forces were

the injustice of not being able to conceive, the raw fact of her infertility, the specific manifestation of being unable to create life, a child, with her beloved Mandel. Her iron rod self was beaten on by the way the world was. Pounded by how I could conceive and she couldn't.[17]

Pounded by how she can conceive and I can't. That underscores the raging current, the envy of the infertile mother toward the woman who will donate her eggs, lend her womb so the mother can have a baby. The green eye of infertility envy burns its way into other types of assisted conception as well. Heather and Betty were a lesbian couple who decided it was time to have a child. They each wanted the experience of pregnancy, but Heather, the older of the two, was to go first. She tried for several months to become pregnant with donor insemination and the boost of fertility drugs. Nothing worked. Tensions mounted between her and Betty. They made a deal that if Heather didn't get pregnant after twelve months of trying, Betty would start trying. Twelve months passed. No pregnancy. So, per agreement, Betty started trying. Just at that time Heather consulted another specialist who saw no reason why she couldn't get pregnant. So for a period of time both women tried to get pregnant, with the agreement that whoever got pregnant first, the other would stop trying. Heather never got pregnant. Betty did, with little effort. That marked the beginning of the end of their relationship. Heather could not tolerate the pain of Betty's doing what she couldn't—bearing a child. Heather's envy was not toward a donor or surrogate, but toward her own lover, who in essence, had been transformed into the surrogate who would carry the child that Heather could never make.

If the pain of envy toward another woman who can do what you can't weren't enough, the plot thickens when some of those envious feelings get translated into rumblings of sexual threat. If you are infertile, not only do you have to confront the feelings of barrenness, you may also have to endure the feelings, if they rise to the surface, of being the odd woman out, the rejected lover who witnesses your partner's liaison with another woman. Not just any woman, but a woman who may be quite a bit younger than you, stoking the fires of the prototypical female fear of being left for a younger woman or a trophy wife. And in the vagaries of unconscious life where anything goes, these rumblings can occur in myriad gender and sexual combinations, creating many variations on the primal scene.

Recall the story of the mother who felt like the odd woman out. Caught up in a quagmire of disquieting feelings, she found it painful to imagine that she would be carrying the fetus of her husband and her college friend in *her* womb. In her inner fantasies she had to confront her feelings about her fertile friend who "got together" with her spouse to do what she was unable to do—get pregnant. But here is another story of a mother whose spouse was not a man but another woman. Georgette and Vicky were a lesbian couple who decided to have a baby together. Since Vicky already had two children, they decided that Georgette should be the biological mother. They solicited a gay friend of theirs to be the sperm donor. After several tries, they discovered that Georgette was infertile. They then decided that Vicky should be the biological mother, as she already had a good track record in conceiving. But age was not on their side, and they soon found out that Vicky, now in her forties, was no longer fertile. They then decided to use an egg donor and the gay friend's sperm. Because Georgette had never carried a child, they decided she would be the gestational mother. This all seemed like a fluid and harmonious decision-making process, until Georgette indeed was pregnant, and all hell broke loose. Georgette grew envious of Vicky's more traditional road to motherhood (if one can consider conception with a sperm donor traditional), resentful that Vicky once upon a time got to birth babies made with her own eggs. She began having uncontrollable fantasies that Vicky and the sperm donor were beginning a romantic liaison with each other. Even though a donor's egg, rather than Vicky's, had contributed to the conception of their child, and it was actually the gay friend and the egg donor who "did it" together, Georgette displaced her jealous feelings onto Vicky. Georgette also had fantasies of Vicky getting together with the egg donor, who was known to both of them. As excited as Georgette was to be pregnant, she also was tormented by her experience of being the jilted woman, suspicious of the sexual intrigues that seemed to be transpiring all around her. Infertility and a challenge to her *feminisma* had both played their hand in injecting sex into reproduction rather than extracting it.

Georgette had many insecurities from her own childhood that fed her anxieties. But the point I want to make here is that so many of the mothers I have met suffer through these anxieties in their own private hells, shamefully believing they are the only ones who ever had such bad thoughts. Distress about being a birth nobody, fueled by *feminisma*, shows up in mothers—both straight and gay—when they find themselves in competition with the other woman, the birth other with viable eggs or womb. These mothers at other times can feel a swell of gratitude and love toward the women who are helping them have a baby. If you are one of these mothers, I hope it will help you to know that the feelings of envy and gratitude are not mutually exclusive, nor crazy to feel toward the same woman. Envy and gratitude are simply two threads that weave together to create the tapestry of feelings of becoming a mother with the help of an egg donor or surrogate. Rather than sweep the bad feelings under the rug, talk about them—with yourself, with your partner if you have one, with the donor or surrogate if she is close to you, and with other women who have gone through or are going through the same experience.

No Dad Wants to Be Shooting Blanks

While mothers struggle with the affront to their *feminisma*, fathers struggle with their own gender "bruising." To date, men cannot get pregnant. In contrast to women, their core definition of self is often less centrally tied to fertility and parenthood. But if *feminisma* is a coined word, *machismo* is not. I know this because as I write these words my computer spell check program redlines *feminisma* but leaves *machismo* untouched. *Machismo*: "strong or assertive masculinity, characterized by virility, courage, aggressiveness, etc." (*Webster's Unabridged Dictionary* definition). Notice that the very first attribute listed for *machismo* is virility. And that is exactly what is challenged when a man discovers he is infertile and must use another man's sperm to sire a child. In contrast to eggs, we may not find an abundance of sperm-related fairytales or toys (unless we want to include toy guns, rifles, and rockets). But the culture is replete with phallic symbols associated with strong and dominant sperm. In our society's rendition we have constructed the story of sperm actively swimming up to passive eggs waiting to be impregnated, even though we have discovered scientifically that these sperm are really rather weak creatures that need the help of the woman's cilia and mucosa membrane to move them along. A man with no viable sperm is no man at all in our cultural myths of masculinity. He is limp, impotent, a discredit to his gender. He holds no power—he shoots blanks.

If you are a man who cannot make a baby, you, too, may be touched by envy. But it's rather different from a woman's. You may be hit with a surge of resentment toward the "real" man who can give your wife or partner what you can't—a child. Recall Charlie's emotional upheaval when Jo forged a bond with the man she believed was their daughter's donor. Your envy might not be as debilitating as a mother's toward a donor. Having a baby might not be as much at the core of your being. Like the egg donor, the sperm donor might be a younger man, but in our culture most husbands don't worry as much about their wives running off with a younger man as wives do about husbands running off with a younger woman. Yet, still, the envy toward the real man persists.

If it is an affront to your masculinity to turn to a sperm donor to have a baby, you may feel not only envy but also shame or humiliation. Women who can't make babies feel shame or humiliation, too, but, alas, for men, infertility quickly becomes equated with emasculation. This can be the catalyst for some very bad feelings or thoughts.

Christopher had been married to Annemarie for five years when they finally decided it was time to start a family. They were both in their early thirties and assumed a baby would come in no time. All their sisters and brothers had at least three kids. But twelve months went by with no baby in sight. Christopher and Annemarie went for a fertility work-up, where it was discovered that Christopher had almost zero sperm count. It was before the days of intracytoplasmic sperm injection (ICSI), where a doctor can help a couple have a baby by taking just one sperm and injecting it directly into a woman's egg in an in vitro procedure. Finding out Christopher was infertile was a blow to both of them, but Annemarie soon reached the conclusion that they should use donor sperm to have a baby. Christopher wasn't so sure. He imagined how he would explain this to his friends and family. There was just no way. He anticipated people's silent judgments, particularly his buff older brother's—"What kind of guy can't even get his wife pregnant?" He had a nightmare about a baby who called him a wimp. The 2003 *New Yorker* cartoon had yet to be published—a boy and a man with a "World's Greatest Dad" T-shirt cross paths with a man with a "World's Greatest Sterile Guy" T-shirt.[18] That might have lightened his load.

When a father can't beget his own child, he may imagine his children will not love him because he is not their biological father. He may imagine being a poor and weak role model for his son or daughter. He may imagine other men deriding him for not being a real man.

One way infertile men like Christopher, with the help of people around them, try to shield themselves from this pain is to hide the fact of their infertility so as to preserve their manhood. Indeed, donor insemination, the oldest form of assisted reproductive technology, was designed as a private and discreet reproductive strategy that no one ever had to know about. A doctor could match a donor's features to those of a husband. This way the child would be protected from aspersion, the family would remain "normal," and last but not least, the father could be protected from the shame of infertility. The effort to preserve the father's manhood sometimes foreclosed any thoughtful examination of the best interests of the family—whether the family secret really enhanced rather than diminished their well-being.

Fortunately, times are changing. Ironically, infertile fathers using sperm banks are benefiting greatly from the actions of their strange bedfellows—single women and lesbian couples, experiencing no problems with fertility, who have become the fastest-growing clientele of sperm banks. They are the ones who have pushed for identity release programs and for openness rather than secrecy about assisted conception. After all, with no male parent, they are going to have to come up with some explanation for how their baby came to be. As these women advocate for openness, insemination, along with infertility, is neutralized from a hidden shame to merely a challenging physical condition. But we're not quite there yet. In the meantime, if you're confronted with male infertility, you may still grapple with angst about your virility, which can so easily be exacerbated when the donor is a young medical student who has not only viable sperm but also high intelligence and high earning potential, maybe more than your own.[19]

Donor insemination's challenge to machismo is not just the purview of heterosexual men. Stephen Byrnes described his and his gay partner Jamie's experience with surrogacy. He and Jamie decided that Stephen would be the biological father. But after three failed inseminations, the surrogate grew restless and suggested they switch to Jamie's sperm, sperm that "tested off the charts." Shot down by a woman and replaced by his partner, Stephen is taken aback by his emotional reaction:

> I feel like I'm about to get bumped from the team, and it feels like every unfair rejection I've ever suffered. I rise to defend my seed and am surprised by the intensity of my feelings. I thought I was immune to silly macho posturings over sperm strength. Obviously, I'm not.[20]

No inoculation exists to provide immunity against such "silly macho posturings"—even if you're a gay man who, by declaring your homosexual identity, thought you had defied gender roles by going against the grain of prescribed cultural norms of masculinity and virility. Instead, any man who has confronted infertility and turns to donor insemination should be prepared to negotiate potential feelings of rejection, dejection, and inadequacy. The man you might be grateful to for helping you have a baby may be the same man you rail against as the Marlboro Man who makes you feel like a wimp and a discredit to your gender. He may be a stranger, he may be your own partner, but whoever he is, he may pop up as the idealized image of the real man you couldn't be.

Like the woman with her envy, insult is added to injury when these feelings of shame, humiliation, and inadequacy translate into sexual tensions. Marsha Levy-Warren, a psychologist in New York, writes about a family she worked with in which the children had not been told they were conceived with a mixture of their father's weak sperm and the more viable sperm of a donor. The father reports that the birth of his son, David, was a constant reminder to him of what he saw as his compromised masculinity, a feeling that appeared to interfere with his relationship with his son from then on. Sitting in a therapy session, he explains to the therapist and to his wife: "It was probably the worst time in my life. I felt like we should get divorced, so she could be with a real man." Embedded in this statement are this father's fantasies of his wife with another man, sleeping with him, having his babies, while the father skulks off into the fading sunset with his nonworking assets. Perhaps in this father's fantasy life the donor played the part of that "real man," the man whose sperm probably outran his in the race to his wife's eggs.

Fortunately, Dr. Levy-Warren didn't leave it at that. Rather than try to move him away from his feelings, she simply bore witness to them. She then suggested that his shameful feelings might be alleviated if he could finally talk to his son and daughter about their conception and relieve himself of his anxieties about being less than a real man in his wife's and in his children's eyes. He did this, and instead of aspersion, he received his son David's compassion: "I was really thinking about how bad you might have felt when you and Mom couldn't have a kid and it turned out to be because you had this problem."[21]

Let's come back to Stephen Byrnes, the gay father confronting possible infertility. He felt like he was about to be bumped from the team. But I can't help thinking that it wasn't just a team that he felt excluded from when the surrogate turned from him to his partner, Jamie, who had sperm that tested off the charts. I can also imagine him as the jilted boy at the school dance who has lost his dance partner as his best friend cuts in to swing her around the dance floor. Gay or straight, the threat to *machismo* reigns supreme in stimulating sexual threats and tensions for the father who must rely on another man's sperm to have a baby.

GETTING BIRTH OTHER FANTASIES A PG RATING

If we weave together the stories I've told you about sexualized experiences with a birth other on the scene, we see a repeated pattern. If you are a nonbiological parent, you may feel threatened. If you are a biological parent, you may find yourself drifting into erotic fantasies. This makes logical sense. After all, it is the biological parent who is "doing it" with someone else. If you are a partnered biological parent, prepare yourself for unexpected feelings of adultery—images of cheating on your partner, doing something illicit, fantasizing about a person you never expected to find in your erotic fantasies, someone you may never even have met. If you are a single biological parent, prepare yourself for being titillated by sexy thoughts about the proper stranger or even about a close friend, someone you start to imagine hooking up with. If you are a nonbiological parent in a couple, prepare yourself for jealous rumblings about the other man or other woman who contributes half the genetic make-up of your child and "gets together" with your loved one, albeit in a laboratory dish or doctor's office, to make the baby that you will then claim as your own. So what do we do with all these unexpected feelings?

Sometimes we totally deny them:

> I [the surrogate] had asked Alycia [the mother] frequently in this process what she thought it would be like, and now what it was like for her to have her husband's child gestating in me. Was there instinctual jealousy? I would expect there would be. Was there anger at me for conceiving quickly and easily? She said no. Over and over she said no. That answer didn't make sense to me.[22]

Indeed, Alycia's actions throughout the pregnancy showed otherwise. She shut herself off from the surrogate. She demonstrated an apparent lack of interest in the baby; she denied any bad feelings; she avoided the scene, all tactics that helped her put a lid on difficult feelings bubbling underneath. Alycia used denial and avoidance to master her feelings of envy and jealousy toward the surrogate. But there's a whole other set of psychological maneuvers we can call on to assuage our anxieties about sex and reproduction when a birth other becomes a strange bedfellow.

It is not easy to have sexual rumblings or envious or jealous feelings toward the person who was generous enough to become a donor or surrogate, particularly when we thought we were taking the sex out of reproduction. So here's a simple solution—shrink the donor to a vial of sperm or a carton of eggs or reduce the surrogate/gestational carrier to the status of an incubator. Get rid of them as people; turn them into things.

In the face of our sexual queasiness and more general uneasiness about the birth other's presence, we have no ready place for the sperm donors, egg donors, and surrogates in the birth drama. What if they show up in our feelings as an interloper, an object of envy, or a sexual threat? Well, we can do a quick trick of the mind by depersonalizing them. We'll be far less threatened by a body part than by a breathing, living human being. In the case of sperm, those tadpole-shaped little creatures are disembodied from the whole person of the man who made them. In the case of eggs, those microscopic particles that are never seen by the naked eye are divorced from the woman whose ovaries created them. It is hardest to do with a surrogate or carrier, who will visibly grow with child, but nonetheless, we can get rid of her as a person by thinking of her only as the temporary housing for the child.

Is the Part the Sum of Its Whole?

We come by such trickery honestly. In the theories of infant development, psychoanalysts have developed the notion of "part-object" and "whole-object" relating. They never intended this to be a tool to understand procreation with the proper stranger, but, actually, it works. Melanie Klein talked about the infant relying on body parts to represent the whole, especially breast = mother. A baby doesn't close her eyes and dream about Mom. The baby imagines the breast that's going to come and feed her. This is called *part-object relating.* It's considered the most primitive form of relating to another human being, one based on innate knowledge. As the infant grows, the baby discovers that mother is more than a breast. She is a whole being outside the baby's control. She comes and goes, with a mind of her own. This is called *whole-object relating* and is celebrated as the entrance to healthy interpersonal relationships and healthy personal development, where people recognize and acknowledge each other with compassion and concern. As life goes on, times of stress may temporarily catapult us back to this earlier time in life, when the whole is not more than the sum of its parts but is actually reduced to a part in our inner fantasies. Whether babies really engage in part-object relating remains to be proven empirically, but in the context of the anxieties stirred up by procreation with the proper stranger, we certainly find a reversion to such reductionism among adults in the new equation: sperm = biological father, egg = biological mother, womb = gestational mother. We had our baby with donated sperm. There is no donor. We purchased eggs to have our baby. There is no donor. We found a womb because mine didn't work. There is no surrogate (this one, of course, is harder to pull off, as the womb doesn't separate from the person as eggs and sperm do). These sleights of mind, shrinking the birth other into a body part, provide a good strategy for keeping that person out of the bedroom. But the strategy also has its problems.

Honey, I Shrunk the Donor

I'd like to move for a moment from the bedroom to the children's room to il-lustrate how we adults indulge in this part-object thinking when we incorpo-rate the birth other into the birth story. Such reduction of a person to a body part unwittingly surfaces in a sensitively written children's book, *Let Me Explain: A Story about Donor Insemination.*[23] The protagonist, a little girl, tells us, "Someone else's sperm, with Mom's ova, started me growing. . . . What the whole thing comes down to is this. . . . The sperm came from someone else, but once that wonderful baby started to grow (Me! Remember?), there was only one dad. My dad." Once he has delivered his goods, the donor no longer exists as a human participant in the child's development. This book offers a good scientific, family-sensitive explanation of donor insemination, supporting the notion that dads are the men who raise you, not the people who make you. But will the explanation successfully function to dispel any questions or fears about the other man who produced these sperm and gave them to Mommy and Daddy? We will put aside for later discussion whether such reduction of the donor to a vial of sperm negates a child's deep desire to know about the person who helped make him or her. For now, let's focus on its function in getting that man out of this little girl's parents' bedroom.

Richard and Catherine were quite open about their daughter Angela's birth history. She was conceived with sperm purchased from The Sperm Bank of California. Angela was having some behavior problems at school, and I wondered whether some of them might be in her inherited "hard wir-ing" or temperament. Maybe she had a genetically based learning problem that was the catalyst for her behavioral difficulties. So I inquired what Catherine and Richard knew about the sperm donor. Richard responded tersely, "As we said, we went to The Sperm Bank and got some sperm." I re-alized I had better back up and be more sensitive in my queries. It turns out

that Richard was extremely ambivalent about going ahead with donor insemination. When a close friend of theirs offered to be a sperm donor after
finding out Richard was left sterile from a case of the mumps at age eighteen,
Richard adamantly refused—no way could he tolerate such intimacy between his close friend and Catherine. He wanted only an anonymous donor,
which was fine with Catherine. But still, whenever she mentioned anything
about the donor, Richard got quiet and withdrew into himself. After a while,
Catherine discovered that if she avoided using the word *donor* and referred
only to *sperm,* Richard calmed down. So instead of saying, "I hope the donor
will make it to the clinic this week," she would say, "I'm worried there won't
be sperm for us this week."

After a while, the word *donor* disappeared completely from their
speech, and both Richard and Catherine thought only about the sperm that
made the miraculous creation of their daughter, Angela, possible. Until it
came time for Angela to have a developmental assessment. It wasn't the
vial of sperm, but the profile of the donor that would provide useful information about Angela's problems. Richard and Catherine both came to recognize that it was counterproductive to continue pushing away any
thoughts about the donor as a person. They needed that person, or at least
as much as they could find out about him, to help understand what was going on with Angela. Something cracked wide open for Richard and
Catherine as they began to acknowledge that the sperm was attached to a
real, whole person.

In Richard and Catherine's case, they needed to reconstruct the donor
as a whole person so they could find out medical facts about him. For other
families, the ploy of reducing the birth other to a body part also negates the
reality of him or her as a whole person with thoughts, desires, and actions
and as a person who will play a part in the fantasies, if not the actual interactions, of the family. Rather than equating a donor or surrogate with a
body part, a useful way to recognize the birth other as a whole person is to
allow yourself the freedom to explore each and every fantasy or thought
you have about this person, whether you know the person or not. If you
find yourself with "dangling parts," reattach them by reminding yourself
that the part came from a person and that that person is a responsible being
who took action so that your child could be born. Some would argue that
such thinking is sure to interfere with the sanctity of the family, but my
own clinical experience is that the sanctity of the family is reinforced,

rather than shattered, by the psychological recognition that an outside person played a part in the family.

If we adults don't turn the sperm, eggs, or wombs back into people, our children will do it for us. This is the story of a nine-year-old girl from a lesbian family. The sperm donor was a gay friend of her mothers. Gabrielle, the daughter, knew the donor, but only as a friend of the family, not as her genetic father. He had asked to remain anonymous to the child. Unfortunately, he was now dying of cancer. The mothers hoped he would change his mind and reveal himself to Gabrielle as her biological father so she would have a chance to know him as such while he was still alive. Up to that time, Gabrielle knew only that her two mothers had gotten some sperm and, with the help of a doctor, joined the sperm with Mommy's ovum so she could be born. The mothers were in the midst of discussing disclosure with the donor, who staunchly held to his position that he did not want to reveal himself to Gabrielle, when Gabrielle burst into her therapy session with me, leaped into her favorite chair, and announced, "I know who my father is!" I was quite shocked because I had just gotten off the phone with one of the mothers, who let me know that the donor was unwilling to disclose himself to Gabrielle and that the mothers would respectfully honor his desire, which I genuinely believed they would do. I could only conclude that Gabrielle must have figured it out anyway, either by overhearing conversations or through unobtrusive observation—I was told that she bore a strong physical resemblance to the donor, a tall, heavyset, muscle-bound, dark-haired man, whom she saw regularly. I took a deep breath and said, "Oh, tell me about him." She launched into an excited tale, "I know it. I know it. My father's a science nerd. He's one of those short little skinny guys with kinky red hair, wire-rimmed glasses, and a white coat. He works in a lab. A real geek."

Gabrielle was not going to tolerate her biological father being relegated to a vial of sperm. Knowing that she had been born through a scientific procedure, she extended this logic to create in fantasy her "whole" father, a nerdy scientist, as her procreator. Gabrielle's fantasy demonstrates a child's resistance to being asked to reduce her biological father to a thing. Once we know that people come in wholes, it can make us very anxious to be asked to return to our earliest infancy when we thought of them only as parts. I believe we make this request unwittingly when, because of our own anxieties, we ask children born with the aid of reproductive technology to think of their donors or surrogates only as a sperm, egg, or womb. Gabrielle needed a whole person, maybe even a whole father, and probably the unconscious timing of this need was no accident, given her mothers' simultaneous quest to have the donor reveal his identity to Gabrielle before his death.

Making a Parent from Whole Cloth

Gabrielle constructed a whole father from parts. Adults do this, too. If you are a single mother who has used donor insemination, you may sometimes find yourself elevating the donor to the status of a family member in fantasy. Even though you may never have met the donor, you might imagine him coming to the house, taking "his" child to the park, and so forth. Rosanna Hertz, who conducted interviews with single mothers who have used donor insemination, reports that as the children grow, the women come to realize that the sperm represents a human being, not just genetic matter. When the donor is anonymous, mother and child engage in a fiction of who this man is. They imagine conversations they might have with him or conjure up fantasies *he* is having about *them*. Sometimes mothers subsequently try to track down more information about the donor, to get a whole picture of him. To the child they might say, "You must have gotten your musical ability from your father; no one on my side is musical."[24] Hertz's interviews with these women document a single mother's anxieties about leaving the father of her child in the status of a part object—a vial of sperm. If you are single, you might long to be able to fill in the missing piece of the family, to have some image of the man who has mixed his bodily fluids with yours and has had genetic input in your child's being. He might even be a sexual partner in fantasy.

In the struggle to take the sex out of reproduction, we witness a paradox between a reduction of people to parts and an illusion of whole people where there are none. As it stands today, we have yet to come up with a new concept of a donor or surrogate who is a participant but *not* a parent and not a sexual(ized) partner in the birth-other family. If you find yourself anxious about the interloper, you may be drawn toward part-object thinking, the reduction of the donor, surrogate, or carrier to a thing, a vial of sperm, a carton of eggs, or an incubator that represents no threat to the family. If you feel the absence of a parenting partner or if you find yourself succumbing to the erotic undertow of procreation with a birth other, you may be more prone to conjure up a whole parent from a thread of genetic material, engaging in the fantasy of creating for yourself another parent, maybe even a sexual partner.

Either is extreme. The truth lies in the middle—the birth other is a person who helps a family have a child. He or she is not a body part, and he or she is not a parent or lover.

OVERCOMING IMMACULATE DECEPTION

So what would I like to say to all of you who are contemplating or have already embarked on the journey of procreation with the proper stranger? We have not yet been able to take the sex out of reproduction. It is entirely possible that you will experience sexual or erotic rumblings, which appear to be not an inevitable but an expectable component of conception with a birth other.

Therefore, be prepared to catch yourself if you find yourself indulging in immaculate deception fantasies, stories that make no logical sense but serve to ease your own queasiness about your child's birth story. It is fine to *wish* such stories were true, such as that you were the other partner in conception because you carried the live sperm under your arm, as long as you juxtapose those longings with the scientific realities of your child's birth. Later on we will talk about how to interweave those realities into the actual story you will present to your child. For now, the first step is to acknowledge fully that those threads are there to be woven. Be prepared to catch yourself thinking, "Honey, I shrunk the donor [surrogate]." Or alternatively, "Anonymous Sperm Donor #234, your father whom I so dearly love, is a wonderful artist with a sensitive soul." Sometimes you can catch yourself by having a dialogue with yourself or with your partner, if you have one. Go back to the questions at the beginning of the chapter. How would you answer them now—in terms of your images of the birth other, the surfacing of erotic feelings, the presence of jealousy, envy, or resentment?

Occasionally it might be too hard to stop yourself from running from the answers or sweeping the feelings under the rug. In that case, getting some professional consultation or counseling can be helpful. Having a trained mental health professional to bear witness to such delicate feelings and help you manage your anxieties and guilt about procreation with the proper stranger can pave the way for thinking more clearly about how you do want to include the birth other in your family matrix. If you can successfully negotiate the fantasies, the longings, and the anxiety, rather than scurrying away from them or allowing them to sweep you away, the feelings will pass and fade into the background as your experience with your child zooms into the foreground.

Your work, as well as the work of those around you, is to hold on to a reality-based image of the birth other as an actual person, perhaps a person you know nothing about or perhaps a person close to you, but either way, a person who helped make your family. This last task, holding on to the birth other as a whole person, is the linchpin in forging a solid relationship with your child and ensuring strong bonds in your family over time. There is a new "mating game" that goes on when we choose a birth other to participate in the creation of our child. How you negotiate the existence of this outside person who participated in the child's conception deeply impacts your ability to lay claim to your child, to trust in your child's attachment to you. It is the phenomena of possession and "laying claim" to which I now want to turn our attention.

You're Mine . . . or Are You?

Jasper knew there were different ways that children became part of a family. Mostly, they were born to their Mom and Dad. But sometimes they were adopted . . . and Jasper knew his Mom went to the doctor who helped her get pregnant with the sperm from a nice man that his mom never met. So there were lots of ways kids came into families.

—A story written by a single mother for her son

Jasper's mom had done what all parents must do sometime while their children are growing—figure out when and what to tell them about how they came to be and how they belong in *this* family. Whether parents do or don't figure it out, children will inevitably pick up the ball: "Where did I come from?" "Am I really yours?" Ideally, every parent prepares, is at the ready to answer these questions as they pop up. That's no easy task. Multiply the challenge by a thousand if you're a parent who has had a child using a donor or surrogate. Do you disclose or not disclose that the baby didn't come just from you? How much do you reveal about the other person who helped make your child? How do you explain the difference between the person who made the child and the person who is raising him or her?

Noelle Oxenhandler, author of *The Eros of Parenthood*, offers an intriguing notion regarding our feelings about our ties to our children—they are "placed" with us. They could have been placed just as easily with someone else or taken away from us.[1] If that feeling is there for any parent, it may be exaggerated for any of you who have had a child with a birth other, the someone else who could have been the other placement for your baby. Abby flew into her bedroom in a rage, screaming at Sharon, "You're not my real mom. Never was, never will be." Many parents could laugh this off as a dramatized display of childish anger. But Sharon couldn't—maybe Abby was right. Maybe Melinda, the surrogate, was Abby's real mom. Maybe Abby knew that she really didn't belong to Sharon.

Laughing or not, traditional parents who have been challenged to prove that their child belongs in their family quickly realize they have to decide what to say about procreation and what their child can understand about genetics and reproduction. My own father tried to skirt the issue of sex by reassuring me, when I was convinced I was adopted, that I must belong to him because I was left-handed like him and had the same bony elbows he had. Any parent who has used a birth other may have a tougher job than my dad or other traditional parents. Before you decide when and what to tell your child about his or her beginnings, you might have to explore your own deepest feelings about your child's placement with you, your child's arrival and position in the family. To do this is to think about two family issues stemming from the word *belong*. The first is the question of who this child *belongs to*. This is a matter of possession—is this child mine, or not? The second is the question of *belonging*. This is a matter of attachment, bonding, and connection—how do we all fit together as a family? In this chapter, I would like to explore possession—does this child belong to me? Then in the next chapter we'll look at the unfolding drama of love and attachment in the family— how do we all belong together?

Ultimately, in a democratic society, children belong to themselves and no one else. And the tales of children used or abused by parents who perceive their children as property rather than progeny make us squeamish about using the word *possession* at all when it comes to parents' relationships to their children. Yet the care nurses take to secure the matching baby–mother identification bracelet on the newborn's ankle just minutes after the baby's first breaths signals the importance we all place on the parent's rightful possession of the right child. And the horror we feel when confronted with stories of baby mix-ups in the hospital only underscores how crucial we think it is to get it right. So who is the *right* child? The child the woman birthed, the child that came from *her* body. But where does that definition of rightful possession leave parents whose child was born another way?

The answer is complicated in the world of assisted reproductive technology, especially when mix-ups involve not babies but sperm, eggs, or embryos. As we have already learned, medical errors resulting in women being impregnated with the wrong embryos or sperm have been uncovered most dramatically when the baby is born a different color from the parents. The case of Mrs. Fasano giving birth to twins of different colors was followed by the highly publicized British case of Mr. and Ms. A, white parents who gave birth in 2003 to biracial twins after a medical mix-up in which the sperm of Mr. B, a black man using the same fertility clinic services as the A's, was mistakenly injected into Mrs. A's eggs. In court proceedings, Mr. and Mrs. A were awarded custody of the children, but Mr. B was awarded parental rights as the children's biological father.[2] The key to this decision was the question "Who does this child belong to?" The answer: to both the social (nonbiological) parent and genetic parents.

When an outsider has collaborated to make a child, three questions (Is this child really mine? Is this child more mine than yours? Is this child more yours than mine?) can reverberate like the refrain of a Greek chorus. And although the questions may seem intended to establish ownership, as if the baby were a commodity, at base what these questions signify are parents' concerns about whether their children really belong to them. Successfully negotiating the answers to these questions lays the groundwork for a sturdy narrative that parents will share with their children over time about their children's origins, their relationship to the birth other(s), and everyone's place in the family. I'd like to see if I can help with that negotiation.

For parents using a birth other, let me refine the three questions of our Greek chorus so you can turn them around in your mind as we consider the questions about the right placement of the children:

- Do I find myself just assuming that my child is more like me than like my partner (for genetic parents in two-parent families), or can I see myself doing this after the baby is born?
- Do I (or will I) accede to my partner because it's more his/her child (for nongenetic parents in two-parent families)?
- Do I (or will I) think about myself as the "real" parent (for genetic parents)?
- Do I (or will I) feel degrees of separation between myself and my child because my genes didn't make him/her (for nongenetic parents)?

- Do I (or will I) feel my child doesn't totally belong to me because there is someone else out there who could lay claim?

THE SLIPPERY SLOPE TOWARD "MINE" PLAYS AGAINST THE UPWARD BATTLE TOWARD "MINE, TOO"

Sally is immensely proud and pleased that her son Jeremy is such a good student. When it comes to doing homework, she insists that she help Jeremy and asks her husband, Matthew, to do something else instead. He would be perfectly happy to share the homework responsibilities and seems to do fine when Sally is not home, but Sally always finds a reason why she should be the one to do it when they're both home. Sally knows her husband was a great athlete but never a good student. She also knows her son's sperm donor was first in his medical class. She herself was an honor student. When it comes to academic performance, she privileges herself over Matthew because she doesn't think he is enough like his son. Her smart son is hers, not his. She and her baby not only left the hospital with matching wrist and ankle bracelets, but she made this baby—Matthew didn't. Whatever part of the baby's intelligence is genetic can be claimed not by Sally and Matthew but by Sally and someone else, a someone that neither parent has ever met but that both know was smart enough to be a top medical student.

The Tug of War between Genes and No Genes

When there is a birth other, the tension "Is this child mine or not?" nags at both the genetic and nongenetic parent. It can become a tug of war.

The parent with genetic ties to the child has to beware of the slippery slope toward "mine, mine, mine." In a single-parent family, particularly with an anonymous donor or surrogate, the mom or dad can easily forget that anybody else was a participant. So "mine, mine, mine" becomes an easy victory because there's no one tugging on the other end of the rope, claiming to be a parent. In a two-parent family, our culture's tendency to subtly or not so subtly perceive biological parents as more real than nonbiological parents can easily reinforce a genetic parent's feeling that this child is "more mine than yours." This certainly gives the genetic parent an edge in the tug of war for possession.

For the parent with no genetic ties, the struggle is to hold on to the rope, to stay convinced that this child *is* mine, even if not of my flesh and blood. This struggle can become particularly intense if there is another parent who is shaking the rope, a parent like Sally who consciously or unconsciously is also not convinced that the child belongs to that rope-holder.

I was surprised to hear the words of one mother whose son was born with the help of an egg donor. Looking slyly at her husband as she took in my query, "How is it for you that you are not Aaron's genetic mother?" she responded, "Actually, it's quite a relief. I don't have to feel guilty about Aaron's neurological problems. *My* genes didn't cause them." In an era when parents are burdened with feeling responsible for everything that happens to their child, such relief is a genuine plus. But the relief is often fleeting, maybe even illusory, easily canceled out by the angst of non-possession or, far worse, dispossession. Finding solace in being relieved of responsibility for genetic problems seldom gives that parent a stronger grip on the rope of possession, especially if there are tugs from another parent who lays claim to being the more real parent because of genetic links.

The Shadows That Lurk: The Birth Other, Infertility, Impossibility of Same-Sex Conceptions

Every family who has had an assisted conception will also have to confront the presence of a "shadow" parent, the donor or the surrogate, for even the genetic parent constantly lives with the knowledge that biologically this child is someone else's as well. In situations where infertility or disease was a factor, the parents will also have to work through the reality that they could not have their own genetic child or could not have a child who was genetically related to both of them (in two-parent families). In gay and lesbian families who turn to assisted reproductive technology, the tensions surrounding possession can flow from a different source—one of the parents will be the chosen one, the parent who will have the genetic ties to the child, while the other will forever remain the social parent for that child, sometimes with legal rights, sometimes not. On occasion, lesbian families have attempted to remedy the situation by having one mother be the gestational mother and the other mother be the egg mother who harvests her eggs to be implanted in her partner's womb.[3] But nonetheless, until new advances in reproductive technology, lesbian and gay couples can't escape the reality dictated by biology that their genes could not come together to make their child and that only one of them possesses the status of genetic parent.

Wondering "Baby, are you mine? Baby, do you think I'm yours?" can bring angst to anyone having a baby with a birth other. Lindsay announced to her mother Trisha, "You know, Mommy, I'm Mama Sandy's, and Brad [her little brother] is yours." Although this was factually correct—Trisha was Brad's genetic mom, and Sandy was Lindsay's genetic mom—Trisha was crushed. It confirmed her feelings that Lindsay just wasn't a part of her, didn't look like her, and would never see her as her real mom the way Lindsay saw Sandy. Every night Miles came home from work an hour after his wife, Gloria. He would slide into his study to check e-mail, leaving Gloria to finish getting dinner together while keeping three-year-old Nathan involved in his art project. Gloria grew increasingly agitated, seeing Miles as a typical man who left all the housework to her. But that wasn't what was going on at all. When Miles walked into the house, all he saw were the blissful moments between Gloria and Nathan, and when he saw the shimmer in the red hair they shared and the glimmer in their green eyes, all he could feel was left out. Miles was a dad with no sperm. Nathan came to them with the help of an anonymous sperm donor. But Miles wasn't so sure Nathan had come as much to him as he had to Gloria. Miles and Trisha were both suffering from the angst about possession.

So why should we pay attention to this potential worry or tug of war over possession? Because, over time, if the children get a whiff of it, they in turn may never feel secure that they really belong to their parent(s). For the welfare of the child, therefore, it is best to begin exploring anxieties or feelings about possession early on, well before the baby even arrives on the scene. At the same time, it is never too late to visit these questions further along in the children's lives, for parenting is an unfolding drama in which you move forward, fall down, pick yourself up, brush yourself off, and move forward again, giving thought to ways of avoiding falling into the same holes.

Is This My Baby? Well, Did You Intend to Have It?

Anxiety regarding "Whose baby is this?" ran rampant in the well-publicized case of Luanne and John Buzzanca, the divorced parents of a child born with the aid of a sperm donor, egg donor, and surrogate. For a period of time subsequent to the Buzzancas's marital separation, which occurred prior to the baby's birth, the child was left in limbo with *no* legal parents. Bound by neither genetic ties nor marriage vows, John Buzzanca disavowed any connection to or responsibility for the child. The surrogate, who as the gestational mother but not the genetic mother temporarily held the legal rights to the child, placed herself in competition with Luanne Buzzanca, a woman who desperately wanted the child that she and her husband had intended to have. In the ensuing struggle, the surrogate mother, fighting for her rights to the child she had birthed, hurled this missile at Luanne Buzzanca, the intentional mother: "She never gave birth to that child. How can she be a mother? I can't be erased. I won't be erased." In other words, the child is *mine* because I carried her, and she will never be *yours* because you have no biological ties to her. In the end, Luanne Buzzanca was awarded parental rights and legal custody while John Buzzanca was held responsible for child support. The court decision was made on the basis that these two people were the ones who *intended* to have this child together.

The media attention and drama of this case laid bare all of our confusion and anxiety about possession in the fertile new world of baby making with birth others. Who can lay claim to a child? The genetic parent? The woman who carried the baby in her womb? The people who provided their egg or sperm to make the baby? Or the people who intended to have the child, the ones who dreamed of having a child of their own and then set out to make it happen? The Buzzancas's tumultuous legal case helped point us all toward a key concept in family building using reproductive technology— the intent to parent. If we want to know who a child belongs to, ask who made plans to have the child. The intent to parent as a criterion for possession has been used actively in lesbian parenting disputes in the courts. Legal experts have called on the intent to parent to defend the parental rights of a nonbiological mother who did not make the baby and because of present laws finds herself with no legal rights, but nonetheless planned with her partner to have a baby and then actively engaged in raising that baby. But this premeditation to parent is not just a guiding light in courtroom disputes. I would like to offer it as the most helpful guideline in untangling the psychological conundrums of possession. In your own family, if you want to know who your child belongs to, ask not what genes made your child but rather who intended to parent your child.

FINDING MR. OR MS. RIGHT:
THE BIRTH-OTHER MATING GAME

One day in the spring of 2003 I opened *Newsweek* to find a feature piece, "Sperm Banks Go Online."[4] The article's description of Internet searches for donors immediately reminded me of the mail-order brides of yore (and still in many cultures today). A man who contracted for a mail-order bride made his choice sight unseen, on the basis of written reports of the delivered spouse's physical, social, and personality features. How different was this from parents' search for just the right donor or surrogate? Of course, the prospective parents have no intention of spending the rest of their lives with the selected donor or surrogate, but they *are* searching for just the right person to become the biological parent of their future child, and they *are* making their choice on the basis of certain personality/temperament/physical and social attributes without ever having laid eyes on the person.

Sophie Cabot Black describes her and her partner's search through sperm banks for just the right donor: "We looked for those [donors] who had characteristics of each of our heritages, facial features, even personalities. We also tried to read between the lines of their answers to questions about favorite color, desire for travel, long-term goals, SAT scores."[5] Even though Sophie's partner, D., would never be a biological mother of this child, both Sophie and D. went on a quest for a donor who would be similar to *both* of them.

Many people have been horrified by the extent to which people using assisted reproductive technology go shopping for Mr. or Ms. Right, seeing it as a narcissistic endeavor to defy the gods and craft the perfect child, as we've already explored. But what's often misunderstood is that these searches are driven by the parents' legitimate desire to have a child who feels like he or she belongs to them. Going on a shopping spree for the perfect donor or surrogate is a way to gain control over the birth process and lay claim to the child they've created. In the early days of assisted reproductive technology, fertility specialists tried to preserve a family's privacy and an infertile husband's sense of virility by finding a sperm donor who looked enough like Dad to make it impossible for anyone, including the child, to know that Dad was not the biological father. But I think something else was going on as well. In matching donors to fathers' characteristics, the doctors were also, perhaps unwittingly, recognizing that similarity helps people feel like they belong to each other and that too much difference can compromise the sense of possession.

If You Look Like Me, You'll Be Mine

We have a far greater chance of looking like one of our blood relatives than resembling a total stranger. Genetic ties serve as an insurance policy that a child will be similar to the parent, and similarity breeds a sense of belonging. But what if you don't have that insurance policy? Well, then you have the mating game. A person exists somewhere out there who might provide enough similarity to both the biological and the nonbiological parent to solidify a sense of the child belonging to the parents.

Adoptive parents, too, may adopt within their own race or culture to foster that sense of belonging to, but the difference is that their own genes are precluded from being part of the process. Also, in contrast to parents using assisted reproductive technology, adoptive parents may reach out to a child very, very different from them. They may do this because there are children already out there who need a home or because international or transracial adoptions are often the most viable route available to men and women, particularly single and gay and lesbian prospective parents, who so strongly want a child. Parents turning to a birth other to have a child, starting from scratch, don't need to consider children already made and have, ostensibly, considerably more control than adoptive parents over who their birth other(s) will be. Given the greater latitude afforded them, they may very well be inclined to search out similarity not as a narcissistic extension of self but as an effort to ensure a feeling that this child belongs to them.

The new mating game is therefore essentially a matching game. It is also the moment in the family's history when the parents begin to cement the idea that the child is theirs. Parents gain a sense of control by having a choice about the birth other. For couples, the joint effort of searching for a donor or surrogate can bring them together in acting on their intent to parent and finding someone who will participate in having a baby for them. This mating game is an important foundation for the parents' ongoing experience of having a child that belongs to them and, as such, will permeate the entire lifetime of the family.

For Mothers, Invasion of the Body Snatchers

But the mating game doesn't eliminate all the hurdles you will need to jump to gain a feeling of possession if you are having a baby with a someone else. Susan Cooper and Ellen Glazer described one mother's anxiety over the physical size of the egg donor she would choose to have a child: "She feared that if the donor was too big, the baby would be too big, and her uterus might rupture. [She] continued to focus on the ways she imagined the fetus could damage her."[6] This mother was suffering from the "invasion of the body snatchers" syndrome. An alien object, another woman's egg, was being placed in her body to grow into a child that would someday be hers. How could a gigantic baby belong in her—or to her? If we dig below the surface, we can detect in this woman's voiced fears about her body the deeper anxiety that a child foreign to her could be a destructive force in her life.

It's not unusual for a traditionally pregnant woman to have somewhat dark fantasies or dreams about a parasite living in and off her body or an intruder who has come to distort the mother's belly and keep her up at night. Still, that woman knows the baby is part and parcel of herself and this knowledge provides a soothing antidote to any disturbing visions, allowing her to easily laugh them off. The mother whose body actually *has* been "invaded" by the egg of another woman or the sperm of a man with whom she's had no sexual relations doesn't have the same ready reassurance. She has to work harder to root herself in the feeling that the baby is hers, even if someone else planted the seed. Matching might make the task easier. If you are using a birth other, a donor or surrogate who is more similar to you may fortify your sense of connection to the baby and ward off any scary feelings of invasion or dispossession. Even though we know rationally that an egg from a tiny woman can carry the genes of a six-foot-six-inch quarterback, a small mother might be able to relax more easily into a feeling of unity and belonging when the donor is small like herself. Similarity becomes important in solidifying a feeling of possession in yet another way—"body politics."

It's Hard to Claim Possession When You Feel Like a Birth Nobody

Frank was ecstatic that he and June were going to have a baby. After discovering that Frank was sterile, they tried for over two years, using donor sperm, until finally it happened. They were open with everyone about June's donor pregnancy, and Frank thought it would only get more exciting as the due date grew closer. Yet he noticed a feeling of deflation and a twinge of envy every time some well-meaning family member patted June's belly and asked how *her* baby was doing. If you're a nongenetic father, will you, like Frank, end up feeling like a birth nobody when it comes to laying claim to your baby-to-be?

Until we figure out a way for men to carry a fetus in *their* body, all fathers are going to continue to feel one step removed from the physical connection with their baby during pregnancy. So fathers in families created with a birth other will be exempt from the feelings of invasion that may confront a mother using an egg or sperm donor. On the other hand, if you are a nongenetic father in such a family, the battle to lay claim to the baby may feel like a Sisyphean struggle. A mother who conceives with the aid of an egg donor can walk down the street pregnant, and everyone will assume she's the genetic parent of the child she's carrying. All who see her will treat her as the real mother, the one who gives birth to the child. In a donor-insemination family, someone else's seed, not the father's, has made the baby, and no one pats his swelling belly or shares stories of labor pains or kicking fetuses. A father who turns to a surrogate to have a child is luckier—he will have his own genes to bolster him as the real father to his child. But still, like the father in the donor-insemination family, someone unrelated to him and perhaps very far away is carrying his child and no one will be patting *his* belly to solidify his sense that this child is his.

Of course, every father lacks the pregnant belly that can signify ownership of a child. The nongenetic father, however, not only can't rest easy in the knowledge that his sperm helped create the child, but also may suffer from the potential great divide between sperm donor and father. As in the story of Sally and Matthew, the donor may be of a different age, class, and educational background from the father. Sperm banks are usually populated with the sperm of young, well-educated men, many of them medical students. Fathers like Matthew watch their child become the brain of the class in their working-class communities while they were only C students. Les, who was sterile, made a pact with his wife to have children using donor sperm and allow everyone to think that the children were biologically both of theirs. But he suffered by knowing inside that his two boys would never be a chip off the old block. He knew that the boys had "super fathers," which made them exceptionally intelligent and special. His wife never looked down on him, but Les, a small businessman, felt that he couldn't hold a candle in the smarts department to the donors, who were probably thriving doctors by now. He hated it when his wife bragged about the boys' intelligence, angry that she was so insensitive to how that made him feel.[7] Alas, everyone, including the wife, glows, while the father shrinks and glowers.

It's only natural that prospective parents look for the most robust, healthiest sperm to boost the chances of having a healthy, robust child. But if you're seeking a sperm donor with your partner, think about how you might feel later about an other who is so different. What would you do if, in your deepest, darkest moments, you and/or your partner felt that the sperm donor was superior to the child's father (or to the nonbiological mother in a lesbian couple)? If you are a nonbiological father, it is not a question of invasion, but rather one of conquest, an internal battle in which you might grow to feel like the birth nobody who has no rights to a child who neither looks like you, thinks like you, nor comes from you. This is why, to establish confidence as a birth somebody, many couples look for donors who resemble *both* of the parents-to-be.

Of course, mothers, too, can become birth nobodies, negating their legitimate claim to their children. What happens when a mother who is seeking an egg donor finds that the eligible candidates are younger, highly intelligent, athletic, and capable of producing viable eggs where she is not? Add to that scenario the feeling that this other person will count as the real mother of the child. For the mother who has turned to a surrogate, the potential to feel like a conquered birth nobody can be compounded by the reality that she did not even carry her own baby inside her. Someone else, the birth other, was having her stomach patted and having people assume that the baby kicking inside belonged to *her.*

Paid surrogacy has been criticized as a means by which wealthier people can exploit poor women's wombs, and this is a legitimate concern, but it is not the reality for most people who turn to a surrogate to have a child. The social criticism blinds people, including prospective parents, from recognizing the reverse psychological experience—the mother's envy of the surrogate's privileged state. While the baby grows in the surrogate's womb, gnawing questions can fill the inner chambers of the mother's mind: "How could that baby really be mine?" and "Doesn't the baby really belong to the surrogate?" Again, the time to think about how you might feel is during the matching process. A feeling of commonality or similarity with the donor or surrogate can help reduce birth-nobody feelings.

Keeping It in the Family: Using Relatives as Birth Others

Lonnie is the proud mother of two sons. One is her biological child, and the other is her partner Fay's biological child. But Fay's biological son is also Lonnie's biological nephew, and Lonnie's biological son is also Fay's biological nephew. That's because Fay's brother is the sperm donor for Lonnie's biological son, and Lonnie's brother is the sperm donor for Fay's biological son—a creative way of keeping it all in the family in which both mothers, Lonnie and Fay, have a blood tie to each of their sons.

Many couples using assisted reproductive technology turn to their relatives to serve as donor or surrogate for their child. We've already discussed the fact that some do not because in parents' hearts and minds that option can border on the sexually illicit or incestuous or just feel too creepy. But many others do and, in the process, solidify a sense of connection and belonging to the child they did not make with their own gametes. Not only will they know in intimate detail the family history, medical history, personality, state of well-being, values, and life experiences of the donor, but the nongenetic parents will also have the opportunity to indirectly inject their own genes into the child they will raise by calling on a blood relative to be the donor for their child. With shared blood comes both the feeling of being the same and the assurance that, in the sense of generative continuity, the nongenetic parent and baby come from the same place. Ergo, "you belong to me."

Ironically, using a relative as donor can also do the opposite—dispossess a parent. The shadow parent will turn out to be anything but a shadow presence. Maybe he's showing up at every family party and wedding. Maybe she lives next door. In couples, nongenetic parents can begin to feel *dis*possessed by their own relative, the man or woman able to provide their partner with the child that they couldn't. Similar feelings can erupt in single parents if, for example, a woman offers to be the egg donor so that her infertile unmarried sister can have a baby using the sister's egg and the donated sperm of a close family friend. In that case, Mom, with no genetic links to her child, can feel displaced by Auntie, her child's real genetic parent, and perhaps by an imagined coalition between Auntie and Close Family Friend, even though the two hardly know each other. These bad feelings often surface unexpectedly, accompanied by shame or discomfort at having negative thoughts about a relative who was kind enough to step in to help make a child for the person or couple. The feeling of dispossession or competition can also open up old family wounds, particularly when the donor or surrogate is a sibling. Long buried sibling rivalries may resurface if the nongenetic parents grow to feel that the baby seems more interested in their sibling than in them or think that their sibling is trying to woo the child away and become the more favored adult in the child's eyes. Painful childhood memories of vying for their own parents' love and attention can easily be restimulated and may need to be renegotiated within the parent and between the siblings.

Ilene and Seth had been trying unsuccessfully for two years to have a child. They discovered that, even with the stimulation of fertility drugs, Ilene could not produce healthy eggs. They were both devastated. They had heard about an Internet site, eggBay, where prospective parents can search for an egg donor and were just about to log on to the site when the phone rang. It was Ilene's older sister, Marian. Ilene was moved to tears to hear Marian offering an alternative route—Marian would donate her eggs so Ilene and Seth could have a baby. Marian herself was a mother of two, and she did not want her sister to miss the opportunity to carry and bear a child of her own. Having already waited two excruciating years with no baby in sight, Ilene and Seth jumped at the chance. Through her sister's egg donation and an in vitro fertilization procedure, Ilene got pregnant and gave birth to a beautiful baby girl, Samantha. Marian attended the birth, and everyone seemed ecstatic about this closely bonded family affair.

Marian and Ilene lived in the same neighborhood and had always dropped in to see each other regularly. Now when Marian arrived at Ilene and Seth's house, she would bounce Samantha in the air and coo over her beauty and precocious development. As Samantha grew into a toddler, she always had a special smile for Aunt Marian and ran right to her lap in a way she never did with any other visitor to the house. Ilene started to feel a knot in her stomach each time her sister arrived. She began to suspect a subterfuge on her sister's part to become the light of Samantha's life and claim her rights as the real mother. This brought up old feelings from childhood— Marian's grades were always better than Ilene's; Marian always had more dates; Marian got more accolades from her parents than Ilene did. Ilene's resentment toward Marian mounted. Ilene felt guilty for faulting the sister who subjected herself to fertility drugs and surgical procedures so Ilene could bear her own child. Yet she could not stop the flow of angry feelings toward Marian. After a while Ilene grew so agitated that she asked Marian to stop dropping by because she was interfering with their family life. Marian was devastated.

Before the situation grew to crisis proportions, Ilene and Marian got themselves to a family therapist. The therapist helped them sort out their hurts and tensions and pave the way for an extended family in which Ilene could lay claim to her own child and Marian could be mindful but included in the delightful development of her niece who was also her genetic child. But truth be told, in retrospect Ilene regretted her and Seth's decision to use her sister as a donor. She wished that she and Seth had gone to eggBay and pursued an egg donor who was a stranger and would not threaten Ilene's feelings that her child was hers and not someone else's. In light of Ilene's experience, it makes sense to consider, before choosing a relative as a donor or surrogate, "Will I be able to handle someone so close to me holding the genetic tie to my child?"

If there are qualms, this does not necessarily mean stopping right there. Marian and Ilene eased their tensions after the fact, not before. Surely, when choosing a birth other, it will be impossible to "crystal ball" with perfect accuracy all the feelings that will potentially erupt after the baby comes. But there is some useful work to be done.

Flora Scrimgeour asked her sister Emma to be her egg donor. Emma had always lived in the shadow of her successful older sister, and now she had the opportunity to be the one with something to give. They, along with their husbands, went through a roller coaster of up and down feelings in the process of going forward with the egg donation. Flora and Emma even got in an old childhood-style quarrel that, much to their husbands' shock, ended in Emma throwing a punch at her older sister. Because they lived in England, they had access to a psychologist from the ethics committee of the fertility clinic they attended. The psychologist stressed the cons of their plan—wouldn't it be confusing that Emma would be both the baby's aunt and biological mother and Flora's baby would actually be her nephew? But for both Flora and her sister the pros—the close relationship between the sisters and their two families and their perception that Emma's eggs were of their shared ancestry rather than belonging solely to Emma—far outweighed the cons. "Sister eggs" were what they wanted.

More important than any psychologist were the open conversations that Flora, Emma, and their two husbands had together—airing their feelings and leaving room for anyone's doubts or concerns. Emma at first was hesitant to move forward with the egg donation, for Flora had just adopted a child, and Emma didn't see the need for her sister to move forward so quickly to have another. Flora knew this and talked to Emma about her need to bear a child of her own, having lost another baby in utero and no longer being able to conceive with her own eggs. In the end, the key component to an unfolding happy and harmonious life with each other and with their two families was Emma's unflappable compassion for all that Flora was going through and Flora's recognition of the generosity, sacrifice, discomfort, and pain her sister endured so Flora could bear a child of her own.[8]

Emma and Flora's story reminds us that not just the parents, but the relative birth others as well should be ensured the opportunity to reflect on their feelings. In the midst of writing this chapter, I opened up the *San Francisco Chronicle* on Mother's Day to see a full-page spread, "Midlife Mommy." It is the story of Ilona, a fifty-six-year-old woman with two grown daughters, who wanted to have a child with her second husband. Forty-six years old, he had always been single and had never had children. He was hesitant to consider marriage with this midlife mommy unless he could have babies with her. Postmenopausal, this would be quite a challenge for her. So she turned to her twenty-eight-year-old eldest daughter and asked her to be the egg donor. She agreed, and baby Monica was born, to whom Ilona is both the gestational mother and the genetic grandmother. With support from her friends and their small northern California community, all was reported as going well for Ilona and her new family. In the proud father's words, "In the store, in the post office, everybody's had an open mind. Even people here who identify themselves as Christians have been okay with it. What we did isn't against any creed or faith or value. It might be against custom in this country, but I just tell people we're living in a technological age." Ilona is so happy with the experience of late motherhood that she's thinking of having a second child. This time she plans to ask her younger daughter to be the donor.

Yet embedded in this happy Mother's Day tale was a darker story—her daughter's experience. First, it should be said that her daughter, Cecilia, donated eggs so her mother could have a child during a time when Cecilia and her own partner were having difficulty conceiving. A happy ending to that piece of the story is that Cecilia did get pregnant soon after her mother did, but nonetheless it gave me great pause as I read about her experience as the donor for her mother. According to the news report, "Ilona is the mom. Cecilia says so herself. 'Yes, and I was happy to do this for my mother. When I first saw [Monica], it did kind of hit me—that baby came from part of me! But it's their baby, and I've made a point of giving them their distance these last few months .. . so they could bond with the baby.' " Indeed, both Ilona and her husband seem fully possessed of their child, he the doting father, she the breastfeeding mother. But letting go does not seem to have come so easily for Cecilia: "One look at Monica, and Cecilia's maternal feelings surfaced. She didn't expect such a reaction. Throughout the pregnancy, Cecilia referred to Monica as her sister. Afterward, she started feeling as if Monica was her daughter. 'It hit me really hard. It was very emotional, and I had really mixed feelings.'" Ilona seemed unfazed by her daughter's unexpected reactions. In her own words, "Maybe she was a little jealous, after seeing Monica. She was bound to have some feelings like that."[9]

I wondered whether Cecilia, along with Ilona and her husband, had ever been afforded the opportunity to consider all the emotional ins and outs of a daughter being an egg donor for her mom, and I felt sad that Cecilia might be struggling on her own to quell her unsettled feelings, without the help of her mom. I could understand how Ilona and her husband might get swept up in the excitement of laying claim to their new little baby and lose sight of the internal struggle that surfaced for Cecilia as she tried to keep in focus that this child was not her daughter, but her sister. Monica is already born, but perhaps this family could make a better go of it the next time before going ahead with Cecilia's sister as the donor for Ilona and her husband's second child. What could they be more mindful of together, either to make the process go more smoothly or perhaps even to decide that a non-relative egg donor might be a better choice?

Parent–child relationships have many dimensions, one of which is power and authority. At an early age, children grow accustomed to doing what their parents ask them. This can last well into adulthood. In the new phenomenon of older women and men in second marriages wanting children of their own and turning to their older children to be donors or surrogates, we need to pay attention to the power dynamics in such an arrangement. Any time a parent asks a child to be a donor or surrogate, exploring whether the son or daughter feels like a free agent versus feeling obliged to do what Mom or Dad asks will help ensure a positive outcome, whether it be to go forward or to turn elsewhere. Making the decision to have a relative, particularly a child, be a birth other will go more smoothly if thought is given to whether the donor or surrogate will regret the loss of his or her right to claim ownership and care is taken to make sure parents can claim possession of their child without compromising the relative's emotional well-being.

Ilene and Marian's, Flora and Emma's, Cecilia and Ilona's experiences all point us in one direction—the importance of psychological counseling as an inoculation against later problems. From what I have learned from talking to mental health professionals who have conducted preconception or prebirth evaluations or counseling, I would make the following recommendation. Anyone contemplating using a relative or, for that matter, any known donor[10] as a birth other should seek out the services of a counselor, consultant, or family therapist who will provide guidance in thinking through the decision to go forth with the conception so that everyone in the family matrix has the opportunity to explore their feelings, share their thoughts, and make an informed decision together. In Flora and Emma's case in Great Britain, where such services are routinely offered to all prospective birth-other families, the two sisters used the counseling to decide *against* the counselor's recommendations not to go forward, but nonetheless the experience afforded them the opportunity to become clear about what they wanted to do. In the future, I hope that all families in the United States will routinely be offered the same opportunity as part of a program's preconception services, rather than have to seek out counseling on their own.

Which Mr. or Ms. Right Will Make the Baby Feel Most Like Mine?

This brings me to the essential piece of the mating game experience. Thinking about who the donor or surrogate will be is the time to explore all the emotions you have or may have about this child really feeling like *yours* and all the ways you might ensure that legitimate feeling of possession. But as you do this, you are not in this process alone. The heart-wrenching case of Baby M in the 1980s brought this home to all of us, as Mary Beth Whitehead went to court to claim rights to the baby she had grown intimately attached to, conceived of her egg and William Stern's sperm and birthed by her, ostensibly for Elizabeth and William Stern. But there are many far less extreme examples. Alan and his wife, Lindy, asked Alan's beloved brother, Philip, to be the sperm donor so they could have a baby and were chagrined to find Philip beginning to refer to the baby planned-to-be as *our* baby. Laura, who agreed to be an egg donor for her very close friend Martha, lay on the table waiting for her eggs to be harvested and suddenly felt a surge of unanticipated resentment—Why should I be going through all this pain and then have to give the baby away to Martha? All of these—Alan's, Lindy's, Philip's, Laura's—are understandable feelings, not to be overlooked but part of the complicated terrain of making babies not with someone else's body part but with someone else with feelings and emotions. It's easy to ignore these emotional undercurrents and shrink from anticipating future feelings of *all* the participants in the mating game. In the search for the right donor or surrogate, the desperate desire to pursue parenthood can be so all consuming that it is blinding. But blind faith that it will all work out in the end isn't enough. It doesn't always work out.

Especially in couples, the process of choosing the right donor or surrogate is the critical time for parents to begin working together in negotiating feelings about possession. In hybrid biological/nonbiological couples, the genetic parent will need to be aware of both his or her own and the other parent's experience of possession and dispossession and think about how this child can be made to feel like "yours" and not only "mine." The nongenetic parent will need to participate by exploring ways to lay claim to the child who will belong to him or her, not by blood but by bonding. How do you do this, especially when emotions are running high? We can never predict or control the future, but we can imagine it. Here I would suggest a form of guided imagery. Imagine together various scenarios you might find yourself in, such as what to do when some unwitting person leans over the stroller and says, "Oh, the baby looks just like you [genetic parent] and not a thing like you [nongenetic parent]." What will you do if you (the nongenetic parent) notice your partner taking over with the parenting, being more in charge? (Here, of course, you will have to separate gender from genetic issues, for if you are in a heterosexual couple, there *is* a tendency for mothers to take over the daily tasks of child rearing, period). How will you (the genetic parent) understand it and how will you respond to your partner if he or she at moments seems competitive, crabby, or withdrawn when both of you are with the baby? Let your creativity take you to whatever other images or scenarios come to mind. Imagine all the things you will actually do to make a baby feel like yours, individually and together.

Exploring in depth the feelings surrounding "mine," "yours," and "ours" sets a firm foundation for future family life. Whereas possession is not nine-tenths of the law when it comes to children, ensuring that parents feel that their child will truly belong to them is often the first step on the way to robust bonding and attachment. And who they choose as a donor or surrogate is a key element in this process.

Feelings of difference versus sameness, invasion, conquest, fears about bonding or laying claim to children who come from somewhere else are challenging but also manageable psychological struggles for parents. I have found in my clinical work that the best way to manage them is to let them emerge into the light of day, rather than storing them in the deep chambers of the mind. Mental health consultation, straightforward and honest dialogue, listening to and interweaving each participant's experience, and stretching to imagine oneself in the future when baby is already made are all helpful management tools. The mating game that occurs when an individual or couple sets out to choose a donor or surrogate is the essential place to begin this work. And a critical piece of the work is exploring whether parents want a donor known or unknown to them.

SHOULD YOU KNOW THE BIRTH OTHER?

Every parent using a birth other will inevitably face the question of if, what, and whom to tell about their child's origins, but before telling comes knowing. Do you want to know who that person is, or would you rather that person remain anonymous? How much do you want to know about that person? Do you want that person to be someone you already know well? Do you want to get to know that person?

Having a baby with the help of a birth other gives parents two main choices. You can choose a stranger as a donor and choose to know or not know who that stranger is, either now or in the future. Historically, sperm banks typically had donors who remained anonymous, but currently some agencies are requesting and others requiring that donors agree to participate in an identity release program, in which the donor's identity is revealed to the child at age eighteen. Alternatively, you can choose a friend, family member, or acquaintance willing to be a participant in the conception. This is typically a known person. Occasionally, an intermediary will function to find a donor for a family, and although the donor might be known to the family, he or she may remain anonymous as a donor, known to the intermediary but not the parents.

On the spectrum from knowing to not knowing, surrogates are almost by definition known birth others, since the process of coordinating conception and transferring the baby from surrogate to parent lends itself to face-to-face contact. It is also a long-term process of involvement, nine months of pregnancy plus the time taken to conceive. Surrogacy, of course, brings other issues that affect the parents' feelings that the child is theirs, and I'll discuss those later in the chapter. Donor insemination is the other extreme. It can be a one-shot deal and, with the exception of live sperm, requires no coordination between donor and recipient, given advanced methods of freezing and delivering sperm to the recipient. It becomes quite easy for the donor to remain anonymous, relegated to a vial of semen. In the case of egg donorship, the transfer of eggs between donor and recipient must be a carefully choreographed dance in which menstrual cycles are matched and donor and recipient coordinate their lives and schedules. It is indeed possible for all of this to remain anonymous, but, like surrogacy, the procedure lends itself to face-to-face contact, even more so because egg donors are often found either through family and friends or through personal ads to which potential recipients respond directly.

People tend to have strong opinions about knowing the donor. Those who question the importance of genetic origins wonder why a family ever has to know the identity of the donor. Those who highlight the importance of genetic origins for either psychological or medical reasons will strongly advocate that a family know something about the identity of the person who will account for half the genetic make-up of the child. In the United States, the balance has definitely tipped away from secrecy and anonymity and toward disclosure and identity release. I think the fact that many genetically related diseases and other conditions can be cured or prevented today is reason enough for a parent to have information about the donor. This becomes important not just at the time of choosing the donor, but over the course of the donor's life, since certain genetic conditions can surface later and may be unknown to the donor at the time of the donation. Such medical information could easily be communicated without revealing the donor's identity using a donor coding system or an intermediary to handle communication between donor and family. The latter seems preferable because it's far more difficult for parents or medical facilities to keep track of a donor who remains a number in a computer system than to stay in contact with a known person. Either way, the main point is that the donor's identity should be accessible in some form for the medical well-being of the child.

Whether the donor's identity needs to be known for the child's psychological well-being is another story. As in debates regarding open versus closed adoption, the jury is still out. Keep in mind that right now I am concentrating on the parents knowing or not knowing who the donor is. Whether the children should know about donors or surrogates is another question, which I will take up in Chapter 6. As long as the jury is still out, the parents' decision—to know or not to know—must be a very personal one, based on a whole variety of criteria.

Reproductive Biology Slants our Feelings about Knowing

It may seem far-fetched, but the fact that we're accustomed to thinking about and directly experiencing semen outside of bodies but have zero experience of eggs in this way can actually make a difference in parents' decision about whether to know the donor's identity. In the sleight of mind I discussed in the last chapter, where sperm donor equals sperm and egg donor equals egg, I have found that when it comes to knowing the identity of the donor, it is easier to use this mental trick of converting people into parts with sperm donors than with egg donors. Vials of liquid or cumbersome cryotanks housing frozen sperm have physical substance and can make parents feel in a subtle way that they have met the donor. Psychologically, it is much trickier to reduce the egg donor to a dish of microscopic material (ova) invisible to the naked eye and have that suffice as a meeting. The egg donor is a person who will take drugs and undergo a surgical procedure so that eggs can be removed from her body and transferred to either the mother's or a surrogate's body. Her personhood feels palpable, and she is therefore more likely to remain a whole person in parents' minds—a person to meet. So parents who are using an egg donor should not be surprised to find themselves leaning toward wanting to know the identity of the donor more than parents who are using a sperm donor.

Biology also lays its stake in another way. We talked earlier about the fact that nongenetic egg-donor mothers may feel somewhat secure in the possession of their baby because at least they have a biological relationship with their child—carrying the baby in their womb. This security may open them up to knowing and having contact with the egg donor. Nongenetic fathers never get the same break. Afforded no opportunity to participate biologically in either the conception or birth of their child, these fathers may feel anything but secure in laying claim to their child. The least they can do, therefore, is keep their distance from the man who holds the privilege of genetics by never knowing him. What better way to do this than by separating the sperm donor's personhood from the vial of sperm that will be used in the insemination?

Feelings about Knowing Can Change over Time

I've always found it helpful to use the concept of "family matrix" to understand the experience of parents using a birth other. We've gone way beyond the two-parent nuclear family and have long recognized that our society is made up of single-parent families, multigenerational families, divorced families, stepfamilies. But none of these terms address the family reality for parents using a birth other. By definition, a matrix is "that which gives origin or form to a thing, or which serves to enclose it."[11] This is a perfect framework for families using a birth other because it embraces both the people who made the baby (origins) and the people who raise or hold the baby (enclosure). Parents who use an outside party for conception must creatively craft the family matrix that feels right for them. They will have to consider how each of the members in that matrix will participate, if at all, in their family life. It becomes a decision-making tree. The first decision is whether the donor or surrogate will be known to the parents and, if so, how. From there we move to the next decision-making tier: If known, how, if at all, will that person be known to the child and how, if at all, will that person be incorporated into family life?

It is not always an easy road to travel. Feelings about knowing can change over time. And, in the uncharted and rapidly shifting terrain of reproductive technology, so can laws and policies, legal and social changes that can in turn radically alter how parents feel about knowing.

Denise and Sarah had been together for several years when the urge to have children came upon them. They both wanted to have a biological child, so they decided to take turns, using a local sperm bank. Sarah went first, and they turned to the regional sperm bank known to be supportive of same-sex families. They found an anonymous donor who had requested that his identity never be released. They had a beautiful baby boy. Three years later it was Denise's turn. They returned to the same sperm bank and requested the same donor, so that the children could be genetically linked to each other. The donor was still a participant, but by this time the sperm bank had changed its policies and required all donors to agree to an identity release program, revealing their identity to the children when the children turned eighteen. The donor agreed to donate again under these conditions, despite his request to remain anonymous three years earlier. In a quirk of circumstances, since there was no grandfather clause to the policy, the donor did not also volunteer to make his identity known to the older child.

Denise gave birth to a delightful baby girl. But now Denise and Sarah were in the absurd position of having an older child who would only inadvertently find out the identity of his sperm donor when his younger sister turned eighteen. This struck both mothers as absurd and unbearable, so much so that they embarked on a campaign to remedy the perceived wrong. Subscribing to the idea that the end justifies the means, particularly when it comes to providing for one's child, they set out on a crusade to uncover the identity of the donor. They hired a private detective and secretly penetrated the donor's private life, taking such drastic measures so they could both know who the donor was now and, at age eighteen, provide their older son with the identity of his and his sister's donor that was to be his younger sister's birthright when she came of age. The mothers grew to feel that they could not claim their family as their own without this information. They also feared that if they didn't take action their older child might disown them for failing to provide the birthright that his younger sister had.

Is it legitimate to violate a person's privacy and civil rights for the purpose of knowing? I don't think so. But Denise and Sarah's story highlights how strong the need to know can become and how far parents might feel moved to go to find out. Ostensibly, such extreme measures are taken in the best interests of the child. But percolating below the surface may be parents' need to sleuth for themselves to assuage their angst about full possession of their child or dispossession by their child because of the child's experience of having a birth other.

Denise and Sarah's experience alerts us to how radically feelings can change as circumstances are altered by new legislation and policies. If you are embarking on this journey into assisted reproductive technology, I can only invite you to use the full power of your imagination to envision how you might feel later about a decision made now if circumstances change. For example, how will you feel if you were assured total anonymity of the donor and then someday a statute is grandfathered in that all donors could voluntarily participate in a national register that would allow donor children to search for their donors? Would you feel okay if your child would never be able to find out the identity of his or her donor but children born in later decades would always be able to find out, as required by new laws?

What Makes You More of a Parent—Knowing or Not Knowing the Birth Other?

Mary, a single parent with a feisty and sometimes testy little boy, sat in my office and shared her thoughts about the donor who made her motherhood possible. Whereas she was grateful that his services had allowed her to have Benjie, she never wanted to know who he was or have him know her son. As she explained it to me, "My family is myself and Benjie. I want Benjie to grow up proud of that. Knowing the identity of his donor might legitimize that man as a parent, either in his own eyes, in Benjie's, or maybe even in my own. And he's not. I am. Not knowing is the best way for me to authorize my feeling that Benjie is mine and no one else's."

As Susan Cooper and Ellen Glazer have said in their own book on the subject, parents may choose to have a donor remain anonymous just to strengthen their feeling that their child is theirs. Parents who have used a surrogate or donor may also worry that their children will suffer from "genealogical bewilderment," meaning that the child will grow confused about who he or she belongs to.[12] Concerned that their child will be confused about who his or her parents are, some mothers and fathers envision that the closer the relationship between the donor and the parents, the more likely that the child will be befuddled. For example, in a heterosexual donor-insemination family, the child may be bewildered by having both a social father and a genetic father. The emotional equation runs like this: The closer the relationship between donor and family, the more likely the confusion. Ergo, anonymity is the best protection against genealogical bewilderment.

Jill and Tamara are delighted that their little girl Lucy was conceived with the aid of their very close friend Gary. Jill is Lucy's biological mother. Gary and his wife Sherry have been close friends of Jill and Tamara's for years. Gary and Sherry have two children of their own. Jill and Tamara have not yet worked out if and when they will tell Lucy that Gary is the donor who helped make her. Partly it will depend on how Gary and Sherry feel about it in relation to their own children and the conservative community to which they have moved. The four adults are all discussing it together, thoughtfully and with great regard and respect for each other's feelings.

In the midst of these discussions something else is going on—Tamara is now feeling it's her turn to have a child. She desperately wants Gary to be the donor for her child, too. He's not sure he wants to donate a second time. Jill and Tamara are very distraught about this. They so much want a genetic connection between their children and a second chance to use a friend they love and trust as the donor. I wonder with Jill and Tamara whether there might be a silver lining to Gary's hesitancy—the benefits of donor insemination by someone they don't know. Such an arrangement would circumvent the complicated negotiations presently going on among four adults trying to accommodate everyone's best interests and perhaps could create an enclosure for the two women as the parents to a second child.

Jill was intrigued by this new way of thinking about it. But I could see Tamara's face clouding over. The thought of an anonymous donor made her sad and uncomfortable. She wanted the same chance that Jill had had and would feel second best if she couldn't conceive just like Jill had. Ironically, she imagined she would have a harder time laying claim to the baby if she did not know the donor like they knew Lucy's donor. The experience of Gary's presence, accompanied by his sensitive and unwavering recognition of Jill and Tamara as Lucy's only parents, would never be duplicated with an unknown donor. With the lack of that personal acknowledgment from a known and beloved donor, Tamara feared she would always feel her biological child would never really be bestowed upon her. Instead, it would remain in limbo as hers and a distant and unknown someone else's.

The effect on parents' feelings of possession is only one factor in making the decision about whether or not to know the birth other. The child's right to know the person from whom he or she came is another absolutely primary criterion, but we'll save that discussion for Chapter 6. Suffice it to say here that no simple formula exists for the relationship between knowing the birth other and the solidification of your feeling that your child belongs to you. Instead, going inside and exploring all the feelings, fears, and fantasies about the birth other and the birth other's role in the family will help clarify whether or not knowing makes sense.

For example, Jill and Tamara seemed absolutely sure they wanted the same known donor for their second child as for their first. Yet when we worked together to explore all their feelings about this, especially in light of Gary's hesitancies to donate again, they could open their minds to another option—using an anonymous donor might be a simpler and more straightforward way to lay claim to their second child, rather than just a second-best choice if Gary said no. Their willingness to go inside shows us that there is no absolute right or wrong, just creative solutions about knowing or not.

In some cases, there is no choice, as when a couple's only means of conception is through a sperm bank that requires anonymity or, conversely, when the only financially feasible road to conception is a friend and a turkey baster. In such cases, it's not a matter of whether knowing (or not knowing) makes sense, but rather of making sense of knowing or not as a necessary given in the child's conception.

Knowing is a complicated word. In the biblical sense, it refers to the sexual union between two people. By its very definition, that will never happen between a donor and parent or surrogate and parent, because the very terms of the relationship are that no sex has taken place. In the social sense, knowing is about friendship and connection ("I know her well"). This constitutes the level of knowing most directly related to the building of a family matrix for the child—who will be in it and how they will all relate to each other, a topic covered in the next chapter, on family belonging. Finally, in the academic sense, *knowing* refers to the compilation of information, both concrete and abstract. That is exactly the kind of knowing I mean when I speak of donor identity as it relates to feelings of possession, the question of knowing that all parents must sort out as they construct the family that will be theirs.

WHERE IS YOUR BABY GROWING? WHO DOES THE LAW SAY ARE MOMMY AND DADDY?

When your growing fetus resides at your address, in your or your partner's womb, you can reach over, feel the baby kick, and watch the baby grow, inch by inch, pound by pound. As we said before, it is also true that when you walk down the street pregnant, the whole world will assume that the baby inside is yours and treat you accordingly. This is the advantage given to parents using egg or sperm donors and a womb of their own. In contrast, when the growing fetus resides at a different address, in someone else's womb, there is fertile ground for feelings of alienation, distance, and a lack of possession. Such feelings are typically overcome as soon as the baby is born and comes home. Nonetheless, they are there to be reckoned with.

With a surrogate, even if one or both parents will be the genetic parents of the child, the process by necessity is one step removed, if not several states or even continents removed. The feeling of possession that evolves from the intent to parent can be undermined when a baby is grown somewhere else by someone else, not you, someone who will be assumed to be the real mother of the baby as she walks down the street pregnant. And if you are a parent using a surrogate, you also know that you have little or no control over your baby's temporary housing. During pregnancy, the medical field has taught us that the mother-to-be has to eat well, sleep well, avoid substances potentially toxic to the baby, and stay stress-free, for herself but, more important, for the well-being of the child. This takes discipline and concentrated effort, and if you can't monitor your baby's prenatal environment, you can be left feeling both helpless and alienated from the birth process. The work during the pregnancy is to hold to the vision that the child is really yours, even if you can't watch the baby grow or feel it growing in your body and even if you can't contribute to the baby's welfare by doing all the right things (eating well, sleeping well) to keep it healthy.

Meanwhile, the surrogate has a hard task, too—to hold to the vision that the child she is carrying in her womb for nine months does not belong to her, even if it is being fed by her body or made by her own egg. The whole country was indeed galvanized by Mary Beth Whitehead's failure to do this as she claimed that the baby she was having for the Sterns was really hers. Not just surrogates, but sperm donors and egg donors, too, can lay claim to their progeny. But geography is not on their side. In body politics, the surrogate may lay claim to the baby on the basis of territorial rights—the baby lives inside her, is birthed by her, and, therefore, is hers. And the intentional parents may face an uphill battle in taking possession of their child as a result of being physically removed, fenced out of the gestational process.

Ironically, the law is also often on the surrogate's side. Typically, the law states that the gestational mother holds the parental rights, unless otherwise arranged. William Handel, director of the Center for Surrogate Parenting, developed a strategy to help parents using gestational carriers claim their parental rights. He has the genetic parents file maternity and paternity suits prior to the delivery, to prove they are the child's parents. Since the surrogates are not pursuing parental rights, the suits are uncontested and the genetic parents get the child, as early as the last trimester of the pregnancy. Despite the happy endings, the reality is that parents have to take an extra step to claim their child as their own, a step that parents having babies the old-fashioned way do not typically have to take, with the exception of paternity suits filed by fathers trying to lay claim to their sons or daughters.

The pain of having to take this extra step toward possession was poignantly brought home in a 2001 court case. Marla and Steven Culliton were going to have twins with the help of a surrogate. They filed a prebirth petition to be named on the birth certificate, and were turned down by a lower court in the state of Massachusetts. Instead, the Cullitons would have to go through an adoption process to obtain the legal rights to their children. They took their case to a higher court, arguing that they were being denied the right to parent their own children and that the surrogate, who never wanted to be the mother, was being forced to be one by the court.[13]

Regretfully, the courts have not caught up with the realities of contemporary family life. How absurd that a woman who does not even want to be a mother is stuck with parental rights while the parents who intended to have a child together have to go to court to obtain them. If you can't even put your name on your child's birth certificate, how will you come to feel that your child is actually yours? And what if the surrogate who holds that privilege decides to exercise her parental rights?

To counteract the dangers of geographic distance—the housing of your child in someone else's womb—you can decide to use a combination of a surrogate and egg donor, to ensure that the surrogate will feel less like the baby belongs to her as it does not come from her own genes. But even that does not always work. In 1993, Anna Johnson became a gestational carrier for Mark and Crispina Calvert. Although she had no genetic links to the child, she still attempted to gain custody of the baby after the delivery. She was claiming her rights as the mother who birthed the baby, and she believed this took precedence over genetic ties. The baby came from her, she had grown attached to it, and therefore it was hers. The ruling, which went to the California Supreme Court, was against her. The court ruled that the people who had intended to raise the child, the Calverts, should be designated as the parents. Here, both intent to parent and genetics trumped geography. But again, possession was not a given for the Calverts, because, even though they were the full genetic parents of their baby-to-be, it was housed somewhere else. Rather, they had to fight for legal possession of their own child.

Several years ago, I began work with a family that started out as a gay couple and a lesbian couple setting out to have a baby. One of the men in the gay couple agreed to be the sperm donor, and one woman, and then the other, attempted to be the donor recipient, but neither could conceive. As a next step, they turned to an egg donor, a woman known to them, and agreed that the mother who had not had children before would be the gestational mother. While the two mothers would be the primary parents, the two men also planned to take on fathering roles, which they certainly did once their son was born.

Regretfully, the arrangement turned sour as the relationship between the two mothers deteriorated soon after the birth of their son. In a sudden turn of events, the gestational mother took the baby and moved out. Because she, as the gestational mother, was the only one of the two women who held legal rights to the child, she barred the other mother from co-parenting with her. As for the fathers, she filed a suit that they had no parental rights. She claimed that the genetic father was just a sperm donor, since the insemination was done in a doctor's office under circumstances that by California law qualified him only as a donor and not as a father (had the insemination been done with a turkey baster by a friend, he could claim parental rights). The court denied her petition and instead granted parental rights to the genetic father and the gestational mother in a joint custody arrangement. The other mother held no parental or visitation rights, and the other father was included as a family member but not as a legal father. Perhaps if they had had a clearly laid-out parenting agreement before the birth of the child, none of this turmoil and familial distress would have ensued. But I tell you this story to highlight how geography (where the fetus grows) and present legal statutes can coalesce to create conundrums and confusion regarding the question "Whom does this baby belong to?"

In contrast to other Western countries, the United States has yet to develop a clear-cut set of statutes and policies regarding assisted reproductive technology. Whereas, for example, agencies now try to fully screen possible surrogates before matching them with parents and help parents draw up prebirth placement contracts, the reality is that these contracts are not legally binding. Beginning with the case of Baby M in which Mary Beth Whitehead challenged the prebirth contract she had drawn up with the Sterns, we are now all highly sensitized to the risks to parents' possession of their children in this fertile new world of assisted reproductive technology. But we should also remember that the risks are there for the surrogate as well. What if the parents decide that the baby does not belong to them; that is, that they don't want it once it's born? Nothing legally binds them to take it. As a consequence of residential address, her womb, will the surrogate or gestational carrier be stuck with children that she did not intend to have and do not belong to her?

In 2001, in the case of Wheeler and Berman, a couple set out to have a baby using the father's sperm, an egg donor, and a gestational carrier. Early in the pregnancy the carrier discovered she was pregnant with twins. The parents wanted her to have a fetal reduction, but she refused, feeling that the parents had taken too long to decide and it was now too far into the pregnancy and a risk to her health. The parents' lawyer offered the carrier two options: fetal reduction or termination of the pregnancy, with full payment for her services. The carrier offered a compromise of seeking other parents for the fetuses, feeling she could not go through with either option. The parties could not decide how other parents would be chosen and what, if anything, newcomers would pay to either the carrier or the parents for expenses. The gestational carrier was British, and in Britain the surrogate holds the legal rights for the first six weeks after birth. However, the prebirth contract was

signed in California, where the parents held the rights. The gestational carrier, who had relocated to San Diego, sued to sever the parents' rights to the
children and claim damages. In the end, the children were born and placed
with their intentional parents. But the battlefield of possession and the rights
of a woman to her own womb and its contents remained at issue for several
months while the question "Whose babies are these?" remained open.

I have told you many of the extreme cases that hit the front pages of the
newspaper to underscore the challenges to taking possession for parents using a birth other. Each tells us that until the intent to parent more systemati-
cally guides our legal system, parents will have one more hurdle to jump in
ensuring their sense of possession of their child, particularly when the growing fetus is housed at another address.

Yet I don't want to throw the baby out with the bathwater, so to speak,
by failing to highlight the creative solutions the majority of parents have discovered to overcome the roadblocks of geography and the legal system.
Cheryl Saban and her husband had two babies using two different surrogates. In each case they developed a close familial relationship with the surrogate, spending time together, meeting the surrogate's family, attending
doctors' visits together. In the end, Cheryl hopes to tell her children "that
their very existence was made possible by a dedicated group effort, specifically by the unselfish, benevolent actions of two of the most charitable
women I know. Kathy and Lori [the surrogates] will always be part of my
life."[14] We could say that the best antidote to geography's distancing and the
law's foibles is relationship—a close, positive, and open one between the
surrogate and the parents. With that in place, there will be little question
about whom the baby belongs to.

NO MATTER WHAT, WILL BLOOD REMAIN THICKER THAN WATER?

When I was a little girl, in a pre-AIDS era, a monumental and exciting ritual
was to become blood sisters. You would only do it with your closest friend;
you would each prick your finger and then mix your blood together. The ritual
completed, you were now more than just friends. You were tied by blood, and
that made your relationship more special and more permanent than friendship. Truthfully, fifty years later I can no longer remember each of my blood
sisters, but for the period in which we lived by the ritual, we were family.

I tell you this story to highlight the salience of blood relations in our culture and to acknowledge how early in life we internalize their importance. On the other hand, it is not just the risk of HIV transmission that has eliminated my childhood game. We have moved into a new era in which bonds of love begin to vie with bonds of blood in family ties. Stepfamilies, adoptive families, foster families, and now birth-other families enlighten us that no blood needs to be drawn or shared to establish that "we are family." We have entered a confusing time when the old and new commingle—blood matters, blood doesn't. How will it affect your feelings that your child is yours if you have mixed your blood with an outsider's or didn't use your blood at all to have a baby with the aid of a birth other?

The tension between "blood matters/blood doesn't" can confuse all of us about whom a baby belongs to. The medical community says that biology is so important that it will do whatever it can at whatever cost to help parents have a baby genetically related to them. At the same time, the experts are telling nongenetic parents that genetics are so insignificant that not having blood ties to their child won't matter at all, no one needs to know about it, and the child will definitely belong to them anyway. And then egg donors, sperm donors, and surrogates are expected to accept that their genetic relationship to the child doesn't matter at all—they will help create but never be a parent or even have any relationship to the child who is connected to them by blood.

Geography and the law may play their hand, but it may be your own deep-rooted feelings about blood ties in the context of this cultural confusion that will be the linchpin in determining how hard it will be to lay claim to your child if you are using a birth other. Adoptive parents have spent many years teaching us about the deep process they have gone through—in support groups, in their own homes, in a therapist's office, in writing books—to work through their feelings that the child that was placed with them belongs to them, even if the child didn't come from them. One adoptive mother put it most poignantly when she explained, "I feel so connected to my daughter that I tell her that the only sadness I feel is that she who is so much mine didn't also come from me." But what adoptive parents can't teach us is what it is like to lay claim to a child who is only half genetically related rather than not at all. We will have to cut a new path here. We as a village all have to scrutinize our own biases about genetic versus social ties in parenting. And for parents, your work is to explore with openness and honesty, both to yourself and with your partner if you have one, whether deep in your heart you actually believe that blood is thicker than water and whether you can truly embrace the opposite belief that bonds of love trump ties of blood. Neither of these is necessarily a fixed or immutable belief, and remarkably, you can find yourself holding both of them at once. That's okay, but if you don't pay attention to them, they may roll in as the biggest roadblocks in your journey to lay claim to your child.

Recall the story of Sally and Matthew. In barring Matthew from being a homework parent for high-achieving Jeremy because Matthew didn't have "smart genes," Sally was exposing her own deeper belief system that blood is thicker than water. In the process, she begins to see Jeremy as more hers than Matthew's. From Matthew's side, he may buy into the same beliefs and hold back from inserting himself as Jeremy's real dad because his genes didn't make Jeremy and he has no right to lay claim to a child who has another man's smarter genes. It's not uncommon in any family for one parent to be more of the homework parent or for parents to divide up the other tasks of child rearing as well. But when that division of labor is tied to a struggle, either internal or interpersonal, and the genetic parent always wins over the nongenetic parent, there might be some work to be done in asking whether blood matters or not. What could Sally and Matthew do? Talk it out with each other, even though it might be quite painful. Sally could admit her feelings that Matthew is not up to the task of grooming Jeremy for success because he doesn't have the right blood ties and lacks the requisite smart genes. Matthew could explore whether he feels both squeezed out and illegitimate. Each would have to hear the other out and then turn their attention to doing the best for Jeremy—providing him with a mother and father who both feel like legitimate parents. We used to worry about the stigma of the illegitimate child. In birth-other families, we instead have to pay attention to the stigma of the illegitimate *parent*—the one who lacks the genetic tie with the child.

Ms. T, pregnant with her first child, struggled with these very feelings of illegitimacy. The baby was conceived with her husband's sperm and an egg donor. Ms. T found herself acceding to her husband's ideas for the baby's name. Why? Because she felt the baby was more his than hers. Why more his? Because the baby was made from his sperm and nothing from her. Even though it was her blood feeding the baby through her placenta, that wasn't the blood that counted. The blood that counted was the kind that determines hair color, height, even temperament and personality. That was her husband's and the egg donor's blood, not hers. She worried that these feelings would carry over into her attitude toward child rearing after the baby was born, perhaps letting her husband's views take precedence over hers because, after all, he was the more legitimate parent.[15]

A colleague and close friend of mine who has been actively interested in my work admitted to me that he grows squeamish when he thinks about babies born with sperm donors, egg donors, or surrogates. For himself, he would have to feel that a child came from him, was part of his flesh and blood. Anything else would feel unnatural. This friend has had the good fortune of having a genetic child of his own and perhaps would feel differently if those avenues had been closed to him, given how much he loves being a father and what a wonderful father he is. But my hat goes off to him for being brave enough to admit what many enlightened people feel but are afraid to say—that they believe blood is thicker than water. It would help all parents who are contemplating conception with a birth other to go where my colleague had the courage to go—the exploration of any internal biases that privilege genetic over nongenetic parent–child ties. Better to know that the feelings and thoughts are there, either to tweak them or to accept that they may be strong enough to warrant thinking more carefully about going ahead with a conception with a birth other.

The fact of the matter is that parenting is really a trial by fire. You discover that you are a real parent the moment you find yourself on the front lines—feeding, bathing, waking to a baby's cries, waiting anxiously for the pediatrician to call back about a high fever, and so forth. Once that baby arrives, it's yours. But the question "How much yours?" remains. Ms. T is worried that her own psychology will diminish her role as a vital and central player in her child's life and lead her to accede to her husband's wishes. Birthing a baby between her own legs is not enough to undo her belief that she is not a real mother because she could not impart her genes to her child. Only her husband holds that privilege. Sally and Matthew were both real parents, but Sally thought of herself as more real because she, along with the donor, contributed the smart genes to her academically advanced son, Jeremy.

Then I'm reminded of a story a colleague told me. She was conducting a heated therapy session with an adoptive family when the adopted preadolescent son hurled the proverbial toxic missile at his adoptive parents: "It doesn't matter. You're not my real parents." The father's face crumbled as he cried in pain in response to these piercing words. But the mother got out of her seat, walked right up to her son, put her hands on his shoulders, looked him straight in the eye, and responded, "Honey, this is as real as it gets."[16] And I would say the same to parents using a birth other—this is as real as it gets.

Yet, still, the significance of blood ties is a very personal matter and varies widely from person to person. As more and more families blend biological and nonbiological ties, blood no longer triumphs over water. Instead, they exist in creative tension with each other: Blood ties matter; blood ties don't matter. The challenge for all parents turning to a birth other to have a child is to examine the importance of genetics to them and to their partner if they have one and to be aware of the significance of genetic ties to the people around them as well. For example, some lesbian mothers have told me that they decided on donor insemination over adoption in part because they believed their own parents would more likely overcome their resistance to a child born to their lesbian daughter if it was a child genetically linked to them. Cultural mores, religious beliefs, and personal psychology must all be thrown into the hopper in coming to terms with one's feelings about genetic links (or lack of them) to a child.

So who possesses the child—the one whose gametes made the child, the one who grows the child inside her, or the one who raises the child? In birth-other families, the potential owners could constitute up to five people for one child. The answer to the question "Who possesses the child?" is simple: The one(s) who intended to have the child are the one(s) who possess the child. The answer may be simple, but the journey to attaining a sense of possession is not. You've got your personal psychology, your internalized beliefs, and your interpersonal struggles with your partner if you have one, to grapple with, along with the realities of biology, legal statutes, and social and family attitudes. With that in mind, how would you now respond to the questions laid out at the beginning of the chapter: Does your child feel more like yours than your partner's (the nongenetic parent) if you have one, or do you think you will feel this way after your child is born? Do you (or will you) accede to your partner (the genetic parent) if you have one? Is your child really yours, even if you weren't the maker? Is your child not totally yours because he or she belongs to the birth other?

I'm recalling the comments of a mother in the audience of a panel on infertility and adoption in which I participated, titled "Where do Babies Come From?" She was an adoptive mother who invited us to consider a Buddhist notion when thinking about the issue of possession and belonging. In the Buddhist tradition, an adopted child is a soul looking for its parents. It is not random. It's an active journey toward belonging that has intent and direction, that was meant to be. I found this such a soothing and generative narrative, one that could as easily apply to a child of parents using a birth other: "You are mine [ours] because you came to me [us] and no one else, with the help of someone's else gametes or womb. Now that we are together, you belong to me [us]."

A babe in arms definitely soothes our qualms about "Where's the baby?" The baby is right here in our arms. No doubt the best reinforcer of possession is a real baby with real needs who looks to a parent for love. So I now want to turn our attention to the sense of belonging that evolves as parents raise the baby that is theirs. It is a story of bonding, attachment, and family building when a child is made with the aid of a birth other.

What's Love Got to Do with It?

What a family looks like to outsiders is not as important as whether adults know what children need to develop positively, and work to fulfill their responsibilities to each other and to their children.

—Hillary Rodham Clinton, *It Takes a Village*[1]

A little girl came to see me for her second therapy session. In addition to telling me that therapists were pointless, she shot me a glaring look and declared accusingly that all we psychologists did was experiment on people. I thought about her experience—pulled into therapy by parents terribly worried about her. I empathized with her understandable discomfort and suspicion, her hesitance to open up her inner secrets to me, this total stranger. Then my thoughts wandered, as they often do these days, to the parallel situation for parents and children in birth-other families. Like my little patient, they, too, often feel under a microscope, subjects in the grand new experiment of baby making in the era of rapidly expanding reproductive techniques. Not just the researchers, but the whole world looks in on these families, wondering "How will the children fare?" and "Are these 'normal' families?" and so forth. What the family looks like to outsiders may not be as important as what the adults within the family provide, but if truth be told, what the birth-other family looks like to those outsiders can range from unusual to unfathomable, from mildly different to totally revolutionary. So many people wonder what or if the parents will tell their children about their origins. Some wonder whether parents will be able to bond with a child made with someone else's eggs or sperm or carried in some other woman's womb. Under this scrutiny mothers, fathers, and children do their family building.

Establishing your feelings of possession of your child is just the first step in forging a lasting bond with that child. More significant is building a sense of belonging together. Once "unto us (or me), a child is born," the compelling realities of caring for and tending to a real, live child take over. As explained by the psychoanalyst and pediatrician D. W. Winnicott, "There is something about having a baby (even preparing for an adopted child) that alters the parents. They become orientated to the special task."[2] The same, of course, is true if you have a baby using a birth other. But you are different, too, because you are faced with three unique child-rearing tasks:

- Bonding with a child who has been conceived with someone else's egg or sperm or carried in someone else's womb.
- Figuring out how those birth others will be included, or not, in your family's life.
- Deciding what, if, and when to tell your children about their origins with a birth other.

Untangling these three tasks from one another is nearly impossible, so this and the next two chapters must go together like a triptych. The first "panel," this chapter, will explore the task of bonding and family building, the second will move to the decision-making process around disclosure, and the third will lay out a developmental map for what and when to tell a child if the decision is made to tell. Together, I hope the three panels will provide us with a full panorama of love, attachment, and belonging in birth-other families.

As we think about the experience of bonding, which may be fraught with anxieties, here are five questions for parents and parents-to-be:

1. Have you ever worried that your child's donor (or surrogate) will compete for your child's affections?
2. Do you ever have the feeling that attachments are stronger if they're based on blood ties?
3. Does your child or your child-to-be feel different from or like you, and how does that affect how close you feel or will feel?

4. If your child has already been born, do you think you bonded to him or her right away, or did it take time?
5. Do you feel comfortable thinking about or talking about the donor (or surrogate), or do you worry that acknowledging this person out loud might weaken the bonds between you and your child?

THE CONNIVING KIDNAPPER

In Western child development theory, the cornerstone of healthy development is strong parent–child attachment. We take the notion of attachment so for granted that when I went through my old texts on child development I was hard put to find a straightforward definition of the term. It seems that the authors just assumed that everyone would know what they were talking about. So I took it upon myself to synthesize a commonsense definition. Attachment is the nature of our ties with one another. It is a two-way street. When speaking of parent–child relations, attachment is formed from the reciprocal interchange between the mother or father and the child and normatively happens without too much conscious effort. Attachment, when successful, is a warm, intimate, and continuous relationship in which both parent and child find satisfaction and enjoyment. Attachment, when not successful, can be a connection fraught with anxiety and ambivalence, even avoidance.

If we put a random group of parents and their babies in a room together, could we tell any difference in the attachment behavior and experience of adoptive parents and their babies, traditional reproductive parents and their babies, and reproductive technology parents and their babies? I suspect not. I couldn't agree more with a mother whose babies were conceived with in vitro fertilization:

> My passionate attachment to my girls [triplets] is the result of my taking care of them, feeding and soothing and spending some very long days and nights with them. The particulars of their conception are merely a medical fact, no more resonant to me than say, their blood types.[3]

Albeit with many variations on the theme, the critical variable in attachment is not how the baby got to you, but that the baby is there. At the same time, a parent's experience in the evolving relationship with his or her child cannot help being affected by the participation of an outsider in the baby's conception. Let me begin with a particular way this experience may uniquely unfold for parents and children in birth-other families—fantasies of the conniving kidnapper.

Birth Other by Day, Conniving Kidnapper by Night

Noelle Oxenhandler, in her book *The Eros of Parenthood*, sheds light on the seemingly universal parental fear of kidnappers or evil strangers coming to snatch our child away, a fear that appears in myths, in fairytales, and in real parents' minds as well. In our wildest fantasies, wolves, witches, Rumpelstiltskin, crazy people, and perverts are all suspects who might steal children away from their parents. They come to take our children away to punish us for not valuing our children enough. At the same time, they come because our baby is so valuable, who wouldn't want to steal her? Oxenhandler refers to that dark stranger as the "evil other."[4] Because we love our children so much yet fear that we can never love them enough, we conjure up the fantasy of the evil other who will come to take them away from us. Our strong attachment to our children is the very reason we worry about losing them.

In parents' psyches a strong bond exists between themselves and the evil other. Both of them want the same child—the parents' beloved son or daughter. Now try substituting birth other for evil other. I read Oxenhandler's discussion about parents' fantasies of child snatchers and immediately thought about parents using birth others as I learned about the relationship of these fantasies to our strong attachment to our children and to the ambivalence that can accompany such intense bonds. What better breeding ground for fantasies of the snatcher, the evil other, than in the struggles to make sense of the presence of a donor or surrogate in a child's life?

Let's review the psychological role of the donor or surrogate in family life to see how it might fuel fantasies of the evil other in parents' minds. Although in this book I have coined the phrase birth other, as a society we still have yet to land on a commonly held term for this person and his or her place in the narrative of a child's life. Whether socially constructed or deeply embedded in the universal human experience of growing up, it seems that we're all interested in an answer to the question "Where did I come from?" When people become parents they must anticipate the same question coming from their children, directed to them. And when the real answer must be "Not from me," then comes the question "Then from whom?" From there, you might be off and running with unsettling fantasies.[5]

Now let's return to universal parental fantasies of the evil other who might come to snatch the baby away and tear asunder the bond between parent and child. If you've had children using a birth other, forget about visions of wolves and witches dancing in your heads. There is a real, live shadow person, the donor or surrogate, who may lay claim to your children because he or she helped make them. And even if that person never steps forward to lay claim to your child, he or she might still lure your child away in your, their, or your child's inner fantasies. Or maybe the snatching will happen not by any doing of the evil other but because your child has set out on a quest to find the person who made him or her.

The angst about this shadow person resonates closely with the experience of adoptive parents, who live with the anxiety that the birth mother may appear to claim rights to their children or, alternatively, that the children may turn their backs on the adoptive parents as they go in search of their real parents. Yet there's one very important difference. In birth-other families, the evil other has fewer degrees of separation from the parents. The birth/evil other is linked biologically to at least one of the parents, either through joining of egg and sperm or by housing an embryo made from at least one of the parents' gametes. If a person regularly sits at your dinner table, intimately shares her pregnancy with you, or personally collaborated with you in donating eggs or sperm, that person may become (or already is) a genuine intimate other in your life. The real and positive relationship can definitely counteract the fantasies of the birth other transformed into the evil other. But, regretfully, the close, intimate connection can also have the opposite effect. The birth other not only has biological ties to your beloved child, but also, indirectly, to you or to your partner, if you have one. Having mixed bodily elements with you (or your partner), the intimately known birth other can feel too close in, perhaps ready to pounce.

Returning to the Eros of parenthood, in contrast to the predominant cultural image of epoxy bonds that characterize parent–child attachment, Oxenhandler plays with the notion that our children are like changelings sent to us only temporarily for their safekeeping. Having spent a chapter highlighting the importance of a sense of possession for birth-other parents, I'm turning around to say that we also have to consider the opposite notion of "the slender thread of ownership" regarding *all* parents and their children. Our children's first steps are typically away from rather than toward us. This reminds us that attachment is a paradox—we are asked to come very, very close to our children only so we can learn to let them go. Our children only partly belong to us. Someday they will leave us to create lives or families of their own. Ergo, the slender thread of ownership that haunts our bonds with our children. I believe those threads may be stretched even thinner when you have had a child with a birth other. Why? Because there really is the ghost or active presence of a person tugging on one end of the thread. That person is the birth other, the one who either lurks in the shadows or makes his or her presence well known in the family. In fantasy, the birth other is ripe to become the evil other, coming to take the child away.

What to Do If the Evil Other Shows Up

So what does any parent do to dispel his or her fears of the evil other? Defuse the terror by facing him or her head on. Recognize that although this is a real person, it is also a figment of our inner experience, our realization that our ties with our children are always tenuous, for someday they will leave us.[6] The chances of getting rattled by fantasies of the evil other decrease if we recognize that the evil other is our own creative work. We love our child so much and yet recognize how precarious it is to pour all that passion into a child whom we may not be able to serve well enough and whom we will someday lose to adulthood. In response, we conjure up a concrete image of a character who will snatch our children from us.

Years before becoming a mother myself, I remember having this exact feeling about my beloved baby brother, ten years my junior. Again and again, I would anxiously run out to check on him, left in the backyard to nap in his carriage in a sleepy suburb of Chicago. I was sure that a creepy prowler was scheming to steal him from us at any moment. Years later I read Sigmund Freud's work and was led to believe that my fears were really a reaction formation against my death wishes toward my brother. That never made any sense to me, but the idea of the conniving kidnapper does. My kidnapper fears had everything to do with the risky business of love and little to do with the darker demons of hate. I imagine it would have been a lot easier for me to dispel or neutralize my kidnapping fears if I had had the psychological tools to make the connection between my intense bond to my baby brother and my fears of having him taken away from me, but I was only ten.

Making this connection between bonding and kidnapping fears is a challenging process not just for ten-year-olds, but for any of you who have conceived a child with a birth other. As the baby sleeps soundly in his or her crib, the threat to the child and to the parent–child bond is not limited to the imagined attack by a kidnapper read about last week, last month, or even years ago in a sensational news report. The evil other is much closer to home—it is the donor or surrogate, whether known or anonymous, who has participated in the creation of your child.

Especially if you have used a surrogate to have a child, the conniving kidnapper (aka evil other, aka birth other) can grow by exponential proportions in your mind. While awaiting your child, you're forced to deal with the loss of control over your baby's temporary housing, because it is someone else's body. Fears can mount about this other person who may have "stolen" your baby into her own body. Once the baby is born and delivered to you, you can take possession and control of your child's care. The powerful force of bonding can override the estrangement of temporary removal. But the haunting presence of the womb that housed the baby becomes prime fertilizer for the universal parental fantasy of the kidnapper coming to snatch the baby away. After all, for nine months, someone already has.

Sometimes you can dilute the evil other into a more palatable image, a "ghost parent."[7] An adoptive mother recalls the tactless queries of her best friend regarding the birth mother's involvement in her child's open adoption: "Don't you worry she'll get too attached? What about afterward? Are you going to stay in touch? Send her photos? Let her visit?"[8] This is not a kidnapping. It's an attempted cooptation. The key question here is "Don't you worry that she'll get too attached?" Like the birth mother in adoptive families, the birth other might get too attached, and then what? Then birth other and parent will be vying for the same beloved child, and parents may lose their baby to the birth other. So whether ghost or kidnapper, an outsider lurks in the shadows, challenging and at the same time reminding parents of the strength of their love for their child.

The experience of Shawna and her partner, Rosemary, illustrates all too perfectly the potential reality of the ghost parent or evil other. Shawna called me on the recommendation of her lawyer. At the time, she and Rosemary had a seventeen-month-old son named Alex. Shawna is the biological mother. They used a known sperm donor, and for reasons that seemed to make sense at the time, they listed his name on the birth certificate and also had him sign a declaration of paternity. Rosemary now wanted to adopt their son in a second-parent adoption. But the sperm donor, Marcus, suddenly announced that he wasn't sure he would agree to it. He decided he was not just a donor. He insisted on his parental rights and wanted the opportunity to visit his child. He told the child to call him Daddy, without consulting Alex's mothers first. During this period he was visiting Alex once every two months. For the time being Marcus was demanding the right to see Alex when he (Marcus) was available. Shawna was distraught and stressed. She felt bullied into agreeing to Marcus's demands so as to preserve Rosemary's option to adopt Alex. She experienced him as black-mailing her and Rosemary. He paid no child support, expressed no intention to, and was not involved in Alex's daily care. She did not trust him as a parent and had never intended to parent with him. She wanted my advice as to what to do.

Unfortunately, she and Rosemary did not receive legal and psychological counseling when they really needed it, before Alex was born. They would have known to get a written declaration of parenting, with everyone's role clearly delineated, and they would not have put Marcus's name on the birth certificate. Although I had not asked Shawna in my first conversation what had brought them to list him on the birth certificate, I later found out that he held citizenship in another country and she and Rosemary wanted their son to have the opportunity to live and declare citizenship in that country.

Marcus, a gay man in a couple, was a coworker of Shawna's. After knowing him for about six months, Shawna had approached Marcus with the idea of his being a donor for her and Rosemary's child. She had enjoyed his company and considered him both intelligent and physically attractive, attributes both she and Rosemary felt important for the donor to have. It came as a complete surprise when Marcus later appeared on the scene to claim his rights to "his" child. Claiming it had always been his intention to be involved in Alex's life as a parent, he wanted to be included in decision making and discussions regarding Alex and to establish the customary postdivorce custody model of visitation every other weekend and Wednesday evenings. Alex's mothers argued that everyone was clear that Marcus was to be a known donor, nothing more. Marcus countered that he was the only father Alex would ever know, and Alex was the only grandchild Marcus's parents might ever have.

Shawna and Rosemary felt trapped in a waking nightmare. Marcus had stepped in to threaten Rosemary's legal standing as Alex's nonbiological parent as well as her emotional position as Alex's other mother. Neither Shawna nor Rosemary had any desire to co-parent with Marcus. They already had a thriving toddler and a harmoniously functioning family with two parents. Alex was strongly bonded to both of them, and they were still in the stage of early parenthood when parents fall head over heels in love with their child. As a donor Marcus was a good choice, but not as a father. And besides, they never were looking for a father. Alex has two mothers. Shawna, in her eagerness to have a child, signed off with Marcus as the sperm donor, but unwittingly, and perhaps with unconscious motivation, also as the father to her child. What was coming never dawned on Shawna and Rosemary until it came. The evil other was no fantasy. He was right at the front door and at the lawyer's office. He took the form of the sperm donor transforming himself into father and tearing asunder the intimate bonds of the family that included Shawna, Rosemary, and Alex.

A year and a half later, the outcome of their conflict with Marcus was an out-of-court settlement in which all three adults, Shawna, Rosemary, and Marcus, would share parent status and Shawna and Rosemary would have physical custody. From Shawna and Rosemary's point of view, it could have been worse—Rosemary could have been denied parenting status. But it could have been better, too. The evil other, Marcus, indeed came to claim his rights and got them and would be showing up every Sunday to see Alex. In the meantime, Shawna and Rosemary have learned to keep their eyes on the prize, to recognize that the everyday care and deepening bonds between them and Alex over time will take precedence over any of the untoward intrusions of Marcus into their life with their child. Whether they will also be able to transform Marcus from the evil other into a positive member of their family matrix remains to be seen.

Children, Too, Can Conjure Up the Kidnapper

Fears of the conniving kidnapper visit not only the parents. Over time the child, too, can begin to fear the evil other, the kidnapper. While you parents may fret that your child will seek out or run into the arms of the birth other who is transformed in your child's mind into the real parent, your child ironically may be grappling with just the opposite fear—that he or she will be snatched away by this interloper. Here is where we have much to learn from the adoption field. In a 1987 case reported by Calvin Calarusso in *Psychoanalytic Study of the Child*, a twelve-year-old adopted boy was embarking on the first meeting with his birth mother. He expressed the fear that his "new" mother would steal him away:

> I'd be scared she might try and make me part of her family. Then I'd lose my own. She might try and steal me illegally. She'd toss me in the car and drive away. . . . She says to me, "Ron, how would you like to live with me?" I say, "no, I 1like my family the way it is!" Then she grabs me and pushes me into a box in the back of her car. I dive out while the car is going and do a couple of rolls to break the fall. She drives away thinking I'm in the car. Then I call my mom and she comes and gets me.[9]

Not just a random stranger, a particular stranger is coming to take the adopted child away—the stranger who gave birth to the baby many years before. The child's fantasy is to fight this conniving kidnapper off rather than run away with her. Why would he want to run off with a mean stranger who would throw him into a box, when he already has a mom he dearly loves?

Child-snatching fears like Ron's may be stronger for the adopted child than for the child created with the aid of either a donor or surrogate. Children and birth others have a whole different dynamic from children and birth mothers. Unlike birth mothers in adoption, donors and surrogates start out with the conscious intent before conception to have someone else be the parents of the baby created. They did not conceive their own baby either intentionally or accidentally and then decide to relinquish it later. Yet we all know from the widely publicized case of Baby M that conscious intent to help someone else have a baby does not preclude a change of mind. Germaine Greer points out that "in Britain at least ART [assisted reproductive technology] practitioners believe that women can never be trusted after giving up their genetic children to forget all about them."[10] And not just women, for Marcus certainly showed us that as a sperm donor he couldn't be trusted either.

This potential for the birth other not to let go does not escape the tender psyches of the children. We see adopted Ron's fears of being snatched by his birth mother mirrored in a seven-year-old boy's worries about meeting his sperm donor. This boy was growing up in a lesbian family and had a "yes" donor whose identity could be released to him when he turned eighteen. As described by the boy's therapist, "He had it in his mind that he could not meet this man until he was eighteen years old; otherwise this man might want to keep him."[11]

Several years ago I worked with a child who did not find out until she was eight years old that she had been conceived with the aid of an anonymous sperm donor. For two years Delaney worked on processing the information about her origins. At age ten she engaged in a new fantasy. She and her parents were climbing a high mountain together. Unbeknown to them, a scraggly man in a spooky hut had staked himself out at the top of the mountain. Climbing ahead, Delaney reached the mountaintop first, only to be lured away by this evil man, who offered her promises of candy and adventure. Fooled by the strange man, she was snatched away from her parents, never to see them again. She spent the rest of her life on the lonely mountaintop, longing for her family. Who was that scraggly man? The conniving kidnapper, the sperm donor.

Did this fantasy reveal a weakened attachment to her parents? Just the opposite. Delaney's real life was not on a lonely mountaintop but in a close and positive relationship with her parents. The security of this attachment was the springboard that allowed her to engage in this cold and dismal fantasy, which in turn helped her dispel her fears and actually strengthen her bonds with her parents. Many years later, Delaney explained it to me quite clearly: "My parents are my parents, no matter what. It doesn't matter that I don't have my dad's genes; I love him just as much—actually, maybe even a little more than my mom."

In my observation, Delaney reflects not the aberration, but the norm—a warm, intimate, and close relationship between parent and child, the hallmark of positive attachment. Her accompanying conniving kidnapper fantasy is also quite normal. As in any other family, the universal fear of the evil other, based on the slender threads of ownership, may surface. But unlike in other families, the fear in birth-other families may be swelled by the worries about real men and women who exist in the child's past or present and who may have good reasons—genetic or biological—to covet the child whom the parents love so deeply and tried so hard to have. What's love got to do with it? Paradoxically, it's love that generates the fears, and it is love that will overcome them.

BLOOD AND BONDING

Before love conquers all, other attachment hurdles may present themselves, either at the moment parents fall in love with their child or somewhere along the path. Most specifically, "blood matters, blood doesn't" comes to the fore again in attachment building. At the very end of Bruno Bettelheim's book *The Good Enough Parent,* he offers parents the following advice

> The good enough parent will always be aware that conceiving and bearing a child and bringing it into this world are the most wondrous events in the life of a child. The more they can enjoy together, each in their own ways, what follows from it—the parents raising the child, the child being raised by his parents—the happier their lives will be.[12]

Directives to enjoy "what follows from it" should be a welcome salve to any parent. But the reference to what *precedes* it—conception and birth as spectacularly unique events in a child's life—might sandblast the salve from your psyche and leave in its stead a chronic irritation if your child's conception and birth involved a birth other. That wondrous event unfolded not by your doing alone. A donor or surrogate was there, too. Not only does Bettelheim's avuncular advice immediately raise the specter of the ghost parent or evil other, it also reminds us that most people automatically assume that babies are made by their parents, not by someone else, and that their happy lives will unfold from that premise.

And if the babies *are* made by someone else, then what? In *Adoption Nation*, Adam Pertman writes that across all nations throughout history people abide by the assumption that individuals not related by blood will never feel totally connected. The belief is reflected in both a country's legal practices—for example, allowing inheritance only through bloodlines—and in its use of language, such as in phrases like "my own flesh and blood."[13] Translated to parent–child bonds, this means parents will never feel as attached to a child not biologically related to them as they will to their own flesh and blood. Nor will the child feel as attached to the nonbiological parent as to the biological parent. By these terms, a father in a sperm-donor family, a mother in an egg-donor or surrogate family, and a nonbiological parent in a lesbian or gay family will always be compromised in their attachments to their children—less attached than their partner with genetic ties and therefore never fully attached. And their children will be compromised as well as they try to bond with their parents. This cultural prejudice is a hurdle nonbiological parents will need to jump as they secure their ties with their children.

Eliza was just two and a half when I met with her and her fathers, Randy and Martin. Randy was her biological father and Martin, Randy's partner, her social father. Samantha was conceived with Randy's sperm and an egg from a known donor and birthed by her third parent in the family matrix, Allison, Eliza's gestational mother. To Eliza, Randy was Daddy and Martin was Papa. That's all she knew about the different status of her two fathers, unless one counts her explanation that Martin has red hair and a moustache and Randy has dark hair and a beard. Martin and Randy were in the middle of a court fight with Samantha's mother, struggling over parenting status and custody issues. Eliza clearly loved both her dads dearly, and they were obviously crazy about her. It only took minutes of observation to assess that this was a successful attachment for all concerned. Just emerging from her toddler years, Eliza soaked up the doting attention of her two dads, still holding her status as "your majesty, the baby." But she was also moving into her Electra years, newly vibrant with the drama of fickle love affairs when one parent was the love of her life and the other (or others) should just take a walk. And who was the current object of her passionate longing? Martin, her nonbiological father. "Papa, let's play puppets." "Papa, I show you my story." "Papa, I will sit on your lap." And who should take a walk? Randy, her biological father. "Daddy, you go away. I'm playing with Papa. Daddy, go sit on the couch and don't say a word."

Randy took all these rebukes graciously. A mental health professional himself, he recognized the developmental meanings of Eliza's love triangle and knew this was just a passing fancy. Martin, as one could imagine, reveled in the new unfolding scenario in which Eliza had eyes only for him. But a deeper, darker current ran through each father's feelings.

Randy could be lighthearted about Eliza's rejection of him because he felt absolutely secure in his attachment to Eliza and hers to him. Eliza was not only his genetic child, but her face was a carbon copy of his. As her genetic father, by California law he and he alone was Eliza's legal father. Blood ran thick, and his name on Eliza's birth certificate solidified the confidence he had in his bond with her.

Martin had neither genetics nor the law on his side. He held his status as parent only by Randy's good graces. If ever he and Randy were to break up, Martin would have no legal rights to Eliza, even though it was obvious from the day of her birth that Martin was as much of a father to Eliza as any man could be. Such equality in parenting was exactly how he and Randy had planned it to be, regardless of California statutes. Randy, on his part, had no intention of going anywhere. He was deeply in love with and committed to Martin and assured Martin that no matter what the courts said, in his heart and in their agreements they were both fathers together—forever. Together, Randy and Martin railed against a legal system that made no accommodations for gay and lesbian families and repeatedly denied parental status to nonbiological parents.

Yet Randy's assurances, Eliza's love affair with Martin, and all of the recognition Martin got from both extended family and friends that he was Papa to Eliza still failed to quell his anxieties that the thread of ownership was indeed slender for him and Eliza and much slimmer than for Randy and Eliza. I watched with sadness as Martin sat on the floor of my office playing with Eliza. His nonlegal, nonbiological parenting status prevented him from totally believing in the bond he had so beautifully established with his daughter. I could feel his angst as he played 'til he dropped, offering the best any dad could to a daughter but showing beads of sweat as he tried to quiet the still, small voice within that whispered, "Your days as a dad could be numbered."

As a clinician, I could worry that Martin's insecurity and compensatory efforts to secure the permanency of his bond with Eliza might impair his ability to execute Bettelheim's directive to "enjoy together . . . the parents raising the child, the child being raised by [her] parents." A parent's anxiety about losing a child can indeed germinate an unsuccessful attachment laced with anxiety, avoidance, or ambivalence. Regrettably, this is always the risk for any nonbiological parent in a birth-other family. The risk grows greater when that parent also has no legal rights, which is typically the case in gay and lesbian families. And the risk can be exacerbated even further if the biological parent in subtle or not so subtle ways reinforces the feeling that the baby is "mine and not yours."

The good news is that these insecurities are rarely at the base but more likely at the fringe of parents' experiences with their children. At the core, overshadowing the doubts is the deep and intense connection that unfolds as parents attend to the day-to-day realities of caring for and loving a child and as children attend to the task of attaching to the ones who love them so. This doesn't mean that parents should ignore these feelings of insecurity if they surface, because they can indeed fester. What it does mean is that such feelings are easily negotiated if biological and nonbiological parent alike remain mindful and supportive of each other in their relationship with their child. Emotional sensitivity is particularly important when the nonbiological parent is also a nonlegal parent, because that parent is denied the palliative of legal rights that soothes the pain of nonbiological status (a palliative more typically operative in heterosexual couples using a birth other).

In the case of Randy, Martin, and Eliza I have had the good fortune of following their family over time. A year after the love affair with Martin, Eliza dumped Martin for Randy. Now it was "Daddy, Daddy, Daddy." Although it was hard for Martin to lose his place in the sun to Randy, he was better able to weather the fickle finger of preschool love because he now had under his belt another year of bonding on the front lines—the day-to-day experience of caring for, playing with, thinking about, and just being with Eliza. The court proceedings had also settled down, and Martin and Randy had been in long-term couples therapy where they worked to better understand their differing experiences with Eliza and identify the supports they needed from each other. Randy had to recognize that his position of privilege, in his case being the genetic and legal father, blinded him to the precarious position Martin found himself in. Martin had to learn to trust Randy more and calm the hair trigger on his assumption that the odds were stacked against him in his attachment to Eliza. Two more years passed, and the roots of their family's bonding had taken even stronger hold. Two years later, with Eliza now seven, the ease and flow of love among Randy, Martin, and Eliza was so palpable that I could hardly remember who was the genetic and who the nongenetic father, even in light of the unchanged phenomenal physical resemblance between Eliza and her father. They all clearly felt they belonged together.

The Invisible Man Can Come to Threaten Your Bonds

In the asymmetry between biological and nonbiological parent–child ties, the nonbiological parent's feelings of insecurity can bleed into feelings of invisibility, as they did for Martin. But the invisible man can also show up as the shadow birth other who hovers at the edge or participates in the center of the attachments being built between parents and child. If, as the nonbiological parent, you ever find yourself to be the invisible man (or woman), that feeling might interfere with the experience of bonding to your child in those moments you sense yourself as not really being there. And if the invisible man should show up as the birth other, especially the unknown donor, the bonding in your family may feel temporarily disrupted as you try to tackle this shadowy intruder who may not be seen but is always there.

In Chapter 3, I introduced Caroline and her parents, Charlie and Jo. Caroline was not her father's biological child, although she did not know it when I first started working with her. I would like to tell you another part of her family story that reveals the effects of invisibility on the attachment scenario when a birth other, in this case a sperm donor, hovers in the family's history. Caroline had spent her early years in a communal household, until her parents' separation. She was brought to me for treatment because of anxiety attacks subsequent to her parents' divorce. In my first session with her parents I was struck by Charlie's insistence on the virtue of having multiple caretakers for Caroline, none related by blood, but all identified as members of her communal family. At the time, I had not yet been told that Caroline was not Charlie's biological child. I took note of Jo's strong objection to Charlie's stance that all these caretakers were significant others to seven-year-old Caroline. Jo only saw that as confusing and damaging to Caroline, although she had gone along with the notion of one big happy communal family in Caroline's early years. I attributed Charlie's tenacious insistence on the value of this communal family arrangement to his adherence to 1960s countercultural political beliefs, which included "smashing the nuclear family."

Then came my first session with Caroline, to which she was brought by her mother. Coming to get her in the waiting room, I was totally taken aback by the striking physical resemblance between mother and daughter. I was then further taken aback that I had had such a strong reaction. I had seen plenty of parents and children who were remarkable look-alikes and yet never reacted so strongly. I wondered why. During this first session, I asked Caroline to do a kinetic family drawing, in which she was to draw everyone in her family doing something. Instead, with tape in hand, she created a spreadsheet four feet wide, with a grid of aunts, uncles, cousins, grandparents, and fictive relatives that went on and on, ending only because the session did. I had no idea what to make of this (again, remember that at this time I did not know she had been conceived with the aid of a donor).

Typically, when children create a kinetic family drawing they include only the people to whom they are most strongly attached. And most often the clinician looks for the immediate family members who are excluded, potentially signifying something awry in those attachment relationships. Yet Caroline's kinetic family drawing went in the reverse direction, with a cast of thousands. At the time I thought that Caroline's family grid revealed her historical experience in a family with no clear boundaries and an unending stream of potential members. Later, when I found out that Charlie was a nonbiological father and that Caroline was a sperm-donor baby, Charlie's celebration of communal life and Caroline's never-ending family grid began to make better sense to me. Charlie had transferred to Caroline his anxious preoccupation with the viability of all Caroline's nonbiological communal family members. And that anxiety was in turn a displacement of his central anxiety about the undisclosed fact about *him-self* as a family member—that he was not Caroline's biological father. If he could convince Caroline that everyone close to her was her family, whether related by blood or not, then she would have no trouble if she found out later that her own father was not related to her by blood either. Charlie's anxiety was so strong that it clouded his thinking. During the court battle with Jo around custody issues, his angst about his attachment to Caroline drove him to defy his attorney's counsel. He insisted on having one of the communal "parents" in Caroline's life write a friendly letter to the court defending her blossoming in her nontraditional communal family and her right to multiple caretakers, a move that could only shoot Charlie in the foot in their custody battle before an extremely conservative family court judge.

Charlie was speaking in tongues. Caroline's real blossoming had more to do with a loving dad who was not her biological father, but a father she adored, than with her communal upbringing. Charlie was fighting all too hard to build up insurance against his feared invisibility and rejection by Caroline were she to discover that he was not her father by blood. And regrettably, unlike Martin with Randy, Charlie did not have the kind support of Caroline's biological parent in helping him negotiate these feelings of potential invisibility and illegitimacy. To the contrary, Jo was suing him for sole custody of Caroline, claiming she was the primary parent.

Aggravated by divorce proceedings, Charlie's angst about his nonbiological parent status was getting in the way of both his judgment as a parent and his daughter's sensibilities about what a family member is. And although, unlike Martin, he was buttressed by his standing as Caroline's legal father, even that was being threatened as Jo took him to court in custody proceedings.

Yet, like the story of Martin and Randy, this story has a happy ending. Because Charlie and Jo were both strongly committed to Caroline and very devoted parents, they were willing to roll up their sleeves and iron out the wrinkles in their family relationships. Through months of working together in therapy, they recognized that not disclosing to Caroline was getting in the way of Charlie's "attachment security" and violated their own social values of honesty and forthrightness with children. They eventually decided to tell her. Jo dropped her custody suit, recognizing how destructive it was to Caroline and to the family ties they had built, and Charlie let go of his preoccupation with communal families and took responsibility for the confusion it had been causing Caroline. Over time, Charlie and Jo were even able to become friends. Again, I have had the good fortune of following Charlie, Jo, and Caroline over time. Caroline has lived in a fifty-fifty joint custody arrangement. She knows that she was born with the assistance of donor insemination; she knows that Charlie is her only father. She's not that interested in the donor. No more family grids. Caroline is now in high school. Running into them all recently at a park, it was heartwarming to watch Caroline move easily between her father and mother, a hand on her father's shoulder, an arm crooked through her mother's.

Don't Surrogates Have Claim to Baby's First Bond?

The invisible parent can feel pushed even farther back into the shadows when a surrogate is involved and questions of how the surrogate could abandon her baby claim the forefront. In the eyes of outside critics, a surrogate has carried a child for nine months in her womb and then turned her back on it. A baby has been abandoned. Stephen Byrnes, the father in a gay couple who used a surrogate to have their daughter, described how people often ask, "How can she give away her baby?" Indeed, one of the readers for this chapter's draft scribbled in a marginal comment that she wondered about it, too. Admittedly, it challenges all of us, if we have never been a surrogate ourselves, to imagine how one goes through the experience of growing a baby in her womb all the while knowing this baby is not intended for her and planning to hand it over to someone else at birth. How does she ever detach enough to do it?

Stephen Byrnes and his partner were fortunate enough to have an extremely understanding and sensitive surrogate. Psychologically, they were also able to stretch their thinking and feeling to counteract this cultural perception of the surrogate abandoning her child:

> I think of this sonogram moment [Tammi, the surrogate, did not look at the sonogram screen at the doctor's office but instead focused on the two

fathers-to-be as they stared at their baby-to-be on the sonogram screen] when Tammi's motivation crystallized for me. She isn't giving away her baby—she is having a baby for us. Tammi has her own family, and I have never felt that she wanted or needed our baby.[14]

Tammi did not abandon her baby; it was never hers. From the moment of conception, she had every intention of relinquishing the baby to its proper parents, Stephen Byrnes and his partner. She operationalized this intention by carefully gauging her actions to remove herself and instead to reinforce the attachment bond between the men and their baby.

Not everyone is as lucky as Stephen and his partner. It does not help a parent's sense of belonging when well-meaning (or not so well-meaning) bystanders remark, "Oh, how could she [the surrogate] give her baby away after carrying it for nine months?" For the parents, this translates to: We have a child who is a changeling—abandoned by someone else and left for us to raise; we have a child with one parent who does not count because the child didn't come from that parent. Even when parents never hear such a remark from a family member, friend, or stranger, the thought might get called up from deep within themselves. Not just the nongenetic parent but the genetic parent as well can be rendered invisible and ineffective in the attachment scenario because his or her strong bond with the child can feel compromised by the belief that this is an abandoned child. And we all know the potential for permanent scarring in a child who has been discarded. If you are carrying a worry that your child suffers a primal wound that may never be healed by the loving bonds of the only family your child has ever known, this can hardly make you feel vital and potent as your child's main attachment figure.

Nor do the threats to the bond necessarily vaporize when instead of an abandoner the birth other is a highly visible, known, and active member of the family matrix. Quite the contrary—the feelings of invisibility can be even more debilitating for the nonbiological parent who watches his or her child jump into the arms of the person whose blood runs thick within the child. It seems as if you can't win for losing. Asymmetrical blood ties, invisibility, and myths of abandonment are mighty forces to overcome. Paying attention to your own feelings and the feelings of the other family matrix members helps transcend these tensions. Martin and Randy are a perfect example of the steps you can take to secure the bonds with your children in the face of all these feelings. But when you try to sweep these feelings under the rug or when thinking gets clouded by anxious rumblings, you risk stretching the tenuous threads of possession that are the mainstay of attachment.

DO OPPOSITES ATTRACT?

One more attachment hurdle remains—the perceived difference between parent and child. We have already explored how similarity facilitates a sense of possession and how too much difference can impede it. The same principle extends to the sense of belonging, of being a part of each other over time.

Psychologist Marsha Levy-Warren describes the case of a Middle Eastern couple who, as a result of a medical mix-up, unexpectedly gave birth to a blond, blue-eyed baby girl, conceived with a mixture of the father's and a donor's sperm and an egg donor and carried by the mother:

> The Desais, who were dark-skinned and dark-haired, had been able to find donors described as being of similar complexion and hair color. They planned to keep their baby's parentage a secret.
>
> In their consultation, they said their world shattered when Leila was born with blond hair and blue eyes. They were concerned about whether they could keep themselves from conveying the degree of disappointment, alienation, and betrayal they felt toward her. . . . "It's hard to admit even between us that we fear that we cannot love this baby because she is so different from us."[15]

For this family, it was not just a matter of hair and eye color. It was the meaning of the color—an obvious public statement that their child, Leila, was of a different ethnicity than her Middle Eastern parents. How could they possibly keep her parentage a secret with such visual disclosure that she was not made by both of them? More importantly, how could they love her? In the Desais' cultural world, a sense of belonging was limited to like-skinned, like-colored people of the same heritage. They were now forced to bond to a child who, through mistaken mixing, felt like a total outsider.

Fortunately, they had a sensitive therapist to guide them across these troubled waters. Dr. Levy-Warren was very sage when she advised Mr. and Mrs. Desai to give the bonding some time. She suggested that they needed to be patient to allow a relationship to unfold, to allow time in which they could get to know Leila and she could get to know them. No doubt many parents need this time to get to know and bond to their child, not just parents who have used a birth other. Just recently, a young colleague of mine admitted that it took at least three months for her even to begin to feel love toward her baby son. The notion of indelible bonding at first sight is more often a myth than a common reality of parents with their new babies. Yet giving the bonding some time might be even more essential if your child is born not just of your genes but of an outsider's as well and when your child feels so very different from yourself. In the Desais' case, Musaf, the father, came back to the therapist and reported, "We're getting to know Leila. She is so beautiful and alert. She follows us with her eyes wherever we go in the room. She quiets down as soon as we hold her. She is really a sweet baby." And Pilar, the mother, added, "We found it very helpful to feel we had some time to get to know her."[16]

In families who have babies the old-fashioned way, gestation often offers the parents the opportunity to get to know the baby, to feel it moving inside or with a hand on the mother's belly and imagine that inside the womb is a baby who was created by both parents. But gestation for parents who have used a sperm donor or an egg donor comes with a potential set of complications that might undermine this early sense of knowing. At a subterranean level parents might feel that the mother's body has been invaded by an alien who has nothing to do with either the mother or the father, or the mother alone if she is a single parent or in a lesbian family. This hardly creates a feeling of belonging. And if the baby comes out bearing absolutely no physical resemblance to the biological parent, bonding indeed may feel like a stretch. People birthing their own biological children plunge into parenting with the driving force of sameness, regeneration through progeny, and intergenerational connectedness dictated by blood and genes to facilitate their bonding with their children. No intrusion of a poltergeist gets in the way of their sense of belonging and bonding with their child. Not so for parents having a child with a birth other.

The poltergeist phenomenon often takes the form of a "not me" experience. The newborn is experienced so much as "not coming from me" that a parent worries about the rejection that might follow either on his or her own part or the baby's. A prospective mother who is considering motherhood using an egg donor admits her fears:

In the back of your mind you're thinking what if I have this completely ghastly, terrible child, who I just won't like. . . . One thing you don't want to reinforce is any feeling you might have that somehow you haven't got a connection with this child, it's the sort of nightmare scenario if you look at your child doing something horrible and you think, oh, that must have come from the mother.[17]

Typically, those fears are easily washed away when a real child is there to hold and care for, albeit not so easily if the child is indeed troublesome or difficult. But, like we learned with the Desais, the gnawing worry of "not-me-ness" must first be dispelled to clear the path for successful bonding with a child who feels or is so different because he or she came from a birth other. The feelings may pop up again later—let's say at a moment when your child begins playing the piano like a virtuoso and everyone in your family is totally tone deaf. Then the not-me feelings will need to be negotiated again, or maybe for the first time—and any time they appear on the interior screen of your parenting life.

Children Like to Be the Same, Too

"Are you like me?" and "Are you not like me?" are questions not just for parents but also for children in the choreography of parent–child attachment. Many theories of child and human development focus on the relation between the child and the people closest to him or her. For the small child to develop a strong identity later on, she must first attach to the people who care for her. In doing so, she negotiates a psychological and existential question: Who am I in relation to the people closest to me? One dimension by which a child measures this is sameness versus difference. The tiny infant is so closely connected with the parent that sameness is not only about likeness but also about a lack of knowledge that there are even two separate people. As the baby grows, her life task is to move from likeness toward otherness— to learn that she is indeed not the same person as her parent(s) and that she is both alike and different, that is, separate from her parent(s).

With the child who starts out being very different from her parents as a result of the presence of a birth other, the process may be partially reversed—she must move from otherness to sameness. Indeed, her parents must do the same. As in the Desai family, the baby may begin life somewhat separate from her parents. She comes in part from another person's body, from a person who will never be her parent. And she may end up looking very different from her parent(s), like little Leila.

As we learned with Pilar and Musaf, a great deal of anxiety may surge through you if you are confronting the challenges of bonding to a baby or child who seems so very much a stranger. Your task is to forge a tie with a baby who does not come totally packaged with the sometimes mythological certifications of "our flesh and blood," "Uncle Harry's hairline," "Grandma Jo's fussiness," perks that often help solidify the connection. From your child's point of view, the partial absence of such certifications can create ongoing angst—"Who *do* I look like? Certainly no one in *this* family!" Infertility doctors who help couples have babies using donated eggs or sperm know about this difficulty and try to remedy the stranger situation for the child by matching the donor's features to those of the nonbiological parent. This way the children will not grow up looking or feeling so other. This way the parents can grow to feel that the child is the same as them, rather than coming, at least in part, from a stranger or from someone who is definitely not me. This way the family can establish a sense of belonging with each other.

Whether it is a socially constructed phenomenon or built into the human condition, we cannot overlook that people struggle when they feel too physically other from their family. Parents struggle, and so do their children. I am recalling the request of my five-year-old daughter to dye her hair black, not to emulate Madonna's ever-changing hair colors, but because she was the only one in the family with blond hair. She wanted to be the same as her dark-haired mother, father, and baby brother. Otherwise, she felt like an outsider.

Wesley was also five years old and, like my daughter, had different coloring from his family; he had many of the dark features of his sperm donor. Neither his lesbian biological mom nor his nonbiological mom nor his brother, born to his nonbiological mom with a different donor, shared his dark features. Wesley came up with a creative solution—he would paint himself lighter. That way he would belong better. His mothers did a beautiful job of showing him all the ways he *was* like his mothers and brother, while empathizing with his sadness that he didn't look more like them. I think it is important to acknowledge this hurdle to attachment created by too much difference if we are to reinforce secure bonds for children who come from a birth other who might be very, very different from the parent(s).

A sense of belonging is based in part on a sense of sameness, and those of you in birth-other families must be mindful of the quest both you and your children will make to find the sense of sameness, a sense that will in turn nurture the connections among you. If you are in a family that has both a biological and a nonbiological parent, the task is not only to forge a sense of sameness with a child who may feel very different, but also to forge a sense of social and emotional sameness between a parent and child who share no genes but do share a life together. I am reminded of a father who was explaining to me that his daughter was as stubborn as he was, and it started her first year of life. His child was born with the aid of a sperm donor. She had no genetic links to him. But the similarities between him and his daughter were profound—not just their stubbornness, but their interests, their moods, even their curly hair and long, slender bodies. The similarities were there to be found, and he found them, and that sense of sameness reassured him that his daughter was indeed his and secured the bond between them.

Sameness does not just come from genes. Nor is it based only on looks. It comes from shared moments together; it comes from common values; it comes from finding yourself in the other person. Just as best friends and lovers seek out their likenesses and commonalities, so, too, can you help yourself and your child forge your bonds to each other if you pay attention to what you have in common rather than what separates you from each other—your different genes.

FAMILY REVERIES

Jumping the hurdles of evil others, biological/nonbiological asymmetry, invisibility, and otherness are daunting tasks for parents who have already spent months or years traversing the world of assisted reproductive technology to have a child so dearly wanted. In addition to taking the time to bond and being mindful of the disparate experience for all the parties involved, there are supports that will facilitate healthy attachment among all the members of the family and ensure a secure sense of belonging. The first has to do with allowing space for reverie and fantasy about *all* the members in the new family matrix and their relationships to one another—children, parents, and, whether disclosed to the child or not, birth others.

All You Have to Do Is Dream, Dream, Dream

Psychoanalyst Ken Corbett coined the term "family reverie." By this he meant the parents' and children's collective fantasies about the donor in

families using a birth other. He recounted the experience of a lesbian family—two mothers, Ellen and R.J., and a seven-year-old son, Andy, conceived with a sperm donor, a "yes" donor whose identity would be revealed
to Andy when he turned eighteen. In keeping with my observations of parents' fears of the conniving kidnapper, Dr. Corbett observed that over time
the entire family had worked to silence their fantasies about this man. To
think about him was to open the doors to the intruder and allow him to interfere with their family bonds.

This code of silence had not always existed in Andy's family. Before
Andy was born, the two mothers had had many discussions about the donor,
colored by lively fantasies. They fantasized the ways they would be similar,
connected to him, and ways he would be familiar. They drew pictures of him
in their minds, created from the little information they had about him, like
his hair color and his interest in mathematics. They even developed a crush
on this man, whom they named Tim. They imagined him as a lovable man.
But the music stopped once the baby came. No more donor fantasies. Both
moms were worried that the reveries might generate a whole lot of questions
from Andy that they could not answer. And they worried that the reveries
might rev up wishes or desires, either their own or Andy's, that could not be
satisfied. More deeply, they were afraid the fantasies might function as an
interloper that would shatter the intimacy of their family and weaken their
family ties. Their worries rendered them unable to think any more about the
donor, the one they used to call Tim.

Dr. Corbett worked with the mothers to help them recognize that rather
than preventing an intrusion, they had unwittingly created one. By putting
their fantasies about the donor in cold storage, they had created an impedi-
ment to family bonding, similar to the fracturing effects of family secrets. He
helped the mothers return to their prebirth imaginings and feel free again to
engage in their collective reveries about the donor. But this time the reveries
would be not just their own, but Andy's as well. Ellen and R.J. rediscovered
the pleasure they once had in their shared daydreams about the donor before
Andy's birth, and now Andy was included in the fun. And through this process they found that opening up to each other about their thoughts and fantasies about "Tim" actually brought them closer together as a family.[18]

The lesson to be learned from Ellen, R.J., and Andy's experience is that
parents need to allow themselves the freedom for such reveries about their
family, both for themselves and also to prepare themselves to help their child
do the same, assuming the child will know that there was a donor or a surro-

gate. Making room for such fantasizing will be the best way to counteract the fears of the conniving kidnapper. Instead, let him or her in the door as a member in the family's daydreams, in the spirit that the family that dreams together belongs together.

Let's go back to the music stopping as soon as the child appears. The gestational period is a time of unbridled fantasy and musing. But then when the baby arrives, the vital, palpable, and concrete love affair with the child takes over. It is at that point that the donor becomes transformed into the evil other, the conniving kidnapper coming to take the baby away. So why not just stick him or her in the closet, out of sight, out of mind once the baby arrives? Because he or she will pop out later. There is a far better way to secure a sense of belonging and attachment among everyone in the family. Rather than stopping the music, let the good times roll. Give room for everyone to have ongoing thoughts and fantasies about the relationship of this real child to the real person who donated his or her genetic material or womb so a child could be born and raised by one, two, or more loving parents. This holds true whether the birth other is an unknown person or a person known to the family, for the person who sits in our living room is often very different from that same person when he or she shows up in our fantasy life. This also holds true in families where parents choose not to disclose to their children that they were born with a birth other. In this case, not everyone will be having reveries, but the parents who made a conscious decision to have a child using the birth other will, and that in turn will facilitate healthy bonds with their child.

We also have to take into account that somewhere out there is a birth other who may be having his or her own reveries about the child that was born. Rather than being threatened by this, parents and children can incorporate that knowledge into their own reveries, imagining what that person might be thinking about them as they think about that person.

Dream On, but Beware Creating Myths

A word of caution is in order, however. Allowing reveries is healthy for family bonding, but creating myths is not. Myth building happens when you transform fantasy into fact and forget that it's just a daydream, even telling it to others as the real story. In the situation of the single-parent family, two simultaneous and opposite myths can evolve that may engender an ingenuous sense of belonging. The first is the Madonna myth—we are one parent and one child; there is no one else on earth. In this case, the myth obliterates the existence of the third party, the other genetic contributor to the child. The second is the One Happy Family myth—our family consists of me, you, and the nice man or woman who helped make you. In this case, the donor, even if anonymous, can be transformed into a glowing figure of heroic proportions—as when a single mother tells her child, "You play piano so beautifully. I'm tone deaf. You have your father's musical genius. You're going to be just like him," this gleaned from the information she received about the anonymous donor from the sperm bank ten years ago.

Recall the love affair with their son's donor reported by Ellen and R.J. prior to Andy's birth. Such passionate musings could happen in any family. Nonetheless, myths created from this love affair are far more likely to occur in single-parent than in two-parent birth-other families. We could say that this would be true of any single-parent family, not just those who create families with the use of donated gametes or a borrowed womb. But the separation of sex from reproduction in the donor or surrogate single-parent family creates a much more fertile ground for the Madonna or One Big Happy Family myth than in other single-parent families who have a child based on a sexual union. Why? Because there is typically no history of a sexual connection or intimacy with another actual person to counteract the fantasies.

The two-parent family can also fall into the trap of myth making, either by denying to themselves that anyone else but the two parents exist in the child's birth history (the suppression of reverie) or by constructing the birth other as an idealized third parent in the family. Whether in one- or two-parent families, the risk of letting minds wander is that they can begin to crystallize into immaculate deception myths. You will know if you have crossed the line from reverie into myth if instead of merely fantasizing about who the birth other might be, you place that person in a role that is far, far from reality and then find yourself beginning to act as if this were true. For example, the birth other becomes the father who will show up one day to lead his child into adulthood or the mother who will always love her child because she carried her for nine months in her womb. Alternatively, the birth other will be obliterated from existence—there is no such person. All of this constitutes delusion rather than reverie. If you find yourself veering off in the direction of immaculate deception, it is probably your anxiety leading you. Reminding yourself and using your other family members as a check that thoughts about the birth other are just dreams that don't necessarily come true will keep the pathways open for playful sharing and creativity, two essential components to attachment building and a sense of belonging together as a family.

Before Andy's birth, his moms had already carved out that creative pathway by playfully indulging in their fantasies about the anonymous donor, "Tim." By keeping those fantasies alive (which they did later with the help of Andy's therapist) while helping each other avoid the trap of converting "Tim" into Andy's real, live dad, they could come close to Andy while he engaged in his own reveries about his donor. Family bonding is built on a bedrock of honesty, realness, and making room for and sharing each other's emotional experiences. Andy and his moms' reveries, balanced by the reality that Ellen and R.J., not "Tim," were Andy's real parents, provided just such bedrock.

THE FAMILY MATRIX

So what have we learned about attachment in birth-other families? Listen to these two stories. The first is told by Stephen Byrnes, the gay father who had a baby with his partner using a surrogate:

> At the park in Virginia [where they are visiting the surrogate and her family], Sammy [their daughter] calls me Mommy, and Jacob [the surrogate's son] laughs at her. "He's not your Mommy, he's your Daddy." Language is inadequate to describe the facts of our lives. Sammy has a lot of names for me: Mommy, Daddy, Daddy Steve, and Poppa. Each name reflects a different aspect of our relationship. Of all the names Sammy calls me, I like Mommy the best and can't think of another name I'd rather be called.[19]

Stephen is Mommy, Daddy, and Poppa. He spends time with the surrogate and her family. Jacob knows that technically Sammy is his half-sister, but it is clear that his mommy is Tammi, and Sammy belongs to Stephen and his partner.

The next is the story of Joan Lunden, a *Good Morning America* TV host. At fifty-two, she is having twins, using an anonymous egg donor, her husband's sperm, and a known surrogate:

> When you have a really nice relationship with the surrogate and her husband, it's great. . . . I was surprised at how the mother–child connection starts to form even though someone else is carrying the children. . . . Our hope is that Deborah and Peter [surrogate and surrogate's husband] remain part of our lives and connected to us forever.[20]

Joan Lunden has no genetic or biological relationship to her babies-to-be, yet feels connected to them and envisions a family life that will include both the surrogate and the surrogate's husband. In both Joan Lunden's and Stephen Byrnes's stories we find no vestige of the traditional Ozzie and Harriet family, but what we do find are families building strong bonds with each other in new and unique ways.

Although no large fund of data exists to support this claim objectively, such bond-building is what I have seen in the families I've worked with. Susan Golombok and Fiona MacCallum, two British psychologists, have made an effort to compile all the studies that we do have to date on families using assisted reproductive technology. Looking across studies, they concluded that parents appear to bond more strongly to their children conceived with assisted reproductive technology than the parents of naturally conceived children do to their children, providing them with a higher level of nurturing in their early years. Also, in all the measures used, the children raised in sperm-donor, egg-donor and surrogate families were doing as well as children in control groups regarding their relationship with their parents.[21] These data seem to confirm my observations that birth-other babies are strongly bonded babies.

If you have used a birth other, you will have some unique tasks in forging a relationship with your child and establishing a sense of belonging. I have taken to using the term family matrix to refer to the family you will build, a family that will either include the birth other in active participation or not, but inevitably will have to take that person into account. Your family matrix may include a sibling who has been a donor or surrogate for your children or an adult son or daughter who has been a surrogate or donor for you, quite a new concept of extended family. With all the combinations and permutations, the family matrix is a critical variable in forging attachment in birth-other families. By definition, the family matrix dictates that you strive to be clear about who belongs in your family and in what way. There is no one right configuration, but the family matrix works best when all the pieces fit harmoniously, at least as much as possible. Rather than a fixed point in time, constructing an harmonious family matrix is better thought of as an ongoing work in progress.

Do parents need to worry about attachment to their children born with the aid of a birth other? Definitively not. It may seem contradictory that I have dredged up stories of conniving kidnappers, evil others, and invisible men while simultaneously underscoring that these children and parents are forging happy, positive attachments to each other. Let me explain. First, in an effort to advocate for families using assisted reproductive technology, I have noticed a tendency to candy coat the experience. Yet my clinical experience tells me that it is not so simple or sweet in practice. So I have taken it upon myself to bring the sleepy underwater monsters to the surface so that we can discover they are not so scary in the light of day and simply need to be negotiated. I also want to put the anxieties and fears in perspective; they become minuscule on balance with the strong love you feel when you wake up each morning and go to sleep every night with your child in your arms or on your mind.

If you don't have to worry about your bonds of love or that the monsters lurking below are a threat to those bonds, you might be freed up to think more openly about our opening questions—your concern that the birth other will compete for your child's affections, that attachment is diluted when the bonds are of water rather than blood, that your child is too different to feel close to or takes time to bond to, or that you think too much or too little about the donor or surrogate for your child's and your own good. You might also feel free to compare your answers to those questions to your partner's, if you have one, to see whether genetic asymmetry creates a difference in your responses.

Recently I was at a meeting where one of the women brought her small baby. All of us were parents ourselves or worked with babies and children on a daily basis. The baby, sleeping soundly in the other room, started stirring and began to whimper. Before any of us had heard even a peep, Veronica, the mom, had already jumped up and swooped her baby into her arms. That's what parent–child attachment is all about, and that is what I have witnessed in all the parents I have met who have had a child with the aid of a birth other.

Along with healthy attachment comes attunement, the ability to zero in on your child's needs and sensitively calibrate your responses to your child based on who he or she is. It is Veronica going straight to her child when she heard him crying. And it is such attunement that will guide you in the next important task—to tell or not to tell, and if telling, how and when to tell your child and others about the donor or surrogate.

Should I Tell?

> I'm a doctor. I know Mariza should grow up knowing her true genetic history, particularly given her medical problems. But my wife feels so terrible about her difficult pregnancy and her family comes from a country that would never accept a baby born this way—she's adamant Mariza can never know. What should we do?
>
> —Father of an egg-donor daughter

Harry and Lynnette sat close to each other on the couch in my office, leaning toward me with furrowed brows. I had just suggested that their four-year-old, Jason, have a neuropsychological evaluation to help make sense of his impulse-ridden behavior and the failure of his little body to read danger signals accurately. I then began to explore Jason's genetic history, asking if anyone else in either family showed behaviors similar to Jason's. There was an uncomfortable pause. Harry looked anxiously at his wife and finally offered, "Well, Jason isn't Lynnette's biological child. She was too old, so we used an egg donor." Lynnette then burst into tears and said, "Jason can never, never know." Racked with sobs, Lynnette poured out her fears that he would be seen as a freak and would stop loving her forever if he knew. Harry just sat silently, patting Lynnette's hand. Having observed Jason with both his parents, I reassured them that the bonds of love were already firmly in place for Jason with both his daddy and his mommy. But more important, Jason would do as well as each of them did with whatever decision they made about telling or not telling.

For many parents, thinking about disclosure may open up a raw and tender nerve as it did for Harry and Lynnette. What should you tell your child about his or her origins when those origins include a birth other? Does Lynnette have reason to be filled with anguish? If she tells Jason, will he become both a stigmatized and rejecting son? Lynnette and Harry have some work ahead of them to convert their raw nerves into resolute calm, whatever their decision—either to hold to not telling or to reconsider their choice.

Why is this work so important? Because what we tell our children about their origins will stick with them throughout their lives. There is no one straight path, yet the common task is to find a creative way to acknowledge the birth other in the story of your family. You will be doing this whether you are straight or gay, coupled or single. You will be doing this whether or not you intend to share that narrative with your children or with the outside world. Deciding what to tell the children is a task that calls for deep levels of feeling, thinking, discussing, and negotiating, both inside yourself and with your partner if you have one. Nowhere is clarity more essential than in sorting out the question of disclosure: Do I want my child (and others) to know about how she was conceived and/or carried to term? What do I want to tell her? How will I tell it? When will I tell it? This is an "if, what, when, and how" question. Right now we will stay focused on the "if."

Disclosure—to tell or not to tell—will be the focus of this chapter, the second panel in the triptych. Then, in the next two chapters, we will explore what, when, and how to tell if the decision is to tell. Disclosure has three tiers: (1) honest disclosure to oneself; (2) disclosure to relatives, friends, professionals, and community; (3) most important, disclosure to the child. Disclosure is neither a discrete event nor a single point in time in family life. It's a work in progress over time. It can include partial information or the whole, full picture. It can be renegotiated over time.

If you are a single parent or a gay or lesbian couple, you may have it easier than if you're a heterosexual couple. You have neither the luxury nor conversely the headache of deliberating whether or not to tell your child about an outsider involved in his or her conception or birth. As soon as your child is old enough to understand how babies are made, you'll have to come up with some explanation about how he or she came to be. But this doesn't exempt you from the dilemmas of disclosure. For you, too, the question remains: *What* are you going to tell the children?

However the communication about origins happens, it behooves all parents—gay, straight, single, coupled—to have a game plan in mind as they build their bonds with their children. There are so many questions to consider. Here are ten that might help shape the game plan:

1. What will be the benefits of my child's knowing?
2. What would be the benefits of shielding my child from the information?
3. Do I think any harm would come to my child by his or her knowing he or she was born with the aid of a surrogate or donor?
4. Do I think any harm would come to my child if he or she did not know that a surrogate or donor was involved?
5. Do I think my relationship with my child will be strengthened, threatened, or unchanged by his or her knowing about being born with the aid of a surrogate or donor?
6. How would I feel about telling my child, and do I know how I would do it?
7. How will my family react if they know?
8. How will people in our community react if they know?
9. What will it be like if other people know but my child doesn't?
10. What will it be like if my child knows but other people won't be told?

These questions apply whether you're going to tell your children there was a birth other or not, for *all* parents should have a plan in mind for what and how to communicate to the children about their origins.[1]

AND WHERE *DO* BABIES COME FROM?

I am now going to invite us on a journey to sort out whether or not to tell a child, or others, about the child's origins. I will cut to the chase and reveal my bias, which follows the millennium flow in the field of reproductive technology, as reflected in the Ethics Committee of the American Society for Reproductive Medicine's 2004 Report: "The Ethics Committee finds that disclosure to the child of the fact of donor conception, and, if available, characteristics of the donor, may serve the best interests of offspring."[2] In the overwhelming number of cases it is better for a child to know the truth about his or her biological origins, for psychological, medical, and family health. Yet I do not want to advocate this model to every family without leaving room for exceptions. There are rare situations in which a family may have good personal, social, even political reasons for protecting their child by not revealing information that the child was conceived with the aid of an outside party. It is important for us not to forget this. In the words of the old rabbis, "It depends."

Before we embark on the journey of disclosure dilemmas, I want to step way back and cast a look through a wide anthropological and cross-cultural lens. I would like us to place the issue of disclosure of a birth other in a child's conception or birth in its very largest context—humanity and creation stories. Most of us experienced the childhood enlightenment that babies are made from the union of a man's sperm and a woman's ovum. We also grew up with the knowledge that this union occurs through sexual intercourse between a man and a woman, the father and mother of the child so conceived. Conclusive *scientific* evidence for this "One Sperm, One Fertilization" doctrine is only a little over a century old. In a lucky coincidence, this science neatly matched Western folk beliefs already in place, stories that preceded the scientific evidence by millennia. But the age-old belief system of one man, one woman, one fertilization is a Western one. It has never been universal. As we scratch our heads and wonder how we are going to amend our scientific creation story to establish a new, more accurate one that will include something other than "one man, one woman, sexual intercourse, makes a baby," we might learn something by looking across our borders to the creation stories of other cultures.

I am not turning to science but to social beliefs from other peoples and the ease with which those people incorporate their birth stories into their family and community lives. In their book *Cultures of Multiple Fathers*, Stephen Beckerman and Paul Valentine warn us we Westerners have a hard time thinking about anything *but* a man and a woman having intercourse to have a baby who will have one mother and one father.[3] But then they invite us to stretch our imaginations. They take us to some lowland South American societies, where people believe the fetus is shaped at more than one point in time by male semen, not necessarily from the same man. This means one man can start off a pregnancy, and another man (or more) can finish the job. This doctrine of paternity, known as *joint* or *partible paternity*, allows for a child to have several different biological fathers. It also allows for two or more men to share a wife. Common throughout the South American continent, the doctrine of partible paternity has obvious social and economic benefits. Survival rates are higher for children who have one primary and one secondary father to watch over them. Women also get the support of more than one man, and are given some control over whom they designate as primary and secondary father, a designation that is fully disclosed and accepted by the entire community.

I read these accounts with fascination. We Westerners know that the multiple biological fatherhood these South American cultures believe in is pure myth. But their story reminds us that we are facing a major shake-up in our own traditional scientific accounts of conception and birth. Intercourse is no longer necessary for conception. We may not have multiple fatherhood, but we do have multiple motherhood. Two women can share the tasks of biological motherhood, one providing the egg, the other the womb. Combining the eggs of two women to make one baby is on the horizon. We have a lesson to learn from our South American neighbors. The human mind is quite capable of incorporating birth narratives that vary markedly from one sperm, one ovum, one baby. People are also able to develop happy, functioning families based on these narratives. If South American families can do it, so can we.

Why is this lesson relevant to the issue of disclosure? Because the question of whether to tell or not throws us off-kilter in our deeply ingrained beliefs about birth and healthy family life. Whether our family life conforms to the norm or not, the birth narrative of our society is that babies are made from the egg of their mother and the sperm of their father through an act of sexual intercourse. Anything else feels strange. Test that out with your own reactions to the multiple-father narrative of the lowland South American societies. How weird did it sound? Contemplate the new birth narrative that includes "the lady who so generously donated her eggs so we [I] could have you" or "the nice man who gave us his seed so we [I] could have you" or "the woman who carried you in her uterus until you were born," none of which requires sexual union between Mommy and Daddy or a daddy or mommy at all. It is a story that may not easily roll off our tongues. It doesn't sound quite right. We worry about what the children will make of it; we worry about what the extended family will make of it; we worry about what the world around us will make of it. If we're the parents, we're not even sure what *we* make of it.

The doctrine of multiple fatherhood in South America can be our guiding light in reminding us that our Western birth story has never been the only birth story in the world. Let's remember the South American story of partible fatherhood so that we can put our own questions about disclosure in broader perspective. Our culture is rapidly changing, indelibly altered by the scientific advances of reproductive technology. Coming at the question of disclosure through a lens of cultural relativity might stretch our thinking and ease our anxieties, giving us room to think more freely about the new birth stories we will tell our children. We now live in a world where it is no longer myth but reality that a child can have more than two biological parents. The South American partible paternity story teaches us that alterations in our birth narrative can be accepted by children and adults alike. But this will happen only if the people telling the story feel comfortable with it, accept its truth, and believe that the new narrative about parents, babies, and birth others makes for healthy family life.

DISCLOSURE: THE SOCIAL TIDES ARE SHIFTING

Marcy is a mother who is now is her late forties. She came to consult with me about her son, Andrew, who is six years old. She is a lovely woman, soft-spoken and kind in her nature, thoughtful and reflective about her only child. When Andrew was a year old, his father, Cary, had had a head injury that left him with severe brain damage. Prior to that, Cary had been a very involved father, active in every aspect of Andrew's daily care. Then he became a paraplegic. For several years Cary remained in the hospital, where Marcy and Andrew visited him regularly. Now Cary was being released from hospital care, and Marcy came to consult with me about forging a bond between Andrew and his father, who was still significantly impaired, both physically and cognitively. Over the course of the consultation I began to wonder about the circumstances of Andrew's birth, given that Marcy was an older mother. With the time running out in our session, I asked Marcy directly. As is often the case in those moments, Marcy squirmed in her chair, sighed, and replied, "Well, that's a long story in itself."

With few minutes to spare, she went on. "Andrew is a sperm-donor baby. Cary's sperm count was so low, and given my age, odds were against us. So we decided on donor insemination, because we desperately wanted a child. We never really resolved if and what we would tell Andrew about being a donor-insemination child, but figured we'd have plenty of time later to sort it out. But then Cary had his accident when Andrew was just a little baby, and the whole issue of what to tell him just got shelved. And now I don't know what to do. Given Cary's limitations and the long separation, it's hard enough for Andrew to connect with his dad right now. Then to tell him that on top of that his dad is not his biological father might just make it worse."

If Marcy had been pondering this question two decades ago and called on the experts in the field to help her, they most likely would have told her to keep the donor insemination a secret. Even before Cary's injury, the medical field would have wanted to protect Cary's dignity, sense of manhood, and feeling of legitimacy as Andrew's father. Attempts would have been made to match the donor's features to Cary's so Cary and Marcy could gaze down at a son who looked like Cary and so no one would ever suspect that Andrew was not Cary's son by blood. Two decades ago experts also believed that disclosure would be damaging not only to the father, but to the child, creating stigma, rejection, and damage to the child's psyche.[4]

In those years assessments of psychological harm and stigmatization of the child were consistently based on assertion, supposition, and belief, rather than carefully conducted studies of sperm-donor children. The experts could have simply said that the jury was out about the effects of the child's knowing he or she was a sperm-donor baby. From a scientific and ethical point of view, given the lack of reportable results, this would have been a wise stance. Instead, disclosure was deemed harmful. It's ironic that this judgment came at the same time that the adoption field was actively studying the harmful effects of nondisclosure on adopted children.

If we forward the clock from the 1980s to the present, Marcy and Cary might more likely be met with an expert opinion reflected in the 2004 American Society for Reproductive Medicine's Ethics Report: Telling the child the truth about his or her origins is *always* beneficial to the child's health and welfare.[5] I will save the reasons for later, but suffice it to say that this assessment about the benefits of disclosure is put forth with as much assurance as was the opposite assessment twenty years ago and with the same lack of conclusive scientific evidence.

The New Vote for Disclosure

Simply put, the social tides have changed. As they have changed, experts have done a 180-degree turn in their thinking about disclosure. Twenty years ago people thought disclosure would be traumatic for the child, humiliating to the parent, and disruptive to the parent–child bond. Now it is believed to be a violation of the child's rights, a denial of reality, and a threat to the integrity of the family *not* to tell a child the truth about his or her birth history.

As we have entered the present millennium and as the new methods of reproductive technology have taken off in so many new directions, we are growing more accustomed to the reality of babies born in alternative ways. The year 2003 marked the twenty-fifth birthday of Louise Brown, the first test-tube baby ever born. Over these twenty-five plus years we have been better able to accept the reality that one egg, one sperm, sexual intercourse is no longer the only conceivable possibility, no pun intended. Having babies with the aid of donors, surrogates, or petri dishes still may leave us squeamish, but the phenomenon is not so far outside the box as it was even ten years ago. More and more of us know at least one person—if not several—who have turned to assisted reproductive technology to have a baby. A week doesn't go by without a featured media story about some aspect of assisted reproductive technology.

While we are becoming more and more acclimated to baby making with assisted reproductive technology, medical studies are simultaneously discovering more and more ways that our physical and mental health are affected by heredity and genetic loadings. Not knowing that information about yourself could in some cases be a matter of life or death (as, for example, in the genetic mutation for breast cancer). So, it becomes more and more critical to our physical well-being and care to have full access to our genetic history. As more and more medical studies come out, we are also hearing about findings from the adoption field that secrecy has not enhanced children's mental well-being. Times have changed, and so have our sensibilities, bringing us to the cultural stance that disclosure is good, nondisclosure harmful.

Disclosure: One Size Does Not Fit All

I want to stress how important it is that we don't throw the baby out with the bathwater by creating a one-size-fits-all model of disclosure. Not every family, community, or religion has laid down a carpet of acceptance to the children created with the aid of a birth other. In their book *Lethal Secrets*, Annette Baran and Reuben Pannor recount the painful story of Judith and Michael, two grown donor-insemination children partially dispossessed by their wealthy paternal grandfather. In his will, in which he left generous amounts of money to his other grandchildren, he wrote the following: "To Judith and Michael, who carry my son Geoffrey's name, I leave the sum of one thousand dollars each. They do not carry the family genetic inheritance, and they are therefore excluded from the family financial inheritance."[6] Geoffrey, the father, had had a vasectomy because he suffered from childhood-onset diabetes and did not want to pass the disease on to his children. It was his very genetic inheritance (from his own father) that made him turn to donor insemination to save his children from lifelong suffering from diabetes. One could ask why Geoffrey would care at all what his father thought, given his father's negativity and punitive actions toward Geoffrey's two children. But the point here is that we really have to take family rejection and hostility into account when deciding whether it makes sense to tell not just the child, but anyone about the child's origins with a birth other. I could certainly understand how parents would think twice about disclosure, at least to the family, if the outcome was a denial of their children's birthrights because of other family members' adherence to the doctrine that blood is thicker than water.

Casting a wider view, Judith and Michael's story serves as a significant reminder that the tides are not the same everywhere. We should not be so shortsighted as to think that because it is increasingly acceptable to have babies in these new ways, this is the case everywhere and under any circumstance.

Returning to Marcy, Cary, and Andrew, I present Marcy's dilemma to you to highlight the rabbis' wisdom "It depends." Andrew is growing up in a liberal community and in an era when disclosure is increasingly prescribed. But Marcy has to weigh significant psychological issues related to trauma, separation, and bonding that might preclude sharing with Andrew the truth about his origins as he reincorporates his disabled father into his home life. In Andrew's best interests, he may be better off not knowing, at least for now. In the United States a pendulum swing has occurred from "don't tell" to "always tell," and as this shift has occurred, we have forgone the more nuanced thinking that is most helpful to parents making the decision regarding if (and then when and what) to tell. We need to remove the pendulum and replace it with weighted scales. Translated into action, this means that each of you who is crafting a plan for telling (or not) will have to do your own calibrating, carefully measuring the pros and cons of disclosing information about your child's birth and then making an informed decision guided by the way the scales are tipped. Some of you, single, gay, and lesbian mothers and fathers, have no choice in the matter. There is nothing to weigh. Still, I think the mental calibrations weighing the positives and negatives will benefit any parent because they give you an opportunity to test your own comfort level when it comes to telling your children a birth narrative informed by alternative conception.

THE UNTHOUGHT KNOWN

Remember Caroline, Charlie and Jo's daughter, the one who drew the family grid that went on and on? I want to tell you another part of her story. Early in our work together, when neither of us yet knew that Caroline had been conceived with a sperm donor (recall that Caroline was being treated for postdivorce anxiety), Caroline, then seven years old, involved herself in some play that greatly confused me. The play involved birthing scenes in which she would repeatedly reenact an immaculate conception scene: A baby doll would drop from her T-shirt, a baby that she, the mommy, created and birthed single-handedly. I thought this might be a communication about her attachment and loyalty to her mother in the recent custody dispute, but somehow that just didn't feel on target, so I kept my thoughts to myself.

Only when Jo revealed to me that Charlie was not Caroline's biological father did her play begin to make sense to me. Like many parents in a similar situation, Jo, and later Charlie, provided the following reasons for deciding not to tell Caroline that Charlie was not her biological father: "That was our deal before she was born"; "It would only confuse her"; "She's too young to understand such complicated stuff about infertility and reproduction"; "It will disrupt her bond with her dad"; "Her dad is her dad; it doesn't matter what sperm made her."

I recalled that Charlie and Jo, in consort with their political ideals, had handled their divorce by being honest and forthright with Caroline, believing that children should be treated with respect and integrity. Remarkably, neither Charlie nor Jo saw any contradiction between their strong commitment to complete honesty with their child in all other matters and their stance that they would not tell her about her donor-insemination roots.

I remembered how shocked I had been to discover the strong physical resemblance between Caroline and Jo before I had ever been told about Caroline's donor-insemination conception. I remembered the family picture that I had asked her to draw in our first session that became a never-ending grid of parents, aunts, uncles, grandparents, the butcher, the baker, the candlestick maker. I then bore witness to Caroline's immaculate conception fantasies—her single-mommy baby doll birthing scenes. This play occurred when neither Caroline nor I had been told of the insemination.

The plot thickened as I continued to work with Caroline. But it was different, because I now knew that she had been conceived using donor insemination, while she did not. At the time, Charlie and Jo were reconsidering their earlier decision to shield Caroline from the knowledge of her birth-other conception, but they were still undecided. Charlie in particular had reservations, fearing that Jo would use the information against him to woo Caroline and fortify her own position as the most viable parent in their custody battle.

I suggested to them that Caroline might very well already know about her conception at an unconscious level. In my mind I was thinking of a concept that I had learned from reading the work of the psychoanalyst Christopher Bollas. He coined the term "the unthought known" to refer to infants' early knowledge of who they are before they can speak or think in words. He regarded this as a sensibility about their "true self." Even before they can think it, little babies start to know who they really are.[7] The unthought known, a knowledge that is not thought of but just there, isn't limited to babies. It shows up well into childhood and even adulthood. How many of you have had the experience of just having a feeling about yourself, but you can't really say why? That may be the unthought known at work.

In my work with children born with the help of a birth other I began to wonder whether this concept, the unthought known, could apply to some subliminal or unconscious knowing that they were made from a parent and, well, a someone else. Marsha Levy-Warren described a family she worked with where the son experienced just such a knowing. David was fifteen and had been conceived with a mix of his father's and a donor's sperm. David was not told this. Like me with Caroline, Dr. Levy-Warren did not know either at first. David and his dad were having big conflicts with each other. David explained, "I feel like Dad and I are from different planets." Later, when David, with the help of Dr. Levy-Warren, was told by his parents about his conception, he had this to say: "I was wondering if I sort of knew this without knowing it." Dr. Levy-Warren referred to this kind of knowing as preconscious knowing—something on the verge of consciousness.[8] I refer to it as the unthought known.

Coming back to Caroline, she not only persisted full force with her single mommies birthing babies fantasy, but she also introduced a new, quite telling game in her play therapy. One day she chose a pink velvet heart-shaped box, decorated with a bow and a flower. First she filled it with sand. Then she took a beautiful little pink quartz stone and buried it in the sand. She then tightly covered the box. Solemnly, she handed me the box and instructed me to put it on a high shelf for one week. When she came back the next week, lo and behold, I would discover that a baby had grown from the single "egg" in the box. As she played she let me know all the ways she was just like her mother, but nothing like her father.

As I worked with Charlie and Jo, I told them about these play themes. I also referred them to published reports from adults conceived through insemination who claimed always to have known that a vague something was not right about their position in the family. They had these feelings despite not being told of the insemination until adolescence or adulthood.[9] I brought up again that Caroline might already know that something was up about her birth. I realized that this notion of the unthought known about one's biological roots might sound far-fetched. Indeed, Charlie's first reaction was to look at me skeptically, flatly rejecting my proposal that Caroline unconsciously or even partially consciously knew something about her sperm-donor origins. He chalked me up as one of those crazy psychoanalytic types who can never see a cigar as just a cigar. Maybe so, maybe not, but I do find the notion of the unthought known compelling, not to suggest some magical, immeasurable process, but to propose that children may know what we do not tell them.

Children Can Be Good Detectives

Children born with the help of a donor or surrogate, shielded from knowing their origins, may figure it out anyway. Careful as you may be, you may still unwittingly communicate to children in innumerable subtle ways what you consciously chose not to tell. As you think about whether or not to tell your child (or other people), you might want to consider the potential for these subtle slips.

In *Lethal Secrets*, Annette Baran and Reuben Pannor tell the story of Nina, who had not been told of her donor-insemination origins as a child but always knew something was off. It seemed that her father held back from disciplining the children, while her mother always had the upper hand. Nina remembers an incident when her mother was lecturing her and her sister to get better grades, to live up to their potential. Her father intervened to soften the mother's harsh lecture. Nina saw her mother shoot a look at her father:

"[the] way Mother had looked at him had somehow been so weird, so strange, so thick with something. Father stopped in the middle of a word, and then he had abruptly left the room."[10] Nina developed a fantasy that her father was not her real father. She imagined that her mother had had two passionate love affairs and become pregnant, once with her sister and once with her. Maybe her father knew the truth about her mom's flings but loved her mother so much he decided to stay with her anyway.

The subtle look, the power dynamics in the family, the aversion of a parent's gaze when a relative, friend, or even stranger says to a child, "Oh, you don't look anything like your mom" are all leakages. They may become clues that fuel the child's subliminal hunches about who she is and where she came from. If a child is left decoding partial information that is never communicated directly by the parent, the field is fertile for wild fantasies. And so Nina whips up a fantastic tale of her mother's passionate love affairs and her dad's unflappable devotion in the face of his wife's obvious adultery. So let us simply hold the concept of the unthought known, that children may know even what we don't tell, as a cautionary tale while we now weigh on the scales reasons to disclose and reasons not to.

WHY DISCLOSE?

Many years ago, a woman came to see me for therapy who was in her sixties at the time. She recalled her mother's death when she was two-and-a-half years old. Her mother had been ill. One day her mother's bed was empty. When she asked where her mommy had gone, she was simply told, "away." It was never discussed again. In today's cultural milieu, it would be unheard of to treat a child like that—books for parents, books for children, books for professionals are all in abundance to assure that a child will be told honestly and sensitively about a parent's death or any other major family event. Parents today are encouraged to be truthful with their children. Families are instructed that keeping family secrets can create interpersonal fissures and festering individual wounds that never heal. Having a baby using a surrogate or donor is considered one of those major family events. Disclosure is deemed essential to avoid the fissures and festering wounds that family secrets engender.

Experts have called on the adoption field to alert us to the beneficial effects of being open to our children about their origins and the damaging effects when we attempt to keep that information a secret. The adoption field previously went through the transformation that has now hit the field of assisted reproductive technology. Two generations ago it was considered standard practice to shield both the adopted child and the community from the information that the child was not the biological offspring of his or her parents. Shame and stigma were associated with adoption. Then three changes occurred simultaneously. First, a new emphasis was placed on children's rights, in this case the right to know their own origins. Second, open adoption, in which parents and children have access to the birth mother, took the place of closed adoption, in which neither parents nor children would ever have access to the birth parents. Third, as adoptions became more common in American society, the stigma receded. In moving toward disclosure and open rather than closed adoptions, emphasis was placed on the toxicity of family secrets. Children sense secrets, feel betrayed if the secrets come out, and never feel fully accepted by the family if they suspect there is something about them that nobody is talking about. Often they'll assume the worst and think there's something wrong or unacceptable about them that remains unspoken. These adoption doctrines have now been extended to children born with the aid of donors or surrogates.

Medical progress has also left its mark. Judith, a twenty-eight-year-old physician and scientist, was herself a child conceived through donor insemination. She reflects, "twenty-nine years ago when I was conceived, nobody paid much attention to genetics, recessive characteristics, diseases in sperm, and so forth. Now we know a great deal more, and we know how important such information can be."[11] When it comes to ensuring the health and safety of our children, what parent wouldn't do anything to guarantee his or her child grows up with every piece of essential information needed to keep that child free from harm and protected against disease? That includes giving the child access to everything known about the child's genetic roots. And it's a little tricky to do that if you don't tell the child that someone else's genes, not yours, are the relevant ones.

It has been pointed out to me that my argument that children need to know their donor or surrogate for their own medical well-being may soon be obsolete. Scientific advances eventually that will allow us to get all the information about our heredity from a DNA reading of our own chromosomes. In other words, we will be able to obtain a complete medical history from our own DNA; we will no longer need to turn to the people who made us. I have two thoughts about that. First, we'll cross that bridge when we come to it. Second, even if we will know from our own DNA whether, for example, we have the gene for certain kinds of cancer, that will not tell us how the people we are genetically related to have managed or survived that disease if they in fact have had it, or what medications worked best for them, and so on. That information will come from knowing about them and their life experience. In short, children's own DNA readings will still not give them a picture of the whole person who is their donor or surrogate.

Sometimes it is a medical crisis that actually forces parents to disclose a birth other to their children. Felicia, now fifty-one, had given birth to her daughter, Julia, ten years earlier. After years of trying unsuccessfully to get pregnant, she decided to use an egg donor in the early days when this procedure was just beginning to be offered to infertile women. She and her husband, Roy, had decided not to tell Julia about her egg-donor conception. One day Felicia felt a lump in her breast. Two weeks later she was diagnosed with breast cancer. Felicia's mother had died of breast cancer several years earlier, and her older sister had been diagnosed with breast cancer three years ago and was now in remission. Genetic testing revealed that Felicia carried the genetic mutation for breast cancer, as did her sister.

Julia, a precocious ten-year-old, had heard that breast cancer was hereditary and that if your mom had it, you could get it, too. Julia told Felicia how worried she was for Felicia and tried to help out around the house in any way she could. One day, when Julia was bringing Felicia some tea on an evening after a chemotherapy treatment, she sat down on the couch by Felicia, cuddled next to her, and asked Felicia in a voice hardly louder than a whisper, "Mommy, am I going to get sick like you, too, when I grow up and get breasts?" Felicia was stunned. She pulled Julia close to her and said, "Honey, you're going to be just fine."

For once Felicia was really glad that her beloved daughter did *not* carry her genes. But later that night, when she and Roy were getting ready for bed, she told him about her conversation with Julia. They both realized that if they never told Julia that Felicia was not her biological mother, she would be burdened for the rest of her life with worries about her heightened risk for breast cancer. Even the absence of a genetic marker in Julia's own testing someday might not reassure her. Both Roy and Felicia decided that it was no longer feasible to keep from Julia the information that she was conceived with an egg donor. It might even be harmful. To give their daughter peace of mind that she did not have to worry about inheriting her mother's genetic predisposition for breast cancer, they opted to tell Julia the truth about her conception. Like Marcy with Andrew, they worried about telling Julia that

Felicia was not her biological mother in the midst of Felicia's illness, maybe overtaxing Julia with too many emotionally charged things or even disrupting the bonds Julia had with her mother. But they decided, rightfully so, that the ties were strong enough to sustain any shaking of the bonds that would occur. Julia was stunned at first, but recouped quickly, and one day said to her mother, "So now I understand why you told me I was going to be just fine. Thanks, Mom."

Often, advocates of disclosure stress preventing damage rather than enhancing growth as the reason to tell. The child must be told or he or she will be at medical risk. The child must be told or he or she will feel betrayed by family secrets and deception on the part of the parents. The child must be told by the parents to make sure the information doesn't come to the child from someone else first. The child must be told to avoid the possibility that the child might someday inadvertently marry a brother or sister. The child must be told because not being told will become an irritant in the child's psyche. The child must be told to insure against the child's filling the void with wild ideas or maybe even wild actions. The child must be told to avoid distorting or stunting psychological growth as the child goes through contortions to respond to troubling murmurs that push to the surface: "Where did I come from anyway?"

I'd like to think that telling children about their origins with a birth other could be an expansive and positive experience, rather than just a preventive measure. In the 1960s the Black Pride movement made its mark in history by encouraging African Americans to stand up and speak their stories and be proud of their roots and their heritage. In contemplating communicating to children that their birth involved the presence of a sperm donor, egg donor, or surrogate, let's consider a story that helps a child feel proud about him or herself. Not one that is candy coated, but one that is proactive and recalls the lessons learned from the South American cultures that children and adults alike can positively embrace stories about their origins that deviate from one sperm, one egg, one child. A group of teenagers in Berkeley, California, have begun to self-identify as "tubesters"—donor-insemination children. They seek each other out: "Are you a tubester, too?" They appear to derive pleasure from their new collective identity. Might this be evidence of a "proud new tale?"

I have identified a strange bedfellows phenomenon in which one of the bedfellows is a group of parents confronting either infertility or disease who turn to assisted reproductive technology following the loss of opportunity to have a baby under the one egg, one sperm, sexual union doctrine. Here disclosure necessarily includes an account of at least one system down— ovum, sperm, uterus, genes, or some combination thereof. So we can wonder how that generates a positive story of the child's origins: "We couldn't _____, so, therefore, we did _____ to have you." The other bedfellow includes single people and gay and lesbian families who have nothing wrong with any of their systems but have discovered that with the help of assisted reproductive technology they can now have their own children. Their story will include no information about damage to their bodies, but rather an account of a missing piece: "To have you we [I] needed an ovum, a sperm, and a uterus, we [I] had a _____, but not a _____, so we [I] found a _____ to put together with our [my] _____, and here you are." How do such stories translate into proud tales?

Underlying all these stories is the bedrock of desire—the strong wish to have a baby of their own and the pursuit of an innovative way to make it happen. Wanting so much to have a baby is the cornerstone of a birth story laced with pride rather than shame. And a birth story laced with pride, even if there's talk of loss or damage or missing parts, goes hand in hand with thinking about disclosure to your child as a *growth-enhancing* rather than *risk-reducing* decision.

We wanted so much to have you, and we found a way to do it. That is exactly the mantra that motivated Crystal and Benson to tell their daughter, Ellie, about her birth. They had tried and tried to have a baby with no success. Each had a fertility work-up, and nothing showed up. Yet they just couldn't conceive. Finally they decided to try donor insemination. It worked, and they became excited, proud parents. Both their doctor and their families counseled them to keep the insemination private, even to Ellie. But they never wanted their daughter to feel anything but proud about who she was. And how could she feel proud if she didn't even know who she was? They told Ellie not to protect her from harm, but to give her every opportunity to be the most authentic girl she could be. They wanted her, they did everything they could to have her, and that's all that mattered.

WHY DECIDE NOT TO DISCLOSE?

The present social currents carry us toward disclosure, but there are opposing currents as well. Put another way, we are in a state of transition in which the trend is toward disclosure, but the preceding dominant trend of secrecy still holds sway. In a study conducted in the 1990s involving interviews with thirty-five parents who had used donor insemination to have a child, the most common reason given for not telling a child is that it would unnecessarily complicate his or her life. Parents also feared that their child would never be completely accepted by relatives. They believed that society still stigmatized donor offspring and that secrecy would protect the child from the harm that might come to him or her if people knew about his or her insemination roots. Families who used anonymous donors thought it best not to tell their children because why tell if their children would never be able to know who their genetic father was? Lastly, parents feared that their child might reject the father if he or she knew the truth.[12] Protection of the parent and protection of the child, but particularly the child, were the key variables that led a parent to decide to maintain secrecy.

In Britain, recent survey data have been collected indicating that a higher proportion of donor-insemination parents than parents who use in vitro fertilization decide not to disclose the nature of their child's origins to him or her. At first I thought this was because, with in vitro fertilization, you don't have to tell the child that an outsider was involved in his or her conception, whereas in disclosing donor insemination, you do. But then I read on to learn that the data also revealed that the incidence of secrecy increased when conception occurred as a result of donor sperm in contrast to donor eggs. Since the presence of an outsider is true for both groups, something else had to be driving the decision not to tell. That something else would be shame about male infertility.[13] It is not just the fear that the child will reject the father; it's also the attempt to preserve an infertile man's ego that makes parents decide not to tell their children or the outside world that their father could not make babies. Many women find themselves motivated by protecting their husbands rather than focusing on their children when the decision is made that the children never need know about an insemination conception.

When it comes to egg donors, women may not need quite so much protection regarding their infertility. Also, historically, egg-donor babies have come around far more recently than sperm-donor babies, "birthing" in an era when disclosure is favored far more than nondisclosure. Sperm-donor families, in contrast to egg-donor families, may still be operating under older attitudes that favored nondisclosure.

I Have No Idea What to Say

I've also discovered another driving force behind the decision not to disclose that gets totally overlooked. I have met so many parents who feel somewhere between hesitant and helpless when it comes to figuring out what to tell the children. The topic brings up squeamishness and more poignantly, it can stir up feelings of total incompetence or inadequacy.

For many of us, telling our children about the birds and the bees is one of our least favorite tasks. It means we have to talk about sex to our children and brace ourselves for a barrage of innocent questions about the most intimate parts of our adult lives. We may start feeling like we've violated the incest taboo—sex between parent and child, even if it's just a discussion, feels verboten or inappropriate. Now add to that the complications of figuring out how to tell a child about the birds and the bees and the test tubes and the nice man or woman who helped us and . . . by the way, your daddy (or mommy) didn't make you, but your mommy (daddy) did. You can see how this might freeze you in your tracks. So far we professionals have not really offered many guidelines or provided avenues for parents to seek out the advice that does exist. Grandparents can hardly be counted on to extend their elders' wisdom, for this indeed is a fertile *new* world. So, "When in doubt, do nothing." Or alternatively, "Don't ask; don't tell."

Recently I was at a large outdoor community celebration for a local childcare referral group. Part of the day's events included an on-site mental health consultant for parents with questions, like about bedtime or allowance. A friend and colleague of mine was taking a shift at the booth. She found me afterwards and said she was at a loss when a mother came up to her and asked for some tips about telling her daughter she was a donor-insemination baby. I smiled, because that is often the most urgent question parents ask me in the consultation room—"How do I do it?" I thought about this mother so hungry for information that she grabbed the volunteer professional at the booth in the park to answer an ever so complicated and personal question in the midst of clowns and jugglers and children's games. No doubt secrecy can become the default position when you have no idea what to say and you don't know where to go for help. If this resonates for any of you who are reading right now, I would hope that the next chapters about when, what, and how to tell the children will give you access to a set of tools for telling that might help you feel more comfortable disclosing.

Three Good Reasons Not to Tell

Honesty is good for families. Children may intuit things about their origins even if they're not told. Nonetheless, under special circumstances three critical factors may tip the scales toward not telling. All three put the best interests of the child over discomfort or pain for the parents. The first has to do with a child's fragility or vulnerability. The second involves threats to the parent–child bond. The third is about threats, physical but more likely psychological, to a child's well-being in a hostile climate. And let me add right here that if you do not disclose based on any of these factors, the research to date, although far from comprehensive, indicates that children who do not know about their birth-other roots do as well as control groups of children born the old-fashioned way in quantitative measures of cognitive development, social-emotional functioning, and parent–child relationships. [14]

Let's just pretend for a moment that Marcy's son Andrew was a child with developmental problems, such as mild mental retardation or a disorder like autism or Asperger's syndrome. Or let's imagine that Andrew himself suffered a significant medical trauma, leaving him indefinitely weakened, vulnerable, and anxious. Under any of those circumstances, Andrew might not be a child who would have the capacity to process the complexity of the information about his origins.

Fortunately, Andrew is a healthy, well-functioning child. But Marcy is still confronted with a daunting decision. She faces a painful dilemma as she figures out what is right for her son. Her critical parenting task right now is to facilitate a positive and engaged attachment between Andrew and his dad. Andrew will have to adjust to a wheelchair-bound father with limited speech and significant physical limitations. That's not an easy task for a six-year-old—children of that age can shy away from things they don't understand, which could include a father who is different. Also, if Andrew has any memories of his earlier life, he'll know that the father he loved then is not the same as the father he has visited in the hospital and who is now returning home after several years' absence. Cary is a loving father and committed to doing anything he is capable of to connect with his son and to allow his son to rediscover him after his release from the hospital. Given the original grim prognosis, it's a miracle that Cary is functioning as well as he is and will be able to do this.

For the time being, the developmental task confronting Andrew, his father, and his mother—to build a loving and connected family after a major medical trauma—trumps any concerns about whether Andrew understands who was responsible for making him. In Andrew's case, I would recommend against disclosure, at least at this time in his life. It would be too much to ask him to rebuild a relationship with his father and include him in daily family life and at the same time process the information that this man who seems so different from the father he once knew is also not his biological father. Marcy and Cary's decision can then be revisited much later, after the bond has been deepened between Andrew and Cary and when Andrew is at a later developmental stage where he could assimilate the information more easily.

A warning here. This variable—threat to the parent–child bond—can be abused by parents who avoid disclosure because they haven't worked through their own anxieties about this child not being "mine" or "ours." In any family it's complicated, maybe even impossible, to disengage the best interests of the child from the well-being of the parents. However, no studies to date have revealed any jeopardy to attachments between children and parents caused by the child's knowledge of his or her birth with a birth other. In fact, as mentioned earlier, so far studies suggest just the opposite—the children are doing fine in their attachments. My own clinical observations lead me to the same conclusion—children I have known whose parents have told them about their origins with a birth other seem positively attached to their parents, regardless of their genetic links or lack of them. I would say that only in very specialized circumstances, such as illness of a parent or fragility of a child, should preserving the parent–child bond prevail as a reason not to tell children about their origins.

I do want to call our attention to one other threat to the parent–child bond and also to the child's psychological well-being that would argue against disclosure—when couples split up. Regretfully, not all marriages or unions last. Sometimes two parents will have a child together using donor eggs, donor sperm, or a surrogate and decide not to tell the child, for any or all of the reasons we've already identified. Somewhere down the pike the couple starts having trouble. In some families the stress and pain of previous infertility makes an indelible smudge on the relationship that cannot be erased, no matter how hard the parents try. In other families, unresolved tensions regarding possession (Is baby mine, yours, or ours?) wear away at the fabric of the relationship. And sometimes parents simply suffer from any one of the typical strains that tear so many relationships apart in our modern age. Occasionally, in a fit of post-separation anger, disclosure is brought out as a weapon. With no bonds of trust or commitment to bind them, one parent may threaten to disclose, take it upon him- or herself actually to do so, or make a "slip" that communicates to the child the truth about his or her origins. Parents sometimes offer the rationale that now is a time when they need to start being totally honest and forthright with their children. Or a parent may feel forced to take fate into his or her own hands and tell the child before the other parent spills the beans first.

A divorced mother in a donor-insemination family responded in panic right after the father's new girlfriend confronted her with the information that the girlfriend now knew that the children were not the father's "real" children. Late at night, the mother rushed in to her children, woke them, and told them for the first time that they had been conceived with donor sperm, lest the information come in hostile form from the new girlfriend.[15]

Rushing to tell a child in the heat of anger and panic could be significantly damaging to all concerned. Although a parent might be thinking he or she is protecting the child, in a court of law such actions could even qualify as an act of parental alienation—the attempts of one parent to alienate the child from the other parent.

The rule of thumb is simple: telling or not telling should be a joint decision by all parents concerned, and disclosure should never be attached to any element of anger toward the other parent. If in doubt about that, it is best to do nothing until you get your bearings. Parents' separation is a destabilizing event in a child's life. At least temporarily, it consumes a great deal of a child's emotional resources. In that moment, a child cannot handle much else. Decisions about disclosure in a post-divorce family where disclosure has not yet occurred should be postponed until everyone rights themselves again and the children have fortified the bonds with each of their parents in a post-separation family. In cases of medical trauma or family shake-ups, the caveat regarding nondisclosure is a temporal one. *Never* disclosing is not the operating variable. Withholding disclosure *at this time* to preserve parent–child bonds and shield a child from an overload of life events is the guiding concept.

Now we come to the third reason not to disclose, threats to the child from a hostile environment. These may not be transient events that require psychological adjustment, like illness or divorce, but rather permanent fixtures in a child's life. Threats could stem from membership in a religion that condemns any tampering with natural means of conception. Threats could come from living in a community that would castigate or cast out any child who was born artificially. Threats could come from even closer to home—

from extended family members who might disinherit or turn their backs on a donor or surrogate child, driven either by religious or moral beliefs or unbridled hatred, intolerance, and prejudice toward anyone different. Although I have just introduced the idea of a narrative of pride about one's origins, any such narrative may crumble in the face of vitriolic harassment or hatred. Just as Jewish parents hid their children in the countryside to protect them from the Nazis, parents in hostile environments may want to hide their children from the facts of their birth to save them from an environment not ready to receive them or intent on doing harm to them.

Tell Here, but Not There

Assessing external threats is where the notion of disclosure/nondisclosure tiers comes in. You might decide that it's fine for your child to know that he or she was a sperm-donor, egg-donor, or surrogate baby, but not fine for others to know. In that case you must be ready to teach your child about privacy and the reasons for it. Parents aware of the hard time their children will face because of their race, ethnicity, religion, or gender-bending already know about the complicated task of communicating to their children pride about who they are while simultaneously preparing them for a world that might not treat them well precisely because of who they are. The same complicated task may face any of you who want your children proudly to know their origins with a birth other but know this information won't be received kindly by family, school, community, or house of worship. For you, however, there is one important difference—the invisibility of your child's birth otherness that could put your child at risk if it was known. Even with the possibilities of "passing" or assimilating, race, ethnicity, religion (when publicly practiced), and gender-bending are characteristics typically visible to others. Not so for your child's birth otherness, which is typically easy to conceal. Such invisibility is a potential advantage in shielding your child from harassment, but it also comes with a price. You might need to teach your children about confidentiality or privacy at a very tender age, communicating to them pride about their roots but also instructing them about the need to keep this information private from people who might take it the wrong way and who aren't able to understand.

Recall Jill and Tamara from Chapter 4, the mothers of Lucy, and Gary, Lucy's donor, an old friend of the mothers who has relocated to a conservative community. Now they are in the process of thinking what to tell two-year-old Lucy about her origins. They would like to tell her the whole truth, that Gary was her donor. But Gary and his wife, Sherry, weren't quite so sure. If Lucy knew, then obviously they would have to tell their children as well—that Lucy was their half sister and that their daddy was Lucy's donor. Gary had taken a position as an educational leader and knew that the people in their new community wouldn't be receptive to the idea that the man to whom they had entrusted their children was a sperm donor. It would just be too weird. He might even lose his job. His children might be teased or harassed by their playmates or rejected by the conservative families where they now lived.

Could Gary and Sherry communicate to their children the truth about Lucy's origins but ask them not to talk to other people about it because it was private? Or would that put too much stress on the children to request that they keep secrets? Could Lucy be instructed to do the same as she got older and visited Gary and Sherry's family?

Jill and Tamara were fortunate. Gary and Sherry were thoughtful and caring friends who recognized this as a shared problem and were willing to roll up their sleeves to work together and come up with a plan that would take care of everyone. The two families had obvious competing needs that could have generated great conflict among the four parents, but did not. After several weeks of talking together, going off to think about it, and then talking again, the four adults decided on the model of tiered disclosure. They would wait until the younger children were old enough to understand about privacy and then explain to them the biological sibling relationship among the three of them and Gary's role as Lucy's donor. They would ask the children to keep the information private in Sherry and Gary's community, explaining it was for only the family to know because others couldn't so easily accept it yet. They thought about telling Sherry and Gary's older daughter first, as she was so much older than the other two children, but decided that it might be asking too much of her to keep a secret from her own little sister and from Lucy.

Invoking the concept of the family matrix helps us remember that *everyone's* needs—parent's, child's, and birth other's—have to be taken into account when weighing the risks of disclosure. Not just harm to the child but threats to other members of the matrix have to be considered in figuring out whether or not to tell a child, or others, that the child was conceived with the aid of a donor or surrogate or, in Lucy's case, with a specifically named donor. In situations like Lucy's, a tiered model—disclosure within the family but not beyond—may be the best way to promote well-being while reducing risk factors for everyone.

Tiering may protect the child, but it does come with some fallout. We are either keeping secrets from the child or asking the child to keep secrets. In the latter case, you may have to do some fancy footwork to help a child realize that this information kept private doesn't equate with a bad thing that must be hidden. We keep it private not because it's bad but to protect our family from some people who might think it is. Maybe we are asking a child to live a double life, pretending to others that one of his or her parents is a biological parent when the child knows otherwise.

Yet perhaps that's a very small price to pay when we consider the alternative. If bodily or psychic harm might come to the child if others knew, what parent wouldn't consider placing the extra burden of privacy on the child to protect the child and family from unfair treatment, rejection, harassment, or even physical attack? Of course, another option is not to tell the child at all so you never have to ask him or her to take on that extra burden. Or, to maintain truth within the intimacy of your home, you could wait until your child is old enough to take on that burden more easily and only then tell the true birth story. Rather than thinking of tiered disclosure as demanding the child live a double life, better to think of the child as living a *layered* life. Until the world is more tolerant of birth differences, in special circumstances parents in hostile environments or with prejudiced or rejecting extended families may feel that nondisclosure, whether total or tiered, is the only option to keep their child safe.

Shawniese and Tony made exactly this decision, calling on the tiered model. They had told Maurice when he was little that he was made with the help of an egg donor because his mommy's eggs weren't working anymore. But they also feared that Tony's extended family would use the information in cruel and taunting ways. So they never told Tony's family, even though Shawniese had told hers. Remarkably, they never instructed Maurice not to tell anyone; he just knew somehow. Unfortunately, Maurice was one of those kids who got the equation wrong. At age nine, he now believed it was a shameful thing and anyone would either laugh at him or think he was weird if he told them about his birth otherness. He believed this even though he went to a progressive school with plenty of other donor children and with a teaching staff that emphasized diversity and tolerance in its curriculum.

Shawniese, Tony, and I discussed this dilemma together, and they began to recognize that Maurice was no longer being protected by their tiered disclosure system. Instead, he was becoming more withdrawn and unsure of himself in the very arena where he should feel safe—school. As I said, the balancing act between protecting your children from harm and providing them with security and good feelings about who they are is a precarious one. Shawniese and Tony revisited their decision to withhold the information about Maurice's donor conception from Tony's family and decided to take the risk of telling them rather than live with the reality that tiered disclosure was no longer working for Maurice. Right now they are in the process of rehearsing what they plan to say to Tony's family to smooth the waters—to let them know that Maurice was conceived with an egg donor, to explain that they hadn't shared the information before because they thought it would be too upsetting to the family, and to offer help to Tony's family in adjusting to the information while at the same time asking their support in continuing to love Maurice just as they always have. They're nervous but bolstered in their confidence as they realize that, in the nine short years since Maurice's birth, times have already changed dramatically. Just that month *U.S. News and World Report*, hardly a bastion of radical reporting and always a favorite of Tony's father, featured a cover story with the headline "Miracle Babies: How Science Is Helping Childless Couples Beat the Odds."[16] In less than a decade from when they first made their decision not to tell Tony's family, the winds had shifted significantly enough possibly to blow the threat away.

So let's review. There are good and bad reasons not to disclose. The three sound reasons, applicable in exceptional circumstances, are a child's developmental vulnerabilities or limitations, risk to the parent–child bond, and potential harm to the child. Feelings of ignorance or incompetence regarding how to tell children about their origins are understandable but not a good enough reason for not disclosing. Better to build your information base and competence and then decide. Your own anxieties or discomfort about your child's birth otherness and your fears of losing your child's love if he or she knows mean it's time to ask, "Who are you doing this for, yourself or your child?" If the answer is yourself, that is not a good enough reason not to tell your child. This may be the time to find a supportive context to talk about and work through these understandable anxieties, either with other birth-other families, with a counselor, or with a trusted friend or family member and certainly with each other, if there is more than one of you.

IN THE BEST INTERESTS OF THE CHILD

What really is best for a child when it comes to disclosure versus non-disclosure? To date, we have no controlled studies comparing children who have been told with children who have not. While it is conceivable to ask children about their experiences knowing they were donor or surrogate babies, it is impossible to ask them directly how they feel about not knowing that they were conceived with a birth other. We could ask others to report on the children, but that would entail asking parents to participate in an arena of their life that has remained very secret.

The most compelling evidence about disclosure versus nondisclosure comes from the reports of offspring who did not know at first but were told later. Some children are angry that they were lied to. They resent that they were left to struggle on their own with the unthought known about their origins, with no one helping them make sense of it. They find no excuse for their parents withholding from them a basic and essential fact of their life. But what has struck me as a more poignant experience for the children who found out later is their empathy with their parent(s), particularly their nongenetic parent.

One father reported that he had decided not to tell his children about his infertility and their conception using a sperm donor because he worried about hurting them but came to realize that he also worried about himself—how the children would feel about him if they knew. Once he actually told his sixteen-year-old son and twelve-year-old daughter that a donor was used, his son mused, "I was thinking about why Dad didn't say anything about it a long time ago. Maybe it would have saved us a lot of years of being at each other."[17] Bruce, a twenty-one-year-old who only recently found out that his father was not his and his two brothers' biological father, felt great compassion for his father: "I guess one of the good parts of all this is that now Pop isn't lugging that awful secret around anymore. Maybe the drinking and misery won't be as bad now that he knows we love him, fertile or not."[18]

Children feel sorrow for all the pain their parent must have gone through in the discomfort of not feeling like a real parent, and they want to reassure their parent of their love and devotion. They both recognize and accept that the parents' decision may have had more to do with protecting one of the parents than protecting them. They can feel compassion because they grew up loving their parents.

Parents may withhold information to protect themselves, but they also may be genuinely concerned that offering the information to the child, particularly at an early age, would be sexually overstimulating or beyond the child's comprehension. So they don't tell. We never want to overload our children with material they can't digest. But just as we start by feeding our children formula, then baby food, then solids, the information fed to a child about his or her origins can be offered in graduated form, matched to the child's developmental and emotional capabilities. The question is not whether or not to tell, but how to tell in a sensitive and comprehensible fashion that will meet the child where he or she is. Are children capable of understanding that the person who cares for and nurtures them is their parent and that another person was involved who helped make them but is not their parent? Yes, over time, even with all the confusions or fantasies that might come along the way.

THIS CHILD IS OUR CHILD: THAT'S WHY WE TELL, THAT'S WHY WE DON'T TELL

Parents who decide to disclose focus on the internal threats to healthy development if the child is not told. Parents who decide not to disclose often focus on the external threats from a hostile environment if the child *is* told. The internal threats if a child isn't told get tangled up with the external threats if the child is told, leaving each family with a conundrum in calibrating whether or not to tell. We now live in a culture that abhors inflicting any harm on children, to a fault. Add the prescription against harm to the entangled "harm if you do tell, harm if you don't," and you can see how the disclosure decision becomes a work in progress over many, many years.

As I have sat with families sorting out their feelings about disclosing or not disclosing, I've come to realize that parents who decide to disclose and parents who decide not to are driven by the very same motivating force. This child is *our* child, whom we wanted very much. In a study reported by Robert Nachtigall and Gay Becker analyzing five hundred written comments by over one hundred fifty donor-insemination parents, both disclosing and nondisclosing parents agreed on one thing: "Our child is our child—that's it."[19] Parents in both groups emphasized the social rather than the biological roots of parenting. Who is a parent? The person who takes care of the child and raises the child, not the person who makes the child. Parents, whether disclosers or nondisclosers, overwhelmingly held to the principle that parental responsiveness, rather than biological relatedness, is responsible for the child's attachment to a parent. Children will love the people who raise them, not the people who made them if they are not involved in raising them.

So it is typical for all parents who have used a birth other to invoke the concept of social parenting in making their decision to disclose or not. If you should decide to disclose, the social parenting principle will protect you from any threats that would come from the child knowing he or she had a birth other. They don't count as parents. If you should decide not to disclose, based on the three exceptional reasons for not telling, the social parenting concept tells you that it doesn't matter if your child knows about having a birth other. What is important is that your child knows that he or she has parents at home who love him or her. As put by one mother who had decided with her husband not to disclose that their children were conceived with a sperm donor, "We both decided it would be best if we never told the kids about this. He would be the father that hugged them when they skinned their knee, or cried on his shoulder when they didn't have a date for the school dance, so he would be their 'father' in every other way except biologically."[20] Bruce, Pop's son, is a sperm-donor child who sees it the same way: "We don't think of Doc [the donor] as our father in any way, shape, or form. Pop is our only father." [21]

The move toward disclosure in adoption has been accompanied by an emphasis on the child's need and desire to know the *parents* who made him or her, who are referred to as the birth mother or the birth father. The question of disclosure in birth-other families emphasizes the exact opposite. A child may or may not know about the birth other, but whether the child does or doesn't, the only parents in the picture are the ones the child resides with, whether genetically related or not. The birth other is neither a mother nor a father, but rather a donor or surrogate. The emphasis is not only on social parenting, but also on *intentional* parents. Intentional parents are the ones who made the decision to have a child and went ahead to have one. Donors and surrogates are the ones who helped them execute their plan. They are not parents. So to disclose to the children (or not) is to talk not about a child's other parent(s), but about an outside party who helped make the baby *for* the parents.

I want to end by returning to Jo and Charlie and sharing what they decided to do about disclosing to Caroline. Recall that Charlie thought I was a questionable psychoanalytic type in suggesting that Caroline may have already had some inkling about her origins. Disclosure was threatening to Charlie. He worried about losing the bond with his child, and he worried about Jo using his nonbiological parenthood against him. Jo, on the other hand, was more inclined to spill the beans and tell Caroline that Charlie was not her biological father. Unlike other fathers confronting primary infertility, Charlie's infertility was secondary to a vasectomy that could not be reversed successfully. Charlie thus experienced fewer affronts to his virility than do men who face infertility caused by their own body's failure to produce sperm. In that regard, Charlie's ego did not need protecting. Further, the somewhat adversarial divorce had left Jo feeling anything but protective toward Charlie, either regarding his manhood or, perhaps more alarmingly, his fatherhood status. So from Jo's point of view, she had nothing to lose and everything to gain in telling Caroline she had been conceived with donated sperm and Charlie was not her biological father.

To both their credit, Charlie and Jo stuck through an extended therapeutic process, loosening their defenses and suspending their antagonism toward each other. They were guided by their genuine commitment to do what was best for Caroline. I have found that fantasies about what's to come or what I call "crystal-balling" can help parents bring their deeper conflicts to the surface so they can look at and think about them and decide whether the feelings are getting in the way of good judgments. So I asked Jo and Charlie each to imagine what it would be like for Caroline to find out much later that Charlie was not her biological father and that she had not been told this throughout her childhood. Could that possibly do as much or more harm to her and to her future relationship with her family than the potential shake-up in her universe if they told her now, particularly given their staunch commitment to honesty and forthrightness with children? What would happen when she was an adult and decided to have a child and the doctor asked for a family medical history? I also validated Charlie's fears that Jo could potentially use Caroline's knowledge of the insemination as a weapon against him and asked Jo to think about the repercussions for Caroline if she were ever to do such a thing, either wittingly or unwittingly.

In our meetings together, Charlie and Jo worked through their anxieties and fears. They also went out and did their own research about insemination and disclosure. Charlie asked for a commitment from Jo that she would not go in search of the actual donor but leave him anonymous. He remained somewhat anxious. He did not trust Jo to hold her boundaries, and he worried she might manipulate the situation to her benefit. However, he now had in hand a professional judgment (mine) that Caroline's bond to him was as strong as epoxy glue. He was also keenly aware of the potentially harmful contradictions between his commitment to honesty and his and Jo's immaculate deception stance, in which they denied Caroline the truth about her roots. All of this led him to agree to tell Caroline about the donor. Jo and Charlie sat down with Caroline together and, after reviewing how babies are conceived, told her that she was conceived with the help of a man who gave them sperm because her daddy did not have any after a vasectomy that could not be reversed.

Caroline took this information in stride and asked very few questions about it. She did not need a family grid to know that her dad was still her dad. She went back to playing with her dolls and throwing herself into her active life as an eight-year-old. Over the years she expressed more interest in finding out who the donor was, and her parents agreed to see if they could help her find him. They did, and she came to refer to him as her "bio dad." But when she talked to me about "Dad," there was only one person she had in mind—Charlie.

I return to our ten questions and boil them down to their essence: What will be healthier for my child—to know or not to know? Do I feel comfortable about telling, if I decide to? Who should know and who shouldn't? I hope that it is now clearer why you would or wouldn't disclose to your child, or to others, his or her birth otherness. I hope that I have also imparted to you the idea that only under exceptional circumstances—a child's developmental vulnerabilities, genuine threat to the parent–child bond, or potential harm from a hostile environment—will it be in a child's best interests not to know. This now leads us to the third panel in the triptych: figuring out when, what, and how to tell a child about mommies, daddies, and the other men or women responsible for the child's coming into the world.

When to Tell

> She'd known the story since she was in diapers: how her mother wanted to have a baby so much that she went to the "store" to buy sperm to make Maggie.[1]

We are now entering the third panel in the triptych—telling the children. After grappling with the question of *whether* to tell comes the next hurdle: the content and timing of the narrative to tell the children and other people, if you have decided to tell. Planning and then delivering an explanation that your child was made with "a little help from our friends" can be the most challenging task of all. We all wonder when is the right time to tell. We stumble as we try to craft the content of the story—the right words, the right tone. If you are the parent, you have to anticipate your child's response to the story. If there's any moment when anxiety can suppress clear thinking, for professionals and parents alike, it's when we're faced with telling the children the story of their origins with a birth other.

Reviewing published guidelines and recommendations for talking to children about their assisted reproductive roots, I was totally struck by one thing: Nobody agrees, but everyone has a strong opinion. To date, we have no longitudinal outcome studies measuring the relative effectiveness of telling a child when she is three years old versus telling her at seven, stressing the participation of the nice man or woman versus limiting the account to the sperm or ova that Mommy and Daddy got so baby could be made, and so forth. With that said, I suppose I'll have to position myself as yet another expert with an opinion. I base my opinion on my training as a developmental and clinical psychologist, my review of the contemporary literature, my consultation with other experts, and my work with the many parents and children who have worked out a family narrative about their children's origins with a birth other. To my mind, there's no boilerplate that applies to every family. For those of you who are or hope to become parents of children born with the aid of a donor or surrogate, I invite you to think with me about the different issues that will help you develop a narrative tailor-made to your own family's needs or allow you to reflect on the one you've already set in place. In this chapter we will focus on the preparatory work—examining our own feelings about telling and thinking about the right time to tell. Then in Chapter 8 we'll focus on the execution of the task—deciding what to tell the children and knowing what to expect when we do tell.

I have seven questions to guide us in this preparatory work, maybe one for every day of the week:

- When you were thinking about the child you would have (or as you think about the child-to-be now), what were you thinking as to when you would tell your child?
- Once the baby came (if that has already happened), did your thinking change regarding when you would tell your child?
- Do you think there are any benefits in telling your child from very early on, at birth or maybe during the preschool years?
- Do you think there are any benefits in waiting until your child is older, maybe school-age or even later?
- Do you think there is any harm in telling your child very early in life?
- Do you think there is any harm in telling your child much later?
- At what age (of your child) will *you* feel most comfortable telling the story?

TAMING OUR OWN WILD FANTASIES

The experts do unanimously agree on *one* thing. Parents will do as well in communicating to their children their assisted reproductive technology roots as they themselves feel comfortable telling the story. We've already identified all the ways this new way of making babies can stir up archaic anxieties. In the winter of 2004, I opened up *The Wall Street Journal* to a piece, "Cancer Patients Get New Hope for Having Kids."[2] I learned that doctors had for the first time created a human embryo using eggs from a frozen ovary implanted in a woman. As of 2005, no baby has yet been born using this procedure, but the hope is that it will soon give female cancer patients the chance to have a child of their own after the completion of their treatment. The procedure could also offer the possibility of motherhood to women whose biological clock is ticking with no partner in sight. Dr. Kutluk Oktay of the Center for Reproductive Medicine and Fertility led a team who implanted fifteen finger-nail-long strips of previously frozen ovary tissue beneath the skin of a woman's abdomen. Drugs were used to stimulate ovulation, and then the eggs were collected through the skin with a procedure described as being "as easy as drawing blood." Leaning back in my office chair as I digested this information, I began to experience a strange sense of vertigo. Here I was, the psychologist writing pages and pages about our need to get a grip on our wild fantasies about assisted reproductive technology, myself conjuring up bizarre mental images. I envisioned myriads of babies spouting from belly buttons; I imagined expectant mothers walking around with bulges on their sides instead of their middles as ovarian tissue grew every which way into babies.

Throughout history we have created birth myths ranging from cabbage patches to storks. My own personal childhood myth was about bread-boards on assembly lines up in heaven crafted into babies by God. I knew from my early religious training that God created humans on the sixth day of creation. Somehow I got "created" and "carved" confused, so I translated it into being "carved by God." I knew that my mother did her meat carving on a cutting board. I got cutting board confused with breadboard. I knew that God would have to be doing an awful lot of carving to make all the people around. My father, who was in the tool business, had taken me to visit factories. So I was familiar with assembly lines and conveyor belts. Ergo, my conclusion that God was busy in heaven carving babies from breadboards on conveyor belts.

It seems we can't stop creating wild myths in our adult minds, even when we know better. That's what happened to me when I read about ovary implants. I didn't stay there. I regained my composure, lost the sensation of vertigo, and then remembered a fairly dense statement by Joan Raphael Leff, a British psychologist writing about egg donation: "In this illusory realm of omnipotent reproductive control not only are generative representations affected, and psychosocial disturbances unleashed, but our wildest fantasies may be actualized, flaunting reality restrictions and taboos."[3] I don't know about taboo, but my reality restrictions definitely flew out the window in my vibrant fantasies of abdominal babies. I was also aware of my anxiety as I clutched my middle and muttered to some inner audience, "Ovaries don't belong in skin implants; they're in the wrong place, and that can't be right."

I share these fantasies with you not to highlight my own limitations, but to point out how susceptible we all are to archaic fantasies and emotional squirminess as we prepare ourselves to tell children a story about babies made with sperm ejaculated into a jar, eggs extracted in a doctor's office, wombs not biologically related to the eggs placed inside them. Ironically, the terrain is shifting so quickly that what used to be fact is now becoming myth. It's no longer fact that all babies are born from their mommies and daddies, unless we perceive surrogates and donors as mommies and daddies. Yet, as I was reading a pamphlet providing guidance to parents for talking to their children about their donor conception I came across the following quote:

> A typical question of a three-year-old may be "Where did I come from?" For such a question, a relatively simple answer such as "All babies are made of an egg cell from their mummy and a sperm cell from their daddy" may suffice until the child at a later stage asks how the egg and sperm cell got together and actually made the baby.[4]

That answer is no longer true and shouldn't suffice. For *all* children, not just birth-other children, we need to be ever mindful and update our narratives on conception and birth as the times change. Until further notice, today's accurate account is that it takes an egg cell from a woman and a sperm cell from a man to make a baby. Daddies and mommies are another story. If experts writing the advice to parents are having trouble articulating an up-to-date, accurate account, we need to be humble enough to admit that all of us are tripping along together as we think our way through this third piece of the triptych— telling the children.

Don't Worry, Be Happy

Let's return to the one thing the experts agree on—parents who've had a child with a birth other must find a comfort level in themselves if they're go-

ing to have a shot at sending their children a positive message about their beginnings. So, to do a good enough job of telling your children how they were
made, you must filter out the discomfort that any parent feels talking to a
child about sex and reproduction and then grapple with any uneasy feelings
that may surface as you explain to your child that she did not come from you
or that she came from you and someone else who is not her parent. Carole
Lieber Wilkins, an expert in the field of assisted reproductive technology,
wisely counsels that children may raise questions about their birth story or
why they do not look like their mother or father. She reminds parents that in
the face of such questions, any discomfort they display may send a message
to the child that this is a taboo discussion. Such a message, she says, could be
damaging to the child, warning the child to stay out of Mom and Dad's life.[5]

It seems to me that advising parents that they may harm their child if
they don't first feel fully comfortable could ultimately backfire. It might
only fuel rather than soothe anxiety, because now you have to be perfectly
relaxed if you're going to get it just right.

I find myself feeling somewhat disturbed about the message "Get it
right." I grow uneasy, thinking about the work I did for my book *Spoiling
Childhood*. There, I analyzed the undue stress put on mothers and fathers today to be perfect parents in every way. It's illusory to think that mothers and
fathers will be capable of expelling all anxious feelings, every vestige of
self-consciousness, and any signs of awkwardness as they talk to their children and field their children's questions on a topic about as sensitive as it can
get—talk of sex, reproduction, infertility, single parenthood, sexual orientation, and so forth. So what's a better message? If you can work through your
own anxieties and discomforts enough to avoid finding yourself tripping
over your own words, feeling like a deer in the headlights, or drowning in
your own emotions whenever you do tell your child, you'll have the opportunity to send a positive message and field your child's questions as they
come up.

I am proposing that it's fine to be a little squirmy, just not apoplectic
and not so nervous that you can't think straight. Further, it's fine to make
mistakes as you tell the tale, then pick yourself up, correct yourself, and
keep going. Mistakes along the way do not necessarily mean irreparable
harm to the child. Think of it as a family affair. You will all negotiate the
terrain together, shaping a family narrative about your child's birth and
making adjustments as you go. There's no shame in sharing with each
other the parts that have been difficult. Your task is not to purge yourself of

all discomfort, but to have the equanimity to lead the way in the discussions with your child.

The best way to do that is to make sure that you yourself have emotionally accepted the way your family was made.[6] I wrote the preceding chapters with exactly that goal in mind. The idea was to pinpoint the trouble spots that come up when baby is made by you and someone else. Once you know what they are, you can think about them, chew on them, and try to smooth them out so you end up with a whole and positive sense of your family.

Giving yourself the freedom first to let loose with all your wildest fantasies is part and parcel of that process. Establishing a sense of emotional acceptance is obviously a work in progress over the lifetime of a family. To ensure that the process goes well, finding in yourself a relatively—and I want to stress *relatively*—stable sense of emotional evenness and self-assuredness will secure the same for your children as you unfold the story of their birth. Dr. Anne Bernstein, a close colleague and expert in the field, has been able to transform the au courant "get it right" admonishment into a positive message to parents. I'd like to share with you her sage advice: "When young children are assured that their questions can be answered without creating parental consternation, they seem to accept information with relative equanimity."[7]

As you prepare yourself to deliver a story to your children, you will be faced with a specific set of your own developmental steps. First, as just said, you need to explore your own feelings about the story you plan to tell. Second, you have to prepare yourself for the moving terrain of your child's development—the story will never be static; it will grow and change as the child grows. Third, you must ready yourself for the unknown—there is no boilerplate or single set of directions; each child is different, and different children will pose different questions or have different responses to the story "Where Did I Come From?"

WHEN

It is difficult to know whether to discuss what to tell before talking about when to tell or to allow the decision of when to tell lead our thinking about what to tell. It is indeed a chicken-and-egg question, but I've decided first to invite us to think together about the timing of the narrative and then, in the next chapter, move to crafting its content, obviously timed to the age of the child to be told.

So when should you tell a child if you're going to tell? Three main schools of thought say three different things. I'm going to describe each one of them and then consider their respective merits.

School #1: Baby's Born, It's Time to Tell

The first school says tell the child from the very first moments of life, even before the child can understand the words. That way parents will get used to telling the story, so by the time the child *can* understand, the story will roll off their tongues and already be a permanent fixture in the family. Telling the children their story right from the beginning helps parents work their way into a kind of casual conversation about donors or surrogates that will eventually be part of talks with their child in the future.[8] That way, no hemming and hawing and no formal lectures.

This school of thought relies heavily on the wisdom of the adoption field, which has found that children fare better when they are told early on about their adoption. A colleague of mine who had adopted her son at birth described how she talked to him in his infancy about his adoption. She knew full well that he would not understand a word she was saying, but she reported doing it for herself to get used to telling the story and also to give herself some space to correct her mistakes and get it right. She did all this in preparation for the time when her son would be old enough to understand. She thought that at that point she'd feel much greater ease telling the story because she'd already been doing it for such a long time. She told a very simple story of where he came from and who made him, without going into any details of sex and reproduction.

A mother who had her baby with the help of an egg donor reported a similar experience to my colleague's:

> We didn't want our daughter to remember a time when she didn't know her origins, and we didn't want her to remember being sat down and "TOLD." . . . We actually told her the first time, the day she came home from hospital when she was just a week old. It wasn't that she needed to know; it was that we needed to practise to become really confident in talking to her about her conception and we needed to find the right words to tell her. It took us quite a few goes before we felt we were doing a good job.[9]

Practice sessions for the parents are not the only reason for telling so early. In a totally different context, David Scott Levin, a clinical psychologist, has written about doing talk therapy with children who do not yet talk or have full use of language. He describes the task of both therapist and parent: to know empathically where the child needs to go and help the child go there. To be able to do this often means being one step ahead of the child, speaking to the child before he or she fully comprehends language but when he or she can understand that something nurturing and caring is happening.[10] Even though he's talking about children who suffer from developmental disorders, I have found Levin's ideas invaluable in thinking about all children. If we apply his theory to the school of thought that advocates talking to children from birth on about their roots with a birth other, the spoken word is not just for the parent; it's also for the child. The baby hears a combination of words that will someday make sense, and by the time they do, the words will already be familiar in sound and tone. More important, the baby experiences the tale "through the skin"—in the warmth and caring of the parent's voice as the tale is told and in the gentleness of the arms that hold the child while the story is delivered. The child is having a preverbal experience of a verbal tale. That experience begins building a firm foundation of emotional equanimity, for both parent and child. That in turn readies everyone for the child's verbal years, when the story will be elaborated and expanded. So if you tell your children early, in loving tones, your children can begin to feel good about their beginnings, and as they grow, they can know that it's fine to ask you to elaborate on the story of their conception.

Mr. Davids is a father who began to tell his son right after birth about his donor insemination:

> Even in the hospital, Mr. Davids began to tell the baby about his birth history. He became involved in the caregiving, and father and son became attached to each other. When the boy could understand language, his father was surprised that he did not seem to really care about his "birth story" but preferred doing the things he loved to do with his father.[11]

I'm struck by two things that Mr. Davids's experience with his son highlights about early telling. First, by the time your child actually understands, it's not just that the story is already familiar, it may not even be of great interest. Second, the son may be showing little interest in the story because of his attachment to his dad. His bond to his father matters much more to him than his roots do.

Ironically, the one caveat to the tell-as-early-as-possible school of thought has to do with this very thing—attachment. Turning again to the adoption field, Adam Pertman points out that adoptive parents may feel threatened about meeting their children's innate need for information about their birth parents. This may be true especially at the beginning, when they have not yet secured a permanent bond with their children. The adoptive parents may feel jealous as they anticipate the affection the child might someday feel for his or her birth parents, or already does, if the child has been adopted not at birth but at an older age.[12] This very same jealousy may surface if you have a child using a donor or surrogate. Forget about intentional parents, forget about birth other having neither "mother" nor "father" in the title. What if your child will want his or her other biological parent more than you? Perhaps it is asking too much to meet your new infant, establish a connection, and at the same time tell a story that pulls at the threads of the bonds that are just forming.

Common wisdom would say that if that's the case, wait until you feel a secure enough bond with your baby before embarking on the tale of origins, whether that takes hours, days, weeks, months, or even years. You might also want to wait until you feel your child has a clear enough understanding about who his or her parents are and how you will be his or her parent no matter what. The only caveat here is that waiting indefinitely might actually get in the way, rather than help build bonds. Waiting might even be a form of stalling. It might be anxiety about attachment rather than attunement to attachment. If you find yourself putting off telling again and again, waiting until you're absolutely sure the bonds are glued tight, you might want to bite the bullet and push yourself to speak the words and tell your child the story. That way you may actually master the anxiety about bonds and strengthen the bonds as you discover, like Mr. Davids, that for your children, the tale was really not such a big deal.

The words you use might also help reinforce attachments, rather than challenge them. For example, in Jane T. Schnitter's book, *Let Me Explain: A Story about Donor Insemination,* the narrator of the story, a school-age girl, explains to the reader:

> My mom says my dad and I are two of a kind except for one thing. We don't look anything alike. And I know why. It's because we don't have the same

genes. This is where it starts to get confusing. . . . I don't have any genes from my dad because I didn't come from his sperm. His sperm don't work the way they need to make a baby grow. I act like my dad sometimes though, watching football, riding bikes, playing rummy, or saying, "Oh, Baloney." That's because I've learned these things from him, not because I have his genes on the inside.[13]

Jane Schnitter's character emphasizes that she and her dad share traits and behaviors, even if they don't look alike, and they share them because her dad has given them to her. For some, the right time to tell might be just at the time when you want to reinforce the sense of sameness and connectedness between you and your child, rather than waiting until the moment when you're sure of the connection to introduce your child to his or her birth story.

School #2: Wait for the Birds and the Bees

Now we move to the second school of thought. School #2 promotes waiting until a child begins to wonder where babies come from and has the cognitive skills to understand a simple story of conception. This would place a child between the ages of two and five. The advantage of waiting until then is that parents and children have already had some years together to solidify family ties, and the story will be nicely timed with the developmental stage when the child is expressing initial curiosity about the birds and the bees. Linda Applegarth, a psychologist who counsels infertile couples in New York, suggests telling children between the ages of two and four something very simple, such as that a helper was involved to help Mommy and Daddy have a child. Then, when children start asking where babies come from, typically in the preschool years, parents can start talking about eggs and sperm.[14]

In the tell-as-early-as-possible school of thought, you don't have to worry about overwhelming an infant or baby with the content of the birth story because the child doesn't yet have the cognitive capacity to be flooded by such information. With infants and toddlers, the story may go over their heads at the same time that it enters their hearts. But it's a different matter when the entry point is two or older. I had been working with two mothers who were as thoughtful as anyone could ever be in contemplating when to start telling their son the story of his donor-insemination conception. Their son was still under a year old, and they had spoken not a word to him about his birth story. We thought together about the possibility of beginning to talk to him by the time he was two. After that discussion, one of the mothers sent me a note: "You noted that offering a relatively complete narrative for a young child is an approach that many adoptive families take. The purpose is to normalize the story for the child at a young age. Is this right? In doing so, what are the risks of overwhelming our little boy—cognitively and/or emotionally?"

Her question underscores why we can't separate the when from the what. Anything you tell your children about their origins has to be tailor-made to their chronological age and, more important, developmental stage. If we tell children a story that is either too complicated or too charged, they may get confused and lost in the details. They might be overstimulated by age-inappropriate information, the obvious being specific details about sex and reproduction. More typically, they may simply tune out and shut down. None of this is what we would want for a child when the intent is to provide him or her with a clear and steady map of his or her own birth and place in the family, a map that will guide a child through all of childhood. And that never has to happen, because you can create simple stories for two- to five-year-olds that will be neither too stimulating nor too confusing. The risks of over-whelming a little child cognitively or emotionally are low when the story is tailored to preschoolers' typical questions about babies, mommies, and daddies.

So you start out by doing a risk analysis to make sure the story told will not overwhelm your small child. The antidote to overwhelming a preschool child with information that is too much or too complex is to operate with what I call the "titration" model—the information about your child's con-ception will be doled out over time. As your child grows, you'll make adjust-ments in the story to match his or her evolving developmental status.

Another family I worked with was concerned not so much about stimu-lus overload but about developmental disruption if they told the story too soon, in their son's preschool years. Their child was conceived with the help of an egg donor. He didn't know this. He was just turning five. Both parents were open to telling their son about his conception with a donor, but his fa-ther didn't think his preschool years were the right time. His mom was wor-ried their son might feel they had tricked him or lied to him if they waited too long to tell him, and she was growing increasingly uncomfortable misrepre-senting herself to her son as his genetic mother. But his dad was adamant that they should wait. Why? Because in the preschool years their son would be in

the throes of the Oedipal drama, working out his love for his mother and father, his jealousies, and his fantasies about each of those relationships. His
dad feared that introducing an outside party, the egg donor, would muck up
his son's negotiation of the Oedipal complex, particularly his "love affair"
with his mother and his feelings of competition with his father. He thought it
was best to wait until that stage was over, when his son moved forward into
the latency stage, which by reputation is a time when children have forged a
firm identification with both of their parents and when their gender identity
is firmly in place.

I've given lectures to mental health professionals about families using
reproductive technology, and many of them express the same reservations as
this mom and dad. Again and again, I'm asked the question "Don't you think
it's too emotionally and sexually stimulating to introduce such young children to explicit stories about sex and reproductive organs beyond their own
thoughts and fantasies?" In answer to that question, I first acknowledge their
legitimate concern but then invite them to consider whether their adult fantasies may be getting in the way. Little children's erotic fantasies get stimulated no matter what we do or don't tell them. Sigmund Freud enlightened us
about this phenomenon a century ago in the story of Little Hans, a tale of a
five-year-old boy's fantasies about babies, genitals, and sex as he witnessed
his mother's progressing pregnancy.[15] At the same time, the story of conception with a birth other does not need to be sexually explicit. It can be kept
very simple for preschoolers, just giving them the facts that their parent or
parents wanted very much to have a baby and found someone to help them
do it, using an egg and a sperm, or an egg and a sperm and someone else's
womb. Even though this tale still may stimulate little children's erotic
fantasies, which will surface regardless, it hardly sounds like an X-rated
movie.

School #3: School Age Is Prime Time

You may still have doubts about introducing such a complex subject of sex
and reproduction to very young children. So do the proponents of the third
school of thought, who advise waiting until a child reaches school age to begin the discussion. Waiting this long is usually not possible for children who
come from single-parent families or gay and lesbian families. By the time
they have finished preschool, they get it that most children have mothers and
fathers and that not having a mother and father calls for some explanation.

But for children who have both a mother and father, the primary school years, somewhere between the ages of seven and ten, are sometimes seen as the best time to begin talking to children about their conception. A sixteen-year-old girl, a sperm-donor baby herself, is a strong advocate of waiting until children reach school age: "Don't tell them when they're too young. It will only mix them up. They have to be old enough to understand sex and birth and all that. Maybe people could figure out how to prepare kids to be told later on."[16] This young woman's position is supported by psychologists Annette Baran and Reuben Pannor, who argue that children under nine or ten will not be able to understand the complicated story of assisted reproductive technology.[17]

Seven to ten represents a stage in which children have the cognitive resources and conceptual understanding to make sense of the complex phenomena of egg or sperm donation, surrogacy, and their own beginnings. School-age children are ready to comprehend the mechanics of reproduction at a more sophisticated level than a preschooler. They can also make meaningful distinctions between people who count as parents and people who came on the scene to help in their conception either because one of their parents wasn't able to conceive or bear a child or because their parent lacked a partner to conceive with. These years are also perceived as the era in which children have emerged from the tumultuous dramas of separation anxieties, terrible twos, and Oedipal love triangles into the quieter emotional terrain of school, learning, rule building, game playing, friendship formations, and team building. I have highlighted emotional equanimity as a requisite for successfully negotiating the birth narrative. In the wait-until-school-age school of thought, this bedrock will be that much firmer because parents wait until the child is emotionally and cognitively ready to receive such complicated information with equanimity. Parents, too, may be more fortified in that bedrock, not because of evolving cognitive capacities but because of all those years under their belt as the real parents of their child.

I've been surprised to notice in my own work that seven to ten also appears to be a common age for the erosion of doubts on the part of parents who, until that time, had decided not to tell their children about their conception with a birth other. Some parents begin to grow uneasy about lying to their children. Someone begins questioning a decision that seemed wise before, either the parents or some outside party involved with or working with the parents. This was certainly the case with seven-year-old Caroline, discussed in earlier chapters. Her own readiness, tagged by me, the outside party, led Jo and Charlie to rethink their agreement not to tell and then tell her at age eight. As with Jo and Charlie, parents may revisit their original decision not to tell because they watch their children's developmental progression into an age when they really want to know something about their roots in some concrete objective terms, as evidenced in their actions and in their questions. So, as taught to us by the children themselves, the wait-until-school-age school of thought may be on to something in its understanding of a child's optimal receptivity to the story as he or she enters the age seven-to-ten bracket.

With all that wisdom about readiness, we still can't overlook the one major pitfall to postponing telling until age seven to ten. By that time children have already formed firmly conceived notions about their family—who their parents are and how they are related to each of their parents and to their brothers and sisters, if they have any. They know enough about the basic tenets of reproduction to assume, unless told otherwise, that their mommy and daddy were the ones who made them (assuming they have both a mommy and daddy) and that they and their siblings were all made by the same people (assuming they live in an intact family). To be disabused of that theory with the amended story that actually, you didn't come from Mommy's uterus, or actually, you're not related by blood to Daddy and only half to your brothers and sisters, can feel like a bomb being dropped and a colossal act of betrayal. Children have been known to accuse their parents of leading them to believe a story that all the while the parents knew was not accurate. Children's trust in their parents can be eroded as they wonder what else the parents have up their sleeves.

These negative reactions are not universal. Some children may have the response Mr. Davids's son had—"Oh, okay, so can we get on with our game now?" Eight-year-old Caroline indeed was not in the least nonplussed when Jo and Charlie explained to her about her donor-insemination origins. As far as she was concerned, her daddy was still her daddy, and nothing would change that. But Ethan, whose parents decided to wait until he was nine and could understand the information about his conception with the help of an egg donor, flew from the room in a rage. An only child, he had been raised in a caring and loving family. On that day, his parents had just finished telling him a carefully thought-out, sensitive account of his mother's infertility and the need to have the aid of a donor egg so they could have the baby they wanted so badly. They also explained to him why they had waited until he was old enough to understand to tell him the story. All of their gentle words did not assuage his vitriolic response: "I can't believe you've been lying to me all these years. You're not my parents, either of you." With time, Ethan got over his initial upset, and life resumed its steady positive course, but he still reproaches his parents for waiting so long to tell him. In sum, the trade-off, waiting until a child is old enough to comprehend the story fully and thereby risking his or her sense of betrayal, may not be worth it—either for the child's overall well-being or for the building of family trust and harmony.

We can't overlook another final risk factor in waiting until children are school-age to tell them the story of their conception. In the model of tiered disclosure, some families have shared the story with others before they tell their child, perhaps even before the child was born. And word gets around. Probably the worst sense of betrayal or breach of trust a child can experience is when the story is leaked to the child by someone else before the parent or parents have had an opportunity to sit down and tell him or her themselves. An aunt or uncle can naively do this, assuming that by school age the child already knows or forgetting that the parents never told the child. Or it might come in some more insidious form as a taunt on the playground: "My mommy says you were born in a test tube and your daddy's not your daddy!" Obviously, you can establish an insurance policy against such inadvertent and hurtful information leakage to the child:

1. Keep the information of your child's conception extremely confidential if you intend to wait until much later to share it with the child or intend never to tell your child at all.
2. Make sure that anyone who knows understands that this is highly confidential information, that you have not yet told the child, and that you will inform them when you do.
3. Always stay mindful about making sure you tell your child before someone else beats you to the punch—that is, watch out for signs of leakage.

Holding Off until Adolescence

There's no school of thought for this one. It doesn't take a rocket scientist to figure out that if trust-breaking is a risk for school-age children, the risk is heightened a hundred-fold if you wait until your child is a teen to tell. This is another area where all the experts agree—adolescence is late to start telling the story of origins with a birth other.[18] Waiting until adolescence to tell confronts teens with jolting information that disrupts their sense of who they are just at the time when they need that baseboard to anchor them for the emotional roller coaster ride ahead. In our culture, adolescence is a time for children when all of who they are will be up for grabs as their body changes and their souls are left temporarily in upheaval. It is a time when they turn away from their families and toward their peers. They need to fit in; they worry if they don't. They are exquisitely sensitive to anything fake or inauthentic. During this stage they will find themselves engaged in what Erik Erikson identified as one of the most important developmental tasks of life: identity. Their work is to establish a sense of who they are and where they are going in life. If the task fails, they are left with confusion, floundering to find their place both within society and within themselves.[19]

There are many reasons the task may fail, but there's no need to set up that failure by removing a child's stable base of family during the identity journey. Telling the child for the first time that the family is not really what she thought it was and that her own genetic roots are not what she thought they were is just such a potential removal. Discovering that everyone has been living a lie can erode any sense of trust the child has had in the integrity and honesty of the family just when the child needs that stable base to move forward in his or her own exploratory journey of self-identity.

And parents are fully aware of this. Jane and Alexander came to see me in a panic. Their son, Kyle, was fifteen and having a rough go of it in high school. They had decided never to tell him about his donor-insemination roots, an assisted reproductive conception that happened because the doctors couldn't successfully reverse Alexander's vasectomy. The problem was that Jane had failed to establish a good insurance policy—word had gotten out, and her friend, Patricia, with whom she had shared the information in strictest confidence, did not honor Jane's request for secrecy. She began to talk because *she* thought it would be better if Kyle knew. So Patricia confided in another friend of Jane's, and she even talked to her own teenage children, friends of Kyle's, but swore them to secrecy. Teens are wonderful, but keeping secrets is not their strong suit, particularly if it means keeping secrets from their own friends. I think you've probably all had the experience from your own adolescence, "So-and-so told me not to tell, but . . . ."

Jane and Alexander are very caring parents, and they knew full well the damage to Kyle if he were to find out from someone else besides them. But Alexander was also terrified about losing his bond to Kyle, because Kyle had been so rejecting of his dad during this tumultuous period. He truly believed that when Kyle found out that Alexander was not his biological father and that both his parents had lied to him all these years, it would be curtains for their relationship. I tried to reassure Alexander that, although there was definitely a risk to Kyle if they didn't tell him soon, it didn't have to be tomorrow. I also shared with him my own observations that, as far as Kyle was concerned, Alexander was his only dad and that would last forever (I had known their family since Kyle was seven). But when they both asked the next question, "What will happen? How will Kyle get through this?" I began by saying, "First, Kyle will do as well as the two of you do in feeling okay about telling him." That was too much for Alexander, and he broke down in tears. "Well, I'll tell you how I'm doing. I'm totally traumatized."

I felt terrible for Alexander and let him know that the very first task was to help him with his feelings because they made complete sense under the circumstances. He knew they were going to have to tell, but he also knew it was going to be no emotional picnic for him, particularly given Kyle's adolescent storms. I have every confidence that they will ride out this storm (to date, it hasn't happened yet), but we can see from Jane and Alexander's predicament why all the experts agree that adolescence may not be the best time to tell.

Recall David, who was brought into therapy not because of his donor-insemination roots but because he was getting into constant fights with his father. With the help of Dr. Marsha Levy-Warren, who suspected these father–son tensions might very well have to do with the untold story of David's conception, David was finally told by his father during his teenage years that he was conceived with a mix of his father's weak sperm and the sperm of an anonymous sperm donor. David was simultaneously relieved and upset when he heard the news, relieved because it finally made sense to him why he felt his father had been overscrutinizing him for so many years, upset because he felt he had been deceived all his life.[20] David's message was loud and clear. He wished his parents had told him much earlier about the sperm donor. But his engagement in family fighting that finally led to telling also highlights two important points about the timing of the story: (1) children will often push the envelope, and (2) better late than never.

During adolescence, it's quite likely that children's subterranean questions about their origins will surface as they struggle to put together their own about-to-be-adult identity. If they suspect something is askew, they might not just sit on their fantasies. They may take action. In David's case, taking action meant butting up against his father, over and over again, desperately trying to figure out why his father was scrutinizing him so much. David was wrong in his conclusions—it was not because his dad thought he was a bad egg, but because his dad was desperately trying to figure out if David had come from his own sperm. Adolescence was the last chance for David's parents to tell him about his donor roots while he was still a child, and David gave them that chance by pushing his parents to pay attention to the relationship between him and his father.

As for better late than never, David was able to use the information about the insemination to reflect on his life and make better sense of it, particularly his tumultuous relationship with his father. The tensions between him and his father subsided once his father felt he was no longer keeping a secret and once David no longer psychologically scrambled to get something from his father that he felt was missing. When I work with therapists in training, I often remind them not to be so hard on themselves if they missed something in a session, because inevitably the bus will come around again. The same is true when telling the children the story of their roots. It might not be optimal to tell a child later rather than earlier, especially if we're talking about adolescence. But if you've missed the boat before, all is not lost. Being ready to tell later rather than earlier simply means you need to be open, forthcoming, and honest with your children. That includes explaining why you waited until now to tell. The rest will unfold as you gauge your own feelings and prepare yourselves to help your children with whatever complicated responses they have.

You will all have work to do as you rethink your relationships with each other based on the new information provided to your children about their conception or gestation. And your children will have their own work to do as they adjust their self-identity based on the new information that they came from you and someone else. It may not be an easy process and may require weathering the storm and doing some repair work, but if done with love, attention, and openness to each other's feelings and experiences, the reworking has the potential to bring the family closer together, rather than splitting it apart.

Is It Best to Wait until a Child Asks?

Although "better late than never" is a wise dictum for parents to follow, one surefire way to risk missing the boat is to decide to wait until the child asks, "Where did I come from?" or "Did I come from you?" to tell the story. Susan Hollander, the director of the Alliance for Donor Insemination Families, told her own son about his origins with a sperm donor when he was five-and-a-half years old. As she did with her own son, she advises parents to be child-centered and wait until their children ask about where they came from. She advocates that by using wait-until-the-child-asks as a guideline, you ensure that telling your children "can be a very natural loving kind of process if the parents are at peace with how they've made their family."[21] And isn't that what we all want for the children?

The risk of this approach is that you might be waiting forever. "Don't ask, don't tell" seems like an ill-conceived plan for the military, and it is equally ill-advised when deciding when to tell children about their roots. For example, David reported to his therapist that although he began to wonder about his origins, he also sensed his father's acute discomfort and wished to protect him from pain. So he purposely did not ask, to protect his father. Other children who suspect something about their origins with a birth other may hold back from asking because they themselves are anxious about the answer and protect themselves by avoiding the subject. And other children simply never express their curiosity directly.

Although waiting for the child to ask may appear to be a more child-centered approach, it runs the risk of putting too much burden on the child to lead his or her her own journey in a search for roots. Children are acutely sensitive to what is okay to ask and what is not okay to ask in the family. Parents' own conflicts about having a child with a birth other may inadvertently leak out and send the message "Don't go there." No parent is a perfect machine. Even if you've made peace with how you've made your family, such peace making is neither linear nor static. As your child grows, you may encounter some doubtful or uncomfortable feelings lurking at the edges or cropping up when least expected. It is just such internal chatter, transferred to your child, that might become a deterrent, holding your child back from asking "Where did I come from?" So my overall recommendation to parents in sorting out when to tell the story of origins is that you take the lead and have a plan in place that doesn't depend on your children asking but comes instead from your own assessment of when your child is ready to know.

THE RIGHT TIME IS THE BEST TIME

Each of you will have to assess your own situation in deciding when that optimal time is. Going back to the seven questions at the beginning of the chapter, it will depend on how you answer each of them for *your* child and *your* family.

I myself would advocate beginning the narrative either very early, in the first two years of life, or in the preschool years, when children first become curious about where babies come from and how *they* were made. This way the child is never led astray with false information or misconceptions that have to be undone later, there are no untoward surprises or feelings of betrayal and distrust, and family life is built on a foundation of honesty and forthrightness. But no matter when one starts the story, it will never be a one-shot deal. It will be a story that will be told over and over again as the child develops and changes. This leads us to our next chapter: *what* to tell as the child grows.

The Birds and the Bees and the Nice Man or Woman

> The story was always that we wanted a baby, that two women couldn't get pregnant together, so we went to this nice lady who was kind of a doctor, and she found a nice man who donated sperm and she put it inside me.
>
> —Laura Werbner, mom[1]

Each time you craft a story to tell your children about their origins with a birth other, you are inventing a new wheel. And anytime you turn to experts for help, you may face a panorama of contradictory advice. Nonetheless, I want to launch our discussion with advice from one of those experts, Anne C. Bernstein: "And so a word about 'experts' and how to use the advice they have to offer. As you cut the suit to fit your body and not your body to fit the suit, take expert advice only when it fits. If what I suggest goes against your grain, trust yourself. You'll be a better parent for it."[2]

Typically, you'll be flooded with a torrent of questions as you roll up your sleeves to write the stories in your head (or on paper) that you'll tell to your child:

- What do I call the donor (surrogate)?
- How will my child know the difference between Daddy and a biological father, between Mommy and a biological or genetic mother?

- How do I follow my child's lead while at the same time imparting the information I want her to have?
- What do I want to tell my child about why we (I) used a donor or surrogate?
- What do I tell my child about the identity of the donor (or surrogate)?
- How do I explain to my child his sibling relationships—with the other child (ren) in the family and to the children of the donor or surrogate?
- How do I explain that she has two mommies (or daddies) and someone else helped make her?
- What do I say when my child asks, "So why don't I have a daddy (mommy)?"
- What if I don't know how to answer a question?

Thinking through any or all of these questions may be just the measuring tape you need to tailor a suit to fit your family situation. This may be the single most important task in raising your children: providing them with a narrative that they can understand, live with comfortably and positively, and use to let other people know who they are and who their family is.

STUMBLING OVER WORDS: REPRODUCTIVE TECHNOLOGY'S TERMINOLOGY

I want to start by talking about the language you choose. All of us seem to be slipping and sliding around, searching for the right words for all the participants in the birth narrative. I coined the term "birth other" fortuitously. It was a typo. I've now become attached to the term and think it works quite well. It might even solve a problem that's plaguing parents and professionals alike—how are we supposed to refer to the woman or man who has provided eggs, sperm, or a womb so a child could be born? But that still won't end our word search for the best language to use with the children and with other people.

Elizabeth and Fred were sitting in my office sorting out what they were going to tell their nine-year-old daughter, Tanya, about her egg-donor conception. Fred suggested that they could point out to Tanya that she probably got her curly red hair and her long legs from her biological mother. Elizabeth visibly winced and, almost in a whine, meekly protested, "Hey, she came from me. Aren't I her biological mom, too?"

Christine and Annette had a child together using an anonymous sperm donor. They later broke up when Camille, their daughter, was only a toddler. Time went by, and Christine, the biological mother, who was Korean, wanted to begin telling Camille the story of her birth. She very much wanted to talk to Camille about her "birth father," particularly because he, too, was Korean, and she wanted Camille to have a full and proud sense of her racial heritage. Anita, who was Caucasian and the nonbiological mother, was apoplectic at the thought of referring to the donor as a father. She was adamant he should be referred to as the sperm donor. The only people in the story who should be called parents were Camille's two mothers.

Is it all in a name? Of course not. Embedded in Elizabeth's claim to the label "biological mom" is her anxiety that Fred doesn't recognize her as the legitimate parent of their child. Embedded in Christine and Annette's dispute—should the man be called a donor or a father?—are divorce issues, the mounting tensions because one mommy is a biological mother and the other isn't, and unresolved questions about racial identity. Agreeing on what to call the donor won't make those issues go away. But Elizabeth and Fred, Annette and Christine aren't the only families struggling to find the right words for the donor. We just don't have a common language for referring to a birth other. Some call them birth fathers or mothers. Some call them "bio" fathers or mothers. Some, like me, call them egg donors, sperm donors, and surrogates, with no attribute of "mother" or "father." If we can't get the terms straight, how are we going to tell a straight story?

Is a Birth Other a Parent?

Anthropologists anticipated the name problem a long time ago. Over a half-century ago, the social anthropologist Alfred Radcliffe-Brown borrowed a concept from our ancient forebears, who made a distinction between the "genitor" (biological father) and the "pater" (sociological father).[3] He thought this distinction would help us understand families across cultures—there are people who make children, and there are people who raise them. In the social world, the pater has always been privileged over the genitor. That's the same in donor-insemination families today—the father is privileged over the donor. So could we now borrow these terms from the anthropologists and have paters and genitors, maters and genitors? Somehow the words don't roll off our tongues. Try it: "Honey, Daddy's your pater, but you also have a genitor." The words may not work, but the concept does. My own experience tells me it's best to come up with terms that clearly differentiate the *parenting* role of mother and father from the *helper* role of donor or surrogate. I'm using "parenting" as a verb, meaning the people who raise the child, in contrast to the people who helped make the child. Children will create their own theories, images, roles, and labels no matter what we tell them. But I think the best help we can offer them is to be clear about the distinction between who is a parent and who is a helper in making the baby.

In *Flight of the Stork*, Anne Bernstein shares my position that children fare best if we provide a clear distinction between social parenthood and biological parenthood. She proposes using two separate terms, "daddy" and "biological father," when telling the donor insemination story. Indeed, I work with a young woman who refers to her known sperm donor as her "*bio* dad," heavily accenting the "bio" over the "dad" as she speaks. When she says "my dad," there is no question about whom she means—the guy, who by Radcliffe-Brown's terminology, is her pater. In translation, we could say she has a dad and a bio. Using the term "biological father [mother]" has the advantage of providing children with appropriate words to use when other children at school say, "Hey, how come you don't have a daddy [mommy]? Everybody has to have a mommy and daddy!" They can turn around and say: "I do have a biological father [mother]—the donor who helped make me."

Children are typically quite clear about who their "real" parents are—they are the people who get up with them in the middle of the night, pack their lunches, and check their report cards—that is, the social parents, who may also be the biological parents but don't have to be. This holds true even in those drama-filled moments when they scream, "You're not my *real* mother! My *real* mother would let me go to the mall!" and even when they're having fantasies of a better mom or dad who's somewhere out there in the universe. But even with such clarity about their real mommies and daddies, young children may get confused if we start talking to them about other "parents" who are part of their life.

If you're a single parent who has used a donor or surrogate, you may want to use the term "biological father" or "biological mother" to assure your children that they're like everyone else—they have both a mommy and a daddy. Yet referring to the "missing piece of the family" as father or mother may be somewhat of a ruse, camouflaging the donor or surrogate as an active parent participant in the family. If you're in a two-parent family, the terms may confuse your child with too many mommies or daddies. The terms may also jangle your own nerves, reminding you of the conniving kidnapper who could steal your child's affections.

This is why I prefer terms for donors and surrogates that do not use the words "mother" and "father." I would rather reserve those terms for the people who are the legal and social parents of the child.[4] You can refer to a donor as just that or, alternatively, you can use the more cumbersome label "the man who gave us sperm so we [I] could have you" or "the woman who gave us eggs so we [I] could have you." I have also heard the terms "gene lady" and "gene man" used to refer to donors. It becomes a bit more complex with surrogates because by present standards that woman *has* been involved in the early primary care of the child—in utero. As in adoption, you could refer to her as the "birth mother." But here's another idea—we can redefine motherhood by differentiating a woman who carries a child (surrogate) from a *mother* who cares for the child from birth on, whether she did so before birth or not. You could refer to the first woman as a surrogate or as "the woman who carried you in her womb."

We're all working to come up with clear and meaningful terms for the children. When we struggle with what to call something, it's not only because the words don't exist yet. It may also be because we're struggling with the concept itself. It's not just finding the right words to use with our children that we find daunting—it's finding the best way to communicate to the children the whole concept of birds, bees, and nice men and women.

What Should We Call Gametes? What Should We Call Uteruses?

Names for donors and surrogates aren't the only words we struggle with. We're going to be talking to children about complicated reproductive procedures of insemination, egg extraction, in vitro fertilization, embryo implantation, and gestational carrying. How are we going to come up with the right language that will make sense to the children?

Some people advise using the word "ovum" rather than "egg," as egg connotes Easter bunnies, Humpty Dumpty, a dozen lined up in cardboard cartons, or this morning's breakfast. Indeed, four-year-old Molly was told that her mommy went to get some eggs from somewhere else to make Molly because her mommy didn't have any eggs of her own. The next time they went to the supermarket, Molly ran to the dairy section, grabbed a carton of

Grade-A large eggs, and ran back to her mother, yelling across the aisle, "Hey, Mommy, I got some more eggs! Let's make another baby—I want a sister."

Little children like Molly are ripe for such mistakes if we use "egg" rather than "ovum" when we tell the story. But "ovum" is not an everyday word for a child. "Egg" is. Mistakes like Molly's can be rectified, and most children possess the language flexibility to know the difference between eggs that fall off walls and eggs that join together with a man's sperm to make a baby.

Some people also advise that you use the technical word "sperm" to refer to the man's gametes when you tell your children the story of their conception. Others think "seed" is a better word to use with young children because it resonates with their experience of seeds and growth and is a word that's been used since antiquity to refer to men's procreative substance. On this one, I would vote for "sperm," since it's more concrete and specific than "seed," and it matches the term "sperm donor"—we have no comparable term "seed donor" at the moment.

Now what about uteruses? Joyce Sukamp Friedman has written a pamphlet for parents, "Building Your Family through Egg Donation." Her advice is to avoid the word "tummy" when you talk to children about implantation and pregnancy because it might confuse them and make them wonder if when mommy eats a carrot, the carrot will fall on the baby's head.[5] Actually, very young children, under five, are going to have fantasies of pregnancy and birth that have to do with eating, digesting, and evacuating whether we call a mommy's uterus a tummy, a uterus, a womb, or a baby sac. My own son, then age two and three-quarters, marched up to our very close friend who was visiting for the evening, looked up at her swollen pregnant belly, and proposed, quite adamantly, "Nancy, go poop." This was quite out of character for our usually well-mannered little boy. So we asked him, "Jesse, why do you want Nancy to poop?" He looked up at us and explained very matter-of-factly, like an adult to a small child, "Because I want to see the baby come out." My granddaughter, age three and a half, came home and reported to her mother some puzzling news. Her best friend, whose mother was about to have a second child, told her assuredly that the way you have a baby is to eat a lot of food. The friend knows because her mommy is eating an awful lot of food, and that's how the baby who's coming out next month got there. My granddaughter, Satya, wasn't so sure about that. She asked her friend how come she, Satya, wasn't having a baby, too, because she eats lot and lots of food. And so does her mommy, and she doesn't have a baby growing either. "Nope," her friend said, "*I* know. That's the way it is. You eat a lot of food to make a baby."

Carrots falling on babies' heads, babies falling into toilets, and gargantuan baby-making diets are the purvey of small children's minds, no matter how carefully we explain to them otherwise. So I think it would be much better, particularly with small children, to choose user friendly rather than technically correct terms to explain how a baby was made with a donated ovum or sperm or with the assistance of a surrogate's womb. The words should resonate to a child's experience and level of language development. If there's any time to be child-focused rather than adult-oriented, it's in choosing the language you will use, so that you avoid a narrative that goes right over your children's heads or sounds more like a medical lecture than a children's story. And, of course, you will need to substitute more sophisticated words as your child grows older.

There are some words, though, that we're not going to be able to adjust. Those words may simply have to remain open to children's wild fantasies as the story of their birth unfolds. One obvious example is "sperm bank." These days children typically know banks as the places where their parents park and dash to the ATM—you put in a card and out spews cash. So five-year-old Antonio explained to me quite earnestly how he was born with a sperm bank: "My mommies went to the bank, put in a card, and instead of money, these seeds came out. Then they drove to the doctor's with the seeds, and she helped them make a baby with the seeds from the bank and Mama's egg." With a term like sperm bank, you might do better to hold off until your child can think more abstractly and not so literally, maybe somewhere between seven and ten. In the meantime, you could refer to the special place where people can go to get the sperm that is given by men who want to help mommies and daddies become parents.

A general rule of thumb in choosing language: stay child-focused and adjust the terms accordingly as your child grows. But the story is not just a string of terms. It's a concept. It's a flowing narrative that incorporates both facts and feelings. And to that story we now turn.

WHAT TO SAY

What you tell your children will of course depend on their ages and stages. But let's start with our Western default position about the birds and the bees. Despite all the innovations brought about by reproductive technology, the standard tale remains unchanged that babies are made from their mommies and daddies. If you're going to stray from that story, you're gong to be telling a tale that sets the record straight so your child doesn't go along with the false assumption that "a daddy and mommy made me." Telling your children about their origins with a birth other means finding the right words to convey the uniqueness of your family. Know that if you don't, your child will fall back on the default position—mommies and daddies make babies.

The Five Key Ingredients of the Story

I would like to share with you the story that a single mother wrote to her five-year-old son:

> Long before Mikey was ever born, his Mom (who wasn't a Mom yet, and so was called by her name Cindy) lived by herself in her house. She had a happy life. She had many friends and she liked her work as a doctor, but she kept thinking, "Oh, I would love to have a baby." Now, mostly when a woman wants to have babies, she waits to meet a man who could be her partner, and they could both create a baby and be a Mom and Dad. And the same with men—mostly they wait to meet a woman that they can love and marry so that they will be a family and raise kids together. But it doesn't always work that way. And it certainly didn't work that way with Cindy, because she didn't want to wait anymore. She was 39 years old and she wanted to have a baby before she was as old as Methuselah. And she wasn't married.
>
> So, Cindy went to the doctor. And she asked, "Dr. Simpson, is there any way I could get pregnant with a baby (a baby, by the way, that she was hoping would be just like Mikey), if I don't have a man to be my partner right now?" and Dr. Simpson was very smart and very helpful and she said, "Yes, I know of a way. There is a place where men give their sperm to be saved so that a woman like you could have a baby. If you do get pregnant, that baby would never know the man who gave the sperm, but he would know that it was a very nice man because he was willing to give his sperm so that the baby could be born. But you must be very sure that you want to have this baby."
>
> So Cindy went home and thought and thought about it. And the more she thought, the more she was sure. She really, really wanted this baby. So she went back to Dr. Simpson and said, "Yes, I do want to have a baby and I

will love him with all my heart." And Dr. Simpson helped Cindy to get the sperm, and after the sperm met Cindy's ovum, Cindy got pregnant.

. . . she told her mother and father (who, of course, were about to become Nana and Poppa). They were surprised, then pleased, then very excited. They wanted to be there when the baby would be born. And they were—nine long months after Mikey grew and grew inside Cindy . . .

Nana, Poppa, and Cindy were so eager to meet baby Mikey and let him know how much he was loved. So Cindy pushed, and pushed, and PUSHED for almost three hours, and out Mikey came at 5 o'clock in the morning of September 21, 1992. And that is why, every year on September 21, we celebrate Mikey's birthday—to remember what a wonderful, precious, perfect boy was born that day—YOU.

The author of this story was a mother who came to me to consult about her son. Several writers have published books to tell children about their births with egg donors, sperm donors, or surrogates, but none surpasses Cindy's story in its warmth, clarity, and honesty. Cindy's story contains the five key ingredients of a finely crafted story about origins for a child: (1) how much she wanted to be a mommy, (2) how she got some help to figure out how to have a baby, (3) who the players were and how the process worked, (4) who Mikey's family was, and (5) how much she loved her son. These are the five key ingredients whether your child is three, eight, or eighteen.

The Never-Ending Story

As Mikey gets older, Cindy will need to revamp the story to talk to Mikey about the reality that he most likely will never know his donor, to explain the technical procedure for joining the donor's sperm with Cindy's ovum, to address Mikey's concerns that he has a mom but no dad, and so forth. As your children grow, you can look for openings to add to or expand on the story. Recall the mother who told her daughter early because she didn't want her to remember being sat down and "TOLD." As her daughter grew, she and her husband used every opportune moment to talk to her about her conception with an egg donor. Because people were always commenting about their daughter's hair, her parents explained to her that "sometimes she looks a bit like Daddy because she grew from his sperm and sometimes she looks a bit like the woman who shared her eggs with us, because she came from her egg."[6] Every time they added to the story, their daughter reacted like something had just fallen into place for her.

Not only will the story need to change over time, but your child's understanding of the same old story may also radically change. Elizabeth Carr was the first test-tube baby born in the United States. Her parents had fully disclosed her in vitro fertilization roots to her when she was a tiny little girl. But Elizabeth said that only at age seven did she first get it. She was watching a *Nova* documentary about her conception and birth. Dr. Howard Jones of the Jones Institute in Norfolk, Virginia, was giving Elizabeth a step-by-step explanation of everything they saw on the screen. Now a young adult, Elizabeth explains: "'That was the first time I realized how different my conception was from all my friends, that it wasn't the norm. It finally sank in how much my parents went through to get me at that time.'"[7] "Finally sinking in" is the operative term here. You may need to tell the story over and over again as your child digests the information with a more sophisticated mind and a more developed psyche.

In the beginning, you'll talk to your very young children about different ways babies can be conceived. Their thinking is very concrete and they'll probably be most interested in the mechanics of conception and birth. As they grow older, they won't be so interested in the technical aspects of reproduction. Instead, they'll have a lot more questions about the things that motivate people to take part in donorship or surrogacy. They'll also be thinking about how their "birth otherness" affects their feelings about themselves, about their parents, and about their donors or surrogates, as they sort out their own identity.[8]

Tales for Tots

The story for the youngest child is a relatively simple one. If you've used an egg or sperm donor, the story begins by telling your child "how much we [I] wanted to have [dreamed about having] a baby—you. It takes ova [eggs] and sperm [seed] to make a baby, and we [I] didn't have any ova/eggs [sperm/seed], so we found someone to help us. That person helped me [us] by giving me [us] eggs [sperm] so I [we] could have you. That person who helped us so much is called an egg donor [sperm donor]. And now we have you and we love you so much." If you've used a surrogate, the story will talk about the place where a baby grows, and explain that "I [we] needed someone to help me [us] with a place for you to grow, so I [we] found a woman who would help me [us] by growing you in her uterus [tummy]." If you know the donor or surrogate and want your child to know that person as well, you can weave that person's name (and relationship with the child, if it is a friend or relative) into the story as the designated helper.

Many of the stories designed for young children emphasize the nice man or woman who donated sperm or eggs or offered her uterus so the parents who so much wanted a baby could have one. It is indeed a nice thing to do. But underscoring "nice" may also leave no room for a child to have bad feelings toward this person. Perhaps you'd be better off sticking with the word "helpful" to describe the donor or surrogate. This takes the halo off that person and places the emphasis on the gift given to you, the recipients, rather than the motivations of the giver. And then, in the story, it's perfectly fine to express gratitude to those people for the gift given so that a baby could be born, whether those people were nice or neutral. Removing the halo will leave a lot more space for the child's own feelings about the donor or surrogate without feeling guilt for hating an angel.

Now I want to switch the focus from the "nice" to the man or woman. I can't highlight enough the importance of talking about whole people rather than body parts when telling a child, even a very young one, the story about his or her origins using a donor or surrogate.

Of course, with a surrogate, it's nearly impossible to avoid referring to a whole person. You're not going to be talking about a disembodied womb, but about a woman who carries the baby for nine months and nurtures it until it is born. That woman's intrauterine environment may even influence the constitutional make-up of the baby, not just inside, but outside the womb.[9] So the surrogate doesn't just provide a womb; she is a woman whose prenatal relationship to the baby has to be factored into the birth story, just as the mother's prenatal relationship to the baby will be emphasized when the baby was made with a donated egg and grew in Mommy's uterus.

When it comes to donors, particularly but not exclusively anonymous donors, it's easy to refer only to the sperm or the egg needed to make the baby, divorcing the gametes from the person. That way, no interloper shows up in the story to threaten the bonds of the family. But limiting the account to getting the eggs or sperm so baby could be made becomes a verbal sleight of hand in which you pretend that there were no real people with minds and hearts who made personal decisions to be involved, either directly or indirectly, in making your child. It's a soothing pretense, but if you start out with a story that talks only about a vial of sperm or a solicited egg or womb detached from their owners, you may be ill prepared for the interest your children will likely express as they grow older, revisit their birth story, and ask the compelling question "Who is this person who is responsible for half my genes?" or "Who carried me in her womb?" So better to start from the get-go with a birth-other story about people rather than just their body parts.

If you are a family with a history of infertility, you may want to include information that "Daddy's sperm didn't work the way they should to make a baby" or "Mommy didn't have eggs that could make a baby" or "Mommy's uterus wasn't able to carry you while you were growing into a baby" and "that's why we went to the doctor and found the helpful man (helpful woman). . . . " Rozanna Nathalie has written a series of books to assist parents in talking to young children about their births using assisted reproductive technology as a result of infertility. The books are colorful picture books aimed at a preschool audience, one about in vitro fertilization (*Our Beautiful Work of A.R.T.*), one about egg donorship (*A Part was Given and an Angel was Born*), and one about surrogacy (*From Out of My Body Your Soul Did Grow*). In the second two books, the texts read, "there was a part in Mommy that just didn't work as it should" (egg-donor story) or "Mommy wanted you in her tummy for good/But her tummy wasn't working as it should" (surrogacy story). The stories go on with happy tales about "a very special lady with a heart [who] said, 'I'll help you, I'll help you, let me give this to you/ I'll share my part so that your dream can come true'" or "this wonderful lady with a heart made of gold [who] said, 'You can put your baby in my tummy to hold.'" [10]

I'm concerned that preschool tales like Nathalie's that include information about Mommy or Daddy's malfunctioning body run the risk of overwhelming the very young child. By the time children hit school age and want to know *why* their parents used a donor or surrogate, giving them information about a parent's nonworking parts is a good thing because it explains the motivation for turning to a birth other to have a baby. But I'm not so sure younger children are ready to hear about "broken parts" of their parents' bodies. Children under five or six are smack in the middle of a developmental period where they're trying to consolidate their own body integrity, where magical thinking leads them to believe boys can turn into girls, girls can turn into boys, people can grow tails, and body parts can fall off. The news that the insides of their parents' bodies weren't working right could be quite unsettling. Sharing that information may raise children's anxiety about broken bodies and render them unable to focus on the more vital initial information—that an outside person who is not their mommy or daddy was involved in their conception or gestation by providing sperm, egg, or a uterus.

By about age seven, children are both cognitively and emotionally ready to digest a more complicated account of their origins. Elaine Gordon and Kate Bourne are two authors who have done a beautiful job crafting stories for young children about their assisted reproductive roots. In Gordon's book *Mommy, Did I Grow in Your Tummy?* a mom and dad are dreaming about having a baby; they've been trying and trying, and then the nice doctor explains to them that they can have a baby another way:

> He explained that all babies are made with a sperm from a man and an egg from a woman. The sperm and the egg join together. A baby starts to grow the minute the sperm and the egg get together! . . . Dr. Preston said, that to make a baby, the sperm can come from different men and the egg can come from different women and not all babies grow in their mom's bodies.[11]

The book then goes on to offer very simple, straightforward explanations of each process—donor insemination, egg donorship, and surrogacy. For example, "Sometimes the dad doesn't have enough sperm to put in the mom so a baby could grow. When this happens, another man, called a *sperm donor,* helps by donating his sperm to the mom and dad to use to make a baby. The doctor puts the donor sperm into the mom so she can grow a baby."[12] The story ends with "surrogates, egg donors, and sperm donors sure are helpful. They are doing something very special for the moms and dads who need help making babies."[13]

Kate Bourne's book is specifically about egg donorship, geared to children ages three to nine. It describes sperm, eggs, and uteruses and explains that mom and dad wanted a baby. Mom's eggs couldn't make a baby, but another woman, called an egg donor, might be able to give them some of her eggs to help them start a baby. At the end of the book, the child is reminded that the story of his or her own birth with an egg donor is not just a fairytale: "Lots and lots of kids begin like this. Instead of just two people (the Mum and the Dad) who made them, there are three—the Mum, the Dad and the egg donor."[14]

Both of these books normalize the processes of conception and gestation with a birth other. They never refer to the donor as a parent. They describe the specifics of conception and gestation in straightforward terms without going into sexually explicit detail about sex and reproduction. Unfortunately, neither author expands the story to include situations when there are two moms, two dads, one dad, or one mom. It's all about heterosexual couples having a baby. And neither book spells out the more complicated assisted reproductive situations when there were both an egg donor and a surrogate or a sperm donor and a surrogate or both an egg donor and a sperm donor. Yet I wanted to bring these books to our attention because the style, tone, and wording provide an excellent template for framing a story for your young children. You can fill in the particulars of your own family configuration, your own reasons for turning to the help of an outside party or parties to have a baby. For example, "Mommy and Mama wanted so much to have a baby. But to have a baby you need a sperm and an egg. And Mommy and Mama only have eggs. So we decided to use Mama's egg and find a helper who would give us some sperm so Mommy and Mama could have you. We went to a special place and found a man who wanted to help us by giving his sperm to join with Mama's egg. We then went to a doctor who helped us put together the man's sperm with Mama's egg so you could grow inside Mama. And we love you so much."

School Days, School Days

By nine or ten, children have moved into an age group where they want the facts, nothing but the facts. Nine or ten is often the age when children begin the existential quest—"Where did I come from?" and "Who am I?"—a quest that we continue in some form throughout our lives. If you have already told your children the story of their births, nine or ten may also be the time they're beginning to wonder or start asking more questions about their donor or surrogate. They may also have started a social living class or sex education curriculum at school. They're beginning to learn the scientific techniques of sex and reproduction.

Now is the time for full disclosure to the child. If you are telling the story for the first time, the narrative should include your desire to have a child of your own, why you needed to turn to a birth other to have one, how you went about doing that, how happy you are to have the child you have, how your child is related to you and to his or her siblings (if there are any), and who the donor or surrogate is, if you know—or, alternatively, if and when your child will be able to know that information. If infertility is part of the story, your child is now ready to take in that information. More sophisticated in their thinking, children at this age are much less likely to get consumed by morbid fantasies of broken body parts or parents whose bodies don't work.

If you've told the story before, now is the time for add-ons. Your children are ready for more scientific information about the reproductive technique that went into making them and more about the donor or surrogate. Joyce Sukamp Friedman, addressing egg-donor babies, offers this script to parents of eight- to ten-year-old egg-donor children:

> I know you remember mom and dad telling you about the nice people at the hospital who helped us, and the person that gave us a special gift so that you could grow in mom's baby sac. That person was your gene lady. This kind lady donated a small piece of her body, called a cell, or a gene cell, to us. People who want to help others donate some of their blood to help other people stay healthy. Some generous people even donate organs such as kidneys because most people have two normal kidneys and one is enough.[15]

Then at ages ten to twelve, she recommends the following additions to the story: "We want to tell you more about the people who helped us so that mom could become pregnant with you. The gift that we told you about that your gene lady donated to us was a gene cell or a piece of her DNA, which you will be studying about in school."[16]

You get the flavor here of the evolutionary progression of the tale as the child develops the cognitive capacities to take in a more complicated explanation. Friedman also offers an alternative label for the donor—the "gene lady." A cautionary note here. The terms egg donor and sperm donor have become almost commonplace in our culture these days. Therefore, I would think twice about introducing another notion, a gene lady. Gene lady evokes images of Johnny Appleseed spreading seeds wherever he goes rather than a woman who went to a medical facility to have eggs extracted so Mommy could have a baby. Also, gene lady is not completely accurate. The lady donates her *ovum* that contained the genes that now belong to the child. The world of assisted reproductive technology grows increasingly complicated every day—now we're on the brink of combining the "shell" of one woman's egg with the "yolk" of genetic material from another woman's egg to create a baby using both women's eggs. Crafting a narrative for the children means keeping up with the rapidly changing times and making sure the story told is accurate, straightforward, and offers clarification rather than confusion. Gene lady doesn't quite work.

Friedman's script also provides a comparison between eggs and other donations of body substances or organs from one person to another. Children, even older ones, are susceptible to wild fantasies based on what we tell them. Adults are, too. Recall my own fantasies of abdominal pregnancies stimulated by a news report on ovarian tissue transplants. So here's my second cautionary note. Beware telling children information intended to normalize their birth story but that ends up clouding the issue or conjuring up darker or confusing images of the process. Friedman associates egg donorship with blood donation or organ donors. I like the positive image of giving a gift of life that both processes evoke. But for many people, not just children, organ donors stimulate visions of people on the verge of death. We imagine heroic, medically risky efforts by generous people or philanthropic forethought by people prior to their death, promising part of their own bodies after they die to help someone else stay alive. Blood donations have similar life-and-death connotations—we give blood to help sick relatives or friends or strangers, to combat epidemics, to help in war efforts. Why not just keep it simple and stay focused on ova or sperm or uteruses rather than muddy it with stories that potentially stir up fantasies of death, risk, and body parts that need to be cut out and delivered to someone else with permanent loss to the original owner?

As a sidebar on the topic of keeping the waters unmuddied when you tell the story, I want to slip back to the preschool age for a moment and refer again to the author Nathalie's stories for young children. In illustrating the full roster of helpers who made sure all the parts were in order to make the baby, the book provides a colorful kitchen scene with an electric mixer, carton of eggs, jar of pickles, pair of socks, and some snail-like candies, which I presume to be sperm. The illustration is labeled "The Sugar-N-Spice Everything Nice Kitchen." Another illustration shows the "crew" who helped the doctor "so we could have you." The crew consists of a baker, a man with a hard hat and a shovel, two medical personnel with stethoscopes (a man in green scrubs and a woman in a pink dress), and a dog with a saddle embossed with the name Petri. Playing to children's whimsical natures is always a plus in delivering communications that might otherwise seem dry, boring, or over their heads. But leaving them with images of cake beaters, dogs, chefs, and construction workers in an area as sensitive and serious as their own conception and birth is an ill-conceived plan, whether the children are three, ten, or fifteen. A simple rule of thumb: Don't try to candy coat the story with childhood whimsy, and don't bring in extraneous images that will confuse rather than clarify. Construct a narrative around the straightforward information that the child was conceived with the help of medical personnel, donors, surrogates, reproductive procedures—in whatever relevant combination applies.

Now back to the older, school-age child. If you're telling the story for the first time, you need to be prepared for your children's initial shock when they find out something about their life is so different from everything they had always thought. Your narrative should include all the ingredients listed above, but you'll also need to talk about why you're telling your child this important information now, rather than before. The best way to help a child understand why he or she is just now being told is to tell the truth. It could be that you felt your child wouldn't be able to understand when younger. It could be that you took this long to decide whether or how you were going to tell. It could be that you changed your mind about an earlier decision not to tell, based on new information or changing times. It could be that circumstances changed in your life that made you realize you needed to tell your child (such as illness or divorce). It could be that you were protecting your children from a hostile environment in their earlier years, when they would have been too young to handle it. Or it could be whatever else the reason is you're telling now and not before. If you haven't or plan not to tell your children in their earliest years but then do later, the same principle, making sure you explain your true reasons for waiting, applies whether your child is twelve, fifteen, or twenty-five—or, for that matter, at any time in your child's life.

If you're telling for the first time in your child's school-age years, it is also important to stress that you are the parent(s), whether you're genetically related to your child or not, and that your attachments to each other are based on the connections you've had since birth, not on genetics. It's fine to start talking about physical likenesses or similarities based on genes as long as you also stress the likenesses and closeness that come from living together in a family or growing in your mommy's womb, even if you're not genetically related.

Teenage Tales

As their own body morphs into its adult iteration, children entering puberty suddenly have more sophisticated questions about who made them and what those people contributed to their changing body. They will also start asking more abstract, existential questions about motivation, intent, and actions: What would motivate someone to donate eggs or sperm or get pregnant so someone else can have a baby? Who was this person who helped make me, maybe even got paid for it? Why did this woman carry me for nine months and then never see me again? Does my donor (surrogate) ever think about me? And so forth. If you've already been talking to your children, this may be the moment to revisit the story and share your own thoughts about the donor or surrogate's motivations and experience. You may also want to share more about the emotional experiences you went through in wanting to have a child and turning to assisted reproductive technology. This may also be a time, if it has not come up earlier, where your children may wonder or muse about half siblings they may have through their donors or about babies who may have shared the same womb if they had a surrogate.

Even though the experts agree that adolescence is not the best time to first talk to children about their conception with a birth other, sometimes it ends up being the time. Sheri Glucoft-Wong, a family therapist in Berkeley, California, recommends that in such situations the parents emphasize to the children that this is a story about the *parents* and their experiences in wanting to have a child and then finding a way to have one. In one situation, she was preparing two parents to tell their two teenage daughters the truth that their father was not their genetic father, that the girls were conceived with two separate anonymous sperm donors. When they first thought of telling the girls, they were in the midst of marital turmoil. The therapist suggested they wait until tensions died down and the family was in a more stable place. She took that time to coach the parents and rehearse with them what they would say to the children. The facts were that the husband had been previously engaged to another woman who already had an older child. He and that woman decided they did not want more children, so the father had a vasectomy. Unfortunately, the relationship didn't last. The father then met the girls' mother, who very much wanted to have children. He agreed but was unable to reverse his vasectomy. And so they turned to a sperm bank to have children. Glucoft-Wong coached the parents to stress that this was not a story about their children but one they were sharing with them about how much they wanted children and what they had done to have them.[17]

There is much wisdom in this approach to initiating a talk with teenagers—or even with adult children—as evidenced by the response of one of the daughters. Right after she and her sister were told, she reached over to

her father and said, "Dad, you're still my dad. It doesn't make any difference." Framing the story this way effectively reminds teenagers that the attachment that has long existed between parent(s) and child is intact; this is a
story about the parents, not the child. Still, parents who choose this approach
must keep in mind that the story is, of course, also about the children—their
nontraditional conception, their genetic make-up, and their true genetic relationship to their parents and siblings. It is a story that provides a crucial
component of their identity. In essence, the story is about the whole family:
It is a story about the parents, it is a story about the children, and it is a story
about the parents and the children together.

In the case of Glucoft-Wong's clients, everyone in the family would
benefit from follow-up conversations after the children have had some time
to digest the information. In these later talks, the focus would shift from the
parents' story to the children's feelings—how they are doing with this new
information, how they're thinking about themselves, about their parents,
about their birth other, and about the way their family fits together. Or maybe
the urgency of the children's concerns would dictate that the follow-up conversation not wait, but piggy-back right on the parents' story about themselves.

The Leaked Story

In Chapter 7, I mentioned the fact that one strong reason to disclose your
children's origins to them is so that they don't find out from someone else.
What do you do if you've waited to tell, and your children find out somewhere else and confront you? Nina put together the pieces when she discovered her AB blood type after an abortion. Already having felt for many years
that something was awry in her family, she spent months in her own private
investigation, educating herself about blood types, sleuthing information
about her parents' blood types, until she discovered that her father was an O
blood type, which meant he couldn't possibly be her genetic father. She
went to her parents and reported what she knew, to which her father replied,
"You're right and I'm sorry. You see, I couldn't have children but I wanted
your mother to have them, so the doctor found donors for you and Zelda
[Nina's sister]. I don't know how you figured it out, because I was so sure
that neither of you girls would ever find out." He then openly talked about
his sorrow over not being their "real father" but at the same time said, "I
know that you are the only daughters I have and that I am so glad that I am

your father." And, like Sheri Glucoft-Wong's patient, the young woman responded, "It's all right, Daddy, it's all right. It will be better from now on. I love you, too."[18]

Although no longer a child, Melody Ward Leslie, a thirty-three-year-old mother herself, was told by her terminally ill godmother what Melody first dismissed as a wild tale—that Melody's mother had had Melody through donor insemination. Her godmother had decided to break the pact of family secrecy. Before she died, she wanted Melody to know the truth about her origins. The truth was then confirmed by Melody's older brother, who had already known for years.[19]

So you can see, the information about a child's birth-other origins can leak out in myriad ways, even with parents' intentions of keeping it confidential. When that happens, the best response is to acknowledge the truth and offer a full explanation gauged to the child's developmental age and stage. If this should happen in your family, make sure you allow room for any of your children's feelings that may surface. They may feel deceived or betrayed. They may be upset that they had to learn the truth from someone else or from their own detective work. As an anchor, hold on to Sheri Glucoft-Wong's approach—talk about yourselves and your journey into parenthood, including the reasons you decided not to tell. Maybe you'll want to talk about what the times were like when you decided to have a child, an era perhaps when doctors and counselors strongly advised parents not to tell and parents followed the medical wisdom of the time. If your child is school age or older, you'll definitely want to share whatever you know about the birth other and whether or not it will ever be possible for your child to contact that person. You'll also have to be prepared to help your children with their reactions if they already knew the birth other, just not as such. If there's ever a time to be honest, forthright, and let clear thinking trump anxiety, it's in responding to sons' or daughters' requests to know the truth about their origins.

HOW TO TELL THE STORY

Professionals and parents have started to put a lot of thought into what and when to tell the children. But sometimes we overlook the process—how to share the information. Any of you who've been through the experience of telling your children know that a well-timed, well-crafted script is not all that is needed. You'll also have to figure out *who* will tell, with what emotional tone, at what opportunity, and so forth. You'll have to sort out what to tell your child about telling others or fielding others' questions.

Again and again, both in my own clinical experiences and in other people's accounts, if there's a two-parent family, the nonbiological or nongenetic parent is often assigned the task of telling the children the story that signifies that he or she is not related to them by blood. It is as if the onus falls on that parent to legitimate his or her standing as the mother or father in the child's eyes. And it often leads to garbled stories fraught with apologies about not being the child's "real" father or mother.

Sometimes the exact opposite happens. The idea of saying "Honey, I didn't make you" renders the nonbiological or nongenetic parent so emotional that it's nearly impossible to get a grip and deliver the information in a calm and thoughtful way. So the job falls to the biological or genetic parent. At an unconscious level, both parents might be bowing to the biological or genetic parent as the more real parent, unencumbered by infertility or lack of genetic ties to the child. It is as if that parent becomes the gatekeeper of the family information. Designating the biological or genetic parent as the storyteller can only widen the subtle divide that may evolve between the two parents based on a difference in blood ties.

What is the optimal solution? Neither parent should be the designated teller. Instead, whenever possible, if you are a two-parent family, make sure both of you are there for the telling, particularly the first time. Both of you participating makes it a story about *our* family and how it was made. By telling together you reinforce the message that *we* are your two parents and this is how *we* came to have you. The principle of telling together holds even when the first time you tell follows a confrontation from your child who has found out or has suspected that something's up. If only one of you is there for the confrontation, you don't have to answer on the spot. It's fine to say, "Let's wait until Mom [Dad] gets home" and also "Give me a little time to think about it."

Telling the story is not a stage production but rather a dialogue with the audience, one that will happen again and again as your child grows. If it were a scripted play, you wouldn't have to get so jittery about unexpected questions and worry about how to handle your child's emotional reactions. Many years ago a three-year-old daughter of a lesbian couple started asking every man who appeared at her day care center, "Are you my daddy?" Her moms asked me what I thought they should tell their daughter. She was conceived with an anonymous sperm donor. I happened to be having dinner with ten other colleagues the same week, so I seized the opportunity to ask them what they would recommend to these two moms. Notably, this was a time when not much had been written yet on the subject, particularly for lesbian families, and few people were talking about it. To my surprise, I got ten different answers from ten different experts. Not only that. We all seemed to be getting pretty anxious as we talked among ourselves. You can only imagine the heightened anxiety when it's not a dinner table conversation among professionals, but your actual child at the dinner table insistently demanding "Where's my daddy?"

That's not the only curveball a child can throw. The follow-up question, "Can I meet him?" can be a real showstopper. And questions like "So you did it with someone else, Mom?" can leave you stagestruck as you face having to talk to your child about your own sexuality. Like any other delicate area of parent–child interactions, you always want to think in advance about how you will handle your child's questions, concerns, and feelings. This advance planning is your best insurance policy in navigating the ongoing dialogue about your child's birth-other origins.

At the same time, like the 1950s Art Linkletter TV show *Kids Say the Darnedest Things*, you can never be fully prepared for what your children might come up with. And no matter how prepared, you still might be caught off guard by one of their questions. Raising children in this fertile new world is uncharted territory for all of us. It is expecting too much to think that you'll be fully apprised, fully informed, and indelibly even-keeled every step of the way in shepherding your child through the experience. If you ever get thrown by an unanticipated question or an unexpected jolt of feeling, either your own or your child's, it's fine to say, "I'll have to think about that one and get back to you" or "Give me a little time to collect myself." Not having a ready answer for everything sets the tone for your children that conception with a birth other is part of your family's experience that requires a steady flow of thinking and rethinking together over time and that comes with no canned or rote answers. Asking for a time-out to think and regain your emotional footing also sets an example for your children: We will all pay attention to each other's questions, feelings, and concerns, and we'll all ask each other to be compassionate with our own.

Since her pregnancy, Karen had practiced telling her daughter, Alexandra, that she and Daddy really wanted to have a baby, but they needed someone else's egg to help them. So they asked Karen's sister if she would help, and her sister said, "Of course," and that's how Alexandra was conceived. They started telling the story as soon as Alexandra was born, and for years everything went quite smoothly until Alexandra, now eleven, came into Karen's bedroom one morning to talk. Karen was completely unprepared for her own well of tears when Alexandra asked her, "Mom, I know you're my mom because I came from you, but do you ever feel I'm not quite as much yours as I am Daddy's? Are you ever jealous that Aunt Bev is my 'real' mother?" Instead of answering, Karen just sat on the bed all choked up. She was finally able to say, with tears in her eyes, "Honey, I guess you really struck a tender nerve here. Give me a little while to think about your questions because they're really important ones and I want to give you the best answer I can. Would that be okay?" Alexandra squeezed her mom's hand and answered, "Sure, Mom, but just don't wait forever, like you did about whether I could get my ears pierced." It took only an afternoon, and Karen came into Alexandra's room later that evening and asked if it was a good time to talk. It was, so Karen shared with Alexandra her feelings of grief about not being able to make Alexandra from her own eggs, her jealousy not of Aunt Bev but of Alexandra's daddy for getting to be the gene parent, and her unwavering feeling that the real mommy was her. Alexandra hugged her mom, asked her some more questions about how Aunt Bev felt about all this, and also apologized for any pain she had caused her mom by asking the questions. Karen hugged Alexandra back and said quietly that no apologies were necessary; sorrow and tears were just part of the process of being open with each other.

Questions that may really throw you off are children's queries about the donor or surrogate. Parents who have chosen known donors or surrogates often emphasize that they wanted to know that person so that they would be able to speak concretely and forthrightly to their child about the person who helped make him or her. They won't have to surmise but will know about this person from their own experience, even if the child never meets the person. A lesbian mother described her search for a known donor before she and her partner went ahead with the insemination that brought them their son: "We don't lie to our boy, we don't make anything up but we can tell him that we know his biological dad is a good and generous person."[20]

If you use an anonymous birth other, you won't have this information at your disposal. You may find yourself tempted to create a whole person from the limited data you do have. This might not be enough for your children. They may push for more. While they're young, they may wonder why the birth other didn't want to be their mommy or daddy, particularly if the birth other was a surrogate who carried the baby to term. As they get older, they may want to know what the birth other is like. And then later, they may begin grilling you about the donor or surrogate's motivations and wonder how someone could bring a child into the world and then show no interest in that child. No matter how sensitively you respond to their questions, children may still demand, "Are you my *real* parent?"

It's easy to handle your anxiety in such potentially pain-filled moments by launching into lecture mode—laying out all the information seamlessly, maybe offering far more than the child needs to hear, and leaving no stone unturned so your child will have no questions left to ask. It rarely works. You typically end up with your children rolling their eyes or simply checking out. A better rule of thumb: As soon as your child is old enough to be a con- versationalist, replace telling the story with having a dialogue. Children need time to ask questions, and parents need time to pay attention to what a child is actually asking. Sometimes our own agendas to reveal the truth over- ride our ability to stop and listen to our children and what they really want to know.

Four-year-old Malcolm finally asked the question that Serena, his sin- gle mother who conceived Malcolm with donor sperm, had been waiting for—"Mommy, where did I come from?" Serena launched into the story she had long prepared about "wanting so much to have him and going to a doctor to help her . . . " when Malcolm irately interrupted her, and said, "No, Mommy, I mean did I come from Alta Bates Hospital like Julie or Summit Hospital like Ollie?" "Mommy, where did I come from?" might indeed af- ford Serena just the right moment to begin talking to Malcolm about his con- ception with sperm from an anonymous donor, but best to start with answer- ing what Malcolm was really asking—a geography rather than a progeny question. Otherwise, Serena runs the risk of being off the mark by misinter- preting her child's motives and providing an answer governed by her own agenda rather than Malcolm's little psyche.[21]

Your communications to your children may also be muddled by the pressure to keep everyone on a happy plane. A lot of the expert advice these days assures parents that telling your child can be a loving and positive pro- cess, as long as parents are at peace with it themselves. I agree, but often no room is left for sad, mad, or conflicted feelings. Even if you are at peace with your decision and have a loving way of communicating to your children their birth-other story, they may still become unsettled in the process. Your children are not exempt from the culturally defined notions of normal fami- lies even as you happily tell them your own family's story. Anywhere along the line, children might get upset about not being the genetic child of one of their parents, about being born in a "funny way," about never being able to know what their birth other looks like, about being deceived by their parents, about not being as real as siblings who were not conceived with a birth other, and so forth. And, anywhere along the line, you may temporarily collapse under the weight of your child's negative reactions to the peaceful story.

Just as Karen needed room for her tears of sadness in the face of Alexandra's questions about her egg-donor aunt, your children need room for the full breadth of feelings that will surface over time as they process their origins, their identity, and their place in the family. The nice man may at moments be converted into the greedy, narcissistic medical student, the nice woman into a callous baby abandoner. Your children need to know that you're sturdily there to help them process any and all of those feelings as the story of their origins unfolds, rather than sweeping the feelings under the rug or negating that they even exist. When it comes to children's doubts about who their real parents are, the challenge for mothers and fathers is to strike a balance between being compassionate about their children's questioning and staying firm with statements like the wise response of the adoptive mother that you read about in Chapter 4: "Honey, this is as real as it gets."

Your children may come to realize that there are other children in the world who share their genes, the children of the birth other or the other children conceived with the help of the birth other. They may want to know more about these people, who might even be considered half brothers and sisters. It's not so hard to explain to your children that parenthood applies to the people who take care of you—not the people who help make you. Parents serve a function in children's everyday lives. When it comes to explaining siblings, it's far more complicated. Aside from rivalry and loyalty, sisters and brothers really don't have a clear-cut functional role with each other. So what makes a sibling? Are you siblings only if you live together or have at least one parent in common? Or do you count as a sibling if you are born from the same man or woman and share genetic make-up? Given our worry that children might unwittingly marry their half siblings in the new age of donor births, how can we then simultaneously tell the children that these other offspring are *not* their siblings?

Recently I sat in a room with a thirteen-year-old girl furious that her father hadn't told her that her godsister was actually more than that—her father had donated the sperm that conceived the godsister, as a gift to his lesbian friends. Her father and the two mothers were trying to explain that nothing had changed; her godsister was still just that, not her sister. Enraged, this thirteen-year-old hurled back at her father, "For God's sake, haven't you ever taken biology class? We have the same genes. We're sisters." In the process of tracking children's questions about their siblings and their relationship to the other offspring of the birth others, I would heed Anne Bernstein's advice that "it is essential to respond to questions honestly and give children permission to count their half-siblings in or out of the family roll call, depending on the child's needs—be they developmental, existential, or idiosyncratic."[22]

As you tell your children the story of their birth, you are also redefining family—for yourselves, for your children, and for all of us. Miriam and Dawn wondered what they would tell two-year-old Tiffany someday when she asked, "Is Pasqual [the known sperm donor] my daddy?" They thought they would tell Tiffany, "No, Pasqual and Nadia [Pasqual's wife] are very special people because they gave us Pasqual's sperm to help make you. They're also your godparents. But mothers and fathers are people who take care of you. Pasqual and Nadia take care of Sidney and Kevin [Pasqual and Nadia's children], but not you. In your family, you have two mothers instead of a mother and father. It's *our* job to take care of you." Cindy wrote another story for her little boy Mikey called "Different Kinds of Families." She wrote it in response to a painful situation in which Mikey's friend Ruthie thought Mikey's male babysitter was his daddy and just couldn't understand when Mikey said, "No, I don't have a dad. I never had a dad." In the story, Cindy listed all the families Mikey himself knew: divorced families, single-parent families, two-parent families, foster families. She also listed different ways children become part of a family: born to their mom and dad, adopted, assisted reproductive technology. She wrote in her story, "How could Mikey explain about different families to kids who didn't know about them? . . . the main things about kids who didn't understand about different kinds of families was they just hadn't learned yet that differences were possible. No one had thought to tell them." In creating a story for Mikey, Cindy is also a trailblazer for all of us—inviting us to rethink family and pass this on to the children.

In her story, Cindy offered Mikey tools for what he might say to his friends when they ask him about his family. He could say, "I have a dad. I just don't know him." Or he could say the truth: "I never lived with a dad. There are all kinds of different families, and I just live with my mom." This brings me to a final thought in the third triptych—telling the children. We tell the children not just so they will know but also so they will be prepared and have a language to tell others. We tell them in a way that will help them answer others' questions, like "You can't have two mommies. You have to have a mommy and a daddy. Where's your daddy?" We coach the children not just in what to say but also in whom to say it to, how much of the story they want to share, and under what circumstances. This is a time when parents might talk to their children about tiered disclosure—helping them think about who they would like to share the information with, who might not be so understanding, and when and where they might want to keep the information private if they so desire. It is also a time for parents to reveal their own thoughts and feelings about sharing the information—who and what they have chosen to tell or not and why.

If there's any situation where it takes a village, it is in talking to children about their conception or birth with a birth other. We often think of telling as a private, insular experience within the family. Yet it behooves extended family, schools, health personnel, and community groups to provide a supportive environment where the story can blossom in concert with all the other children's stories about their families and their family roots. For example, if schools routinely introduced a curriculum in line with Cindy's "Different Kinds of Families" story, children from assisted reproductive families would become normative rather than alternative. They could more easily tell their tale to others without someone shouting, "No way. You have to have a mommy and a daddy, and they're the only ones who can make you." All the children would already know, "Yes, there's another way." I have invited every one of you who is a parent to think through the questions at the beginning of this chapter to guide you in telling your children. I would now invite the whole village to do the same. Go back to the questions and think about your answer to the overarching question "What should we tell the children?" Do this so we can all create a supportive and accepting world for the children, for the parents, and for our relationship to them.

In shaping a narrative to tell the children over time about their origins using assisted reproductive technology, it is important to help children develop as benevolent an image as is honestly possible of all the people involved in their conception and birth—parents and birth others. But that's not all. It is also important to help children develop a positive image of *themselves*. This brings us to our final area of investigation: And how *do* the children fare?

How Do the Children Fare?

> Your children are not your children.
> They are the sons and daughters of Life's longing for itself.
> They come through you but not from you.
>
> —Kahlil Gibran, *The Prophet*

No matter how we bring our children into our family, someday they will leave us and go on to lead lives of their own. As they launch themselves, how they were conceived is unlikely to be the deciding factor in their destiny. More poignant will be their own hopes, dreams, and personalities as they embark on their journey into adulthood. And what will be most important is not how they came *from* us, but how they came *through* us; that is, how we helped them become the people they are.

This does not mean, however, that we can ignore a salient factor for some of the children—that they were brought into this world with the aid of birth others. These may be your children. So, now, as we come to the end of our journey together, it is time to reflect on what we already know and what we need to think about in answering the question "How are the children doing?" Imagine for a moment that you are one of those children. Perhaps you are. Here are the questions you might be asking yourself:

- Am I different?
- Who do I belong to?
- Who am I?

I'm going to ask each of you to put yourself in the shoes of a child as we walk through these questions. But before I do, I want to highlight our central guideline for this discussion. In a family formed with the aid of a birth other, there is no child without the child's parent or parents, the child's birth other, the spouse or partner of the birth other, the other children of the parents, and the other children of the birth other. Although it makes the process messy and complex, we can know how the child is doing only by considering how everyone in that family matrix is doing—not only how they are doing, but how each holds the others in his or her mind.

Let's go back to the thirteen-year-old girl introduced in Chapter 8 who found out her godsister was her half sister. She struggled to keep herself from taking it out on her godsister: "It's not her fault. I don't want to take it out on her. But they lied to me and they tricked me." She feels tricked because for two years she went along thinking her half sister was her godsister, while wondering from time to time how come her little godsister looked so much like her own father.

Sperm are attached to men who may be fathers of children who could then feel attached to other children created by that same father's sperm. It sounds like the answer to a riddle, but I'm just trying to make the point that when a child is born with the help of a birth other, many people may be having feelings about the child, whether that child knows it or not. And many people may have lives affected by this child's birth. So we have to take all these people's experiences into account when we ask, "How do the children fare?"

Although donor insemination is now over a century old, systematic studies of children born with donor insemination, egg donorship, or surrogacy are few and only very recent. With the exception of studies of lesbian families, most of the findings are based on families where children were not told about their birth-other origins. And no study has yet followed a group of children from birth into adulthood. The lesbian family studies that *do* include children who know their donorship origins do not separate out the effects of having a birth other from the effects of having two mothers and growing up in a lesbian family within a homophobic culture. That means that until further studies are conducted, we have to be humble enough to acknowledge that the jury is still out. Many questions about the children's development from infancy to adulthood—cognitively, socially/emotionally, and even physic-ally—cannot be answered because the research has not yet been done.

I will share with you scientific data that we *do* have to date. But I also want us to use a different way of knowing—the knowing that comes from people's reported, lived experiences, both in their daily lives and in the of-fices of people like me. To answer our questions, I'm going to weave to-gether the objective (the research) and the subjective (the daily lives of fami-lies as evidenced in their own hearts and minds). I don't pretend to know all the answers. So I may leave you with as many questions as answers. My hope is to provide you with a road map to think about your children's growth and development. What I do know for sure is that you cannot look at a child in isolation. How your child fares is integrally related to how you (the par-ents) fare, to the experience of the donor or surrogate, to the experience of the donor or surrogate's family, and to the attitudes and responses of the world surrounding the child. It not only takes a village to raise a child; the village has a strong effect on how the child grows.

AM I DIFFERENT?

Ramie is five years old. She has two moms and a sister. She has a "yes" donor, someone she'll be able to contact at age eighteen. She always knew this, but only at age six did she suddenly grasp that she was actually made with the sperm from a *man* and her mommy's egg. She expressed great shock. "You're kidding, Mommy. I thought I was all girl. I didn't know I had any boy in me!" Ramie had developed her own theory of gender based not on biology, but on her family composition. She was different from her friends' families because her family was all girl. Until scientific fact disabused her of that theory, she had no problems with her misinformed difference. "I am all girl." It was just a fact.

We have talked about the anxiety that can get stirred up when we start playing with Mother Nature and make babies in new ways. The babies go along their own merry way, playing soccer, doing their homework, getting into fights with their sisters and brothers, begging for cell phones, and so forth—just like all the other kids. Most, like Ramie, are perfectly comfort-able with who they think they are—in Ramie's case, all girl. Yet we can't help but wonder, is there anything unique in the child's development? Any differences we should be concerned about? Special life circumstances we should be aware of to shepherd them through their childhoods? To boil it down to its essence, if you're a mother or father, what you really want to know is "Is my child doing okay?"

What Does the Research Tell Us?

Recently a series of scientific reports have been released alerting us to potential developmental or neurological problems in babies born using various forms of assisted reproductive techniques. These studies have concentrated on two specific procedures—in vitro fertilization (IVF), when fertilization takes place in a petri dish, and intracytoplasmic sperm injection (ICSI), when a single sperm is injected into an egg and then implanted in the womb. These two procedures apply to some but not all conceptions or gestations with a birth other. But the findings do give us pause, making us think about potential risks to the baby when we bring the egg and sperm together outside the body, in a medical laboratory or even with sperm from a turkey baster, so that a baby can be made.

First, let me say that most of the news is good. A study of IVF and ICSI babies presented at the 2003 European Society of Reproductive and Embryology meetings concluded that "Overall, the results are reassuring and lay to rest fears about the health and welfare of children conceived through IVF and ICSI." They followed close to a thousand children up to age five. No differences were found in intelligence, language skills, motor skills, or temperamental difficulties when compared to a group of children conceived naturally. But when it came to physical health, there were greater risks for malformations, mostly in the genital and urinary tracts.[1]

A study in Australia found that infants conceived with either one of these two procedures were at higher risk for being delivered by cesarean section, had lower birth weights, and were more likely to be born before term than a comparison group of naturally conceived babies. They were also more than twice as likely to have a major birth defect diagnosed by one year of age—in their urinary and genital systems, their muscles and bones, their vascular systems, or their chromosomes. Here are the possible causes: advanced age of parents, underlying causes of infertility, fertility drugs, or medical procedures such as freezing and thawing of embryos, fertilization with more than one sperm, or delayed fertilization of the oocyte (fertilized egg).[2] A study in the United Sates found similar results. Looking at different assisted reproductive procedures in which both fertilized eggs and sperm are handled outside the body, the study found a risk of low birth weights in these infants that was 2.6 times that in the general population. They came up with the same possible causes as the Australian study.[3] A study in Sweden found that two percent of children born through in vitro fertilization ended up being treated at a disability center for neurologically related problems, nearly double the rate of such complications found in a control group of children born to mothers who conceived naturally. In the Swedish study, problems were attributed to the high frequency of twins, low birth weight, and preterm births. The recommendation in the Swedish study was to transfer only one embryo to the uterus to reduce the risks of neurological complications.[4]

A study at Johns Hopkins University linked in vitro and intracytoplasmic sperm injection with a four- to six-fold increased risk for a condition known as Beckwith–Wiederman syndrome, a disorder typified by children with enlarged tongues and other organs. In January 2003, *Lancet* reported a four- to seven-fold increase in the rate of a disease called retinoblastoma, a rare cancer of the eye, in children conceived through assisted reproductive technology. Again, the possible cause is the culturing of eggs and embryos outside the body in a lab. Gene alteration, which is the cause of these rare diseases, may occur because of the changed salt or amino acid in the culture in which the eggs or embryos grow. The longer the eggs grow in the culture, the higher the possibility of these alterations in the genes. Ironically, scientists have moved to keeping eggs longer in the culture to assure sturdy embryos and increase the chances of successful implantation, but this very insurance policy for conception could put your child at higher risk for disease.[5]

Some of you parents may have had your own suspicions, wondering if the way your baby was made is connected to any medical problems that have surfaced. One mother whose son was diagnosed with Beckwith–Wiederman syndrome went on-line to find parents of other children suffering from the disease. She quickly noticed how many of the parents who responded to her had also used assisted reproductive technology. Parents of older children born with egg or sperm donors have talked to me about language, learning, or attentional problems they've noticed in their children. Some have asked me whether I thought these problems might be correlated with their child's conception with an egg or sperm donor. Many of us in the mental health field have had our own suspicions, making note of the frequency with which we see developmental or behavioral problems in the children conceived with assisted reproductive technology. Recently, I was talking to a colleague on the phone, and she wondered with me what was happening. She was working with three families, all of whom had a child conceived with assisted reproductive technology—one family had twins with heart problems, the second had a child with hearing impairment, and the third had a child with significant motor and learning problems.

Are we affecting the natural order of development in untoward ways in scientifically altering the way babies are conceived? Well, the children may have a chance of being different by a very small margin. In every study I know of, the actual risks are infinitesimally small or the diseases extremely rare, and the investigations are only of babies and small children, with no follow-up into adulthood to study any long-lasting effects. By these studies' own measures, the vast majority of children conceived using in vitro or intracytoplasmic injection were normal. So let me suggest that we not get unduly alarmed. Instead, we can let the studies give us a heads-up. We all need to be aware of and fully informed about any possible effects on a child's physical and neurological development when we manipulate eggs and sperm outside the body or use fertility drugs. This way we can take whatever precautionary measures are available, such as reducing the number of embryos transferred to the womb or limiting the number of days the fertilized egg remains in a dish.

A child's physical status is important but not the only thing that counts. How are the children doing socially, emotionally, and academically? It's not so easy to answer that question thoroughly because the vast majority of the children studied have not been informed that they are donor babies. Also, most of the research is based on parent self-reports and global quantitative measures, rather than systematic outside observations or in-depth clinical investigations. And none to date have followed children from birth all the way to maturity, which is particularly important because some factors can disappear over time and others may surface only much later in childhood, or even adulthood.

Susan Golombok and Fiona MacCallum have provided a comprehensive review of the studies to date on outcomes for parents and children following nontraditional conception, including IVF families, ICSI families, sperm-donor families, egg-donor families, and surrogate families. You will be reassured to know that the children raised in sperm-donor, egg-donor, and surrogate families were doing as well as children in control groups when it came to their relationship with their parents, their cognitive development, and their social and emotional development.

I thought it particularly interesting that donor-insemination children have been found to be more advanced than their peers with respect to intellectual, psychomotor, and language development. Researchers attribute this finding to the strong genetic load from the donors, who are typically medical students, college students, or high-functioning professionals, not to mention doctors who have been known to slip their own sperm into the mix.

Studies on egg-donor babies are still rare, but the few that have been done found no problems in sleeping or eating and no evidence of emotional or behavioral problems.[6] One study of surrogacy found no evidence of speech or motor impairment in only children born after IVF surrogacy and no difference between surrogacy, egg-donor, and natural-conception children in assessment of temperament (fussiness in mood, adaptability to new situations, general activity level, or predictability of reaction).[7] And a study investigating psychosocial adjustment in donor-insemination children from lesbian and from heterosexual mothers found that children in each group were well adjusted, regardless of whether their mothers had partners.[8] In this study both teachers and parents assessed the children, and the children had knowledge of their donor-insemination roots. And, so far, no negative effects on development have been found in the children who haven't been told about the circumstances of their conception, at least by the measures used.

To date, I've discovered only one study that delivered disturbing news about the psychological adjustment of children conceived by donor insemination. A survey of Dutch children found more behavioral problems among donor-insemination children than among children naturally conceived. In the Dutch study, the authors suggested that the results were caused by the lower socioeconomic status of the parents in the donor-insemination group in comparison to the naturally conceived group, rather than their donor-insemination status.[9]

So there's no objective evidence that your birth-other children are any different from their peers born the old-fashioned way when it comes to academics and behavioral and social/emotional adjustment, with one exception. Your donor children may be smart children, with the help of the donor's genes.

Researchers have been interested in one more thing—how you parents are doing and how your children relate to you. Susan Golombok and her colleagues have been involved in a longitudinal study of children conceived with in vitro fertilization. When it comes to parent–child relationships, a history of infertility was more important than how the baby was conceived.

Sensitive responding and reasoning with their children decreased when parents had a history of infertility. On a more positive note, mothers who had experienced infertility were perceived to be more dependable than mothers of naturally conceived children. Like the studies reported above, no differences were found in children at early adolescence across all family types regarding psychiatric disorder, social adjustment, and pro-social behavior. Put differently, all the children seemed to be doing just fine, and the authors concluded that parents using assisted reproductive technology have nothing to worry about regarding their parenting or the psychological adjustment of their children.[10]

Another study of childrearing after in vitro fertilization found that these parents appear to bond more strongly with their children than the parents of naturally conceived children, providing them with a higher level of nurturing in their early years.[11] For any of you who have waited and waited for your child's arrival, maybe following a long and arduous stint of intensive medical intervention, this makes sense. When your desire is strong, your baby is special.

What could be bad about all this bonding and nurturance? Only one thing—the difficulty of letting go as your child grows up. Logically, we could say that the more love to go around, the better for the child. But British psychologist Diane Finiello Zervos suggests a darker side to the strong bonds within birth-other families: "Will these parents be able to let [their children] go as they become adolescents and young adults?"[12] So far, we have no studies measuring children's transition into adulthood, but it doesn't hurt to ask yourself, "How will it be to separate from my child? Are there any signs I might hold on too tight?" Attachment may go smoothly, but we want to make sure that the appropriate separation that allows the child to go independently into the world won't be fraught with difficulties.

I Have No Birthrights

I would now like to leave the world of research and enter the lives of the children. What's unique about their experience? First, we know that many of them have no legal rights to know the person who contributed half of their genes. Donor offspring who try to search for their donors may be told by doctors or sperm banks that this is not possible. Some of the clinics are long gone by the time a donor offspring sets out on a search, and no records have been kept. Throughout the world, advocacy groups have been lobbying for the rights of donor offspring, parallel to the struggles of adopted individuals to have access to their birth parents. In England in 2002, Joanna Rose, conceived by donor insemination, along with an unnamed five-year-old claimant, were given leave by the High Court to act under the Human Rights Act to ask the court to order the setting up of a register that would allow all donors to provide identifying information on a voluntary basis. The register is now in place. Although donors still hold the rights to decide whether or not they will provide the information, Joanna Rose stated that this ruling had created "a legal foothold on which to establish our rights and identities. This is an important and heartening event on a long road to recognition of us as people—just like everyone else, with social and genetic roots—rather than as products."[13]

Unfortunately, most children around the world do not have such a foothold. Canadian filmmaker Barry Stevens, born through donor insemination in 1953, asks how genetic heritage could be so deeply embedded in our culture while donor offspring are expected to accept that for them it doesn't matter: "Everyone was so keen to tell us it didn't matter. . . . And then I felt this enormous anger—that was for me to decide."[14] Another man in his fifties who found out nineteen years ago that he was conceived with a donor because his father was sterile seconds Barry Stevens's emotions: "It's infuriating that most banks remain wedded to the idea that sperm donation has to be anonymous. They want to protect the donor as though he is a victim of some sort. But why should the medical profession have the power to deny someone his or her full genetic history? It's not fair to allow a child to be deluded about who they are."[15]

Denying their birthrights and frustrating their desire to know their genetic roots may very well affect how the children fare, as they find themselves in the same boat as adopted children whose access to their genetic history is permanently blocked. How is it for your children if half their genetic history is blocked and the other half is there for the asking? If you have a child in this situation, you may not be able to change the circumstances, but you can help your child negotiate the frustration or disappointment that might surface for him or her, either as a child or later on in adulthood. You can do this simply by understanding how your child might feel different if he or she can never know and holds no rights to know the identity of the donor or surrogate.

Asher is seventeen. He has known since he was old enough to talk that he was conceived with anonymous donor sperm. He's now heavy into dating. But unlike all of his friends, he has an extra worry about "getting together" with someone. What if she is his sister? So Asher asks every girl he meets if she's a sperm-donor child, just in case. Of course, this doesn't take care of the remote possibility that she is in no way a donor child, but that her own father could have been Asher's donor, or maybe nobody ever told her that she is a sperm-donor baby. So what's he to do—ask every date to take a DNA test? Of course not, but what sets Asher and any other donor child apart is that they have to worry about unwitting incest, a minuscule yet real possibility. If you have no access to your donor records, how would you even know if your date might be a relative by blood? And if you've never been told you're a donor child, your parents will be the anxious ones—hoping against hope that such mistaken incest will never come to pass.

In the novel *The Sperm Donor's Daughter*, Jessica, the protagonist, does her own successful sleuthing to find her donor father, now a gynecologist in a different state. Jessica, in her twenties, confronts the donor: "Can you imagine if you had examined me? Can you imagine if we slept together? I've slept with men as old as you and I've wondered if I might sleep with one of my brothers by mistake. You know, there's no central registry in this country." The donor responds, "Yes, I know that. Still, it is a remote possibility." To which Jessica retorts, "Strictly speaking, yes. But you've never felt what it's like to wonder about it."[16]

The lack of rights of the vast majority of donor children to know their roots, accompanied by the worry that they, along with all of us, have about unwitting incest, is indeed something that many of us have never felt or wondered about. In this respect, the newfangled forms of reproduction have created a burden for the children. We have now lost hold of our old insurance policies against incest that remained in place as long as children were born the old-fashioned way. Granted, adoption has always confronted us with this conundrum, as have parents' indiscretions that created "love children" outside the family. But now, with the possibility of a donor contributing to the creation of many children, the danger feels greater as the odds go up that one could fall in love and even have babies with one's sibling. We cannot forget that this worry, even if slight, creates a significant difference for donor children.

When a Piece of the Puzzle Is Missing

Some children who know they had a donor or surrogate but don't know who that person is experience themselves as a puzzle with a piece missing. In a publication of a conference on donor conception in Australia, the audience, composed of donor offspring, was asked, "Do you feel different?" One of the participants responded:

> I think the way I feel different is sometimes when I go into family houses and I see photographs of the grandmother and the great grandmother and great grandfather did this and grandfather wrote poetry and I just think, wow, I would just love to have that information from my biological father's side. . . . Yes, I suppose I feel different in the sense that most people have the history of both sides of the family.[17]

Like adopted children or foster children or children conceived in a liaison with a stranger never to be seen again, your children may feel different because they suffer from genealogical bewilderment—the lack of knowledge of part of their biological roots.

At the same time, children conceived with a birth other are very different from adopted, foster, or one-night-stand children. Birth-other children are far less likely to feel they've been let down or rejected by a parent—a person who was supposed to take care of them but then didn't or couldn't. Donors and surrogates enter the conception contract with no intent to parent the child born. Of course, your children may not see it that way. A colleague told me about her six-year-old daughter, conceived with an egg donor, who popped up with the searing question "So, Mommy, why was it that the egg donor didn't want to keep me?" This was asked after many years of careful explanation about Mommy and Daddy and the nice lady who gave her egg so Mommy and Daddy could have her. Children's fantasies have a life of their own. Still, in reality, your child has never been subjected to parental rejection by a person who intended to parent but didn't or who engaged in sex but wasn't willing to take responsibility for the results of those actions.

If you're a single parent, you've also insulated your child from family break-ups. Recall Cindy, the single mother who wrote two stories to her son Mikey. In her second story, "Different Kinds of Families," she reminded him, "Although some of his friends' families changed if the Dad and Mom stopped living together, there was no way his family—which was her—would ever change. She would just keep on loving him." Mikey, a donor child with a single mom, was lucky—he would be assured a stable family free from divorce, split custody, and desertion. Statistically, that makes him different from approximately half the kids on his block.

Sierra is another one of those lucky children. She is now nine, has a single mom, and was conceived with the aid of an anonymous donor. Her mother told me that Sierra felt bad about not having a father. When I asked Sierra directly about her feelings that she didn't have a father, she had an eloquent response: "Oh, when I was little, like two or three, I used to go to the swimming pool and felt bad when I saw all the kids with a mother and a father. But then I discovered that my godfather Terry could be like my dad, and I don't feel bad anymore. And besides, there's some good things about not having a dad. You never have to put the toilet seat back down, you don't have to bring a guy beer, you don't have to see your mom and dad fighting about stuff or watch them get a divorce, and, well, you get a whole half of the bed to sleep in, you don't have to be squished between a mom and a dad." Not only is Sierra reveling in her escape from marital discord, divorce, and two-household post-divorce families, she has completely normalized her experience. She may be different from other kids she knows, but what she has feels just right. Of course, Sierra could be caught up in a defensive strategy, masking deeper, uneasy feelings about what she does *not* have, about something she wished for once upon a time and realized she would never get. But Sierra's account is not unique. Her acceptance of her life and comfort with her differences is mirrored in so many of the other children I have seen who are conceived with a birth other.

Knowing you are different but wanting exactly what you have was highlighted most poignantly in a lesbian couple who came to me for a consultation because one of the women in the couple was going through a sex change operation and they wondered how their three-year-old daughter, who was conceived with donor insemination, would adjust to the change. They had thought she would be happy to finally have a daddy, like all the other children in her preschool. My first thought was that she would do as well as her parents were doing with the change. My second thought was based on what they reported to be their daughter's first response when they began talking to her about it, explaining that one of her mommies would be becoming her daddy and then she would have a dad like all the other kids: "I don't want a daddy. I have two mommies. I want my two mommies." This little girl's response demonstrated that when it comes to family, children can easily embrace the ways they are different from other families. Trumping any of the discomforts of difference is the security in holding on to what the children already have and know.

Whatever I Have Is Normal

"Normalizing" is the key variable. Caroline, the girl with a never-ending grid of family members, is now sixteen. At age eight she found out she was conceived with donor sperm. At age twelve she asked to know who her donor was, as she wanted to know her biological roots. Her parents were able to confirm that Caroline's donor was a family friend, who was now willing to be identified as her donor. He now became her bio dad. She also discovered that the children of her bio dad, whom she had been babysitting for, were actually her half siblings. They now call her "sis." Caroline in no way sees this as a complication in her life. Instead she says, "Oh, it's great. I like my bio dad. And I like having a sister and brother. I never had one before." As a therapist, I know that it may not be as wonderful as Caroline makes it out to be, but at a conscious level Caroline has readjusted her sensibilities to take this in as normal information about herself and her family. It just is.

How do children digest all the carefully thought out information you give them about their birth? Does it make them feel like freaks, different from all the other children? Here again, the concept of normalizing is key. Emma is the egg donor for her sister, Flora, who gave birth to Seth. Flora also has an older adopted daughter, Melody, who was adopted in infancy. Both children have been told about their origins. One day Emma was driving the two children, who were sitting in the back seat. Melody, Flora's adopted daughter, announced: "Emma, you know, Seth and I both have two mothers. I have my mother and Flora is my mother and Seth has you and Flora is his mother, too." As far as Emma was concerned, "It was said with absolute certainty and without a trace of confusion."[18] Seth and Melody's mother, Flora, agrees:

> He [Seth] and Melody both know their stories. We have stressed the common ground between them, so they both think of themselves as having two mums. . . . Seth is very matter of fact. It isn't particularly clear that he understands how he came to be, and it is harder to explain his arrival to him because the biological detail is still difficult for him to grasp at his age. . . .

It is of course not clear whether the fact that Seth's life would have been unthinkable shortly before it became commonplace will matter to children like Seth or not. I expect we will be upbraided for bringing him about when he's an adolescent and no doubt Melody will have much to say about our interference in her life, but I don't expect the invective to be much more poisonous than the things more routine children think and say of their parents in adolescence.[19]

Josh was a school-age boy with two lesbian mothers, conceived through donor insemination. His mother recalled him coming home from school complaining about his teacher's insensitivity. The teacher had given the class a homework assignment, to interview all the members of their family—mothers, fathers, brothers, and sisters. He had no problem for himself, because he had learned to translate mother and father into "parents." But he was outraged for his friend who was a single child with a single mother. Why didn't the teacher think about how that would make his friend feel, a boy with only one parent and no siblings? His mother, Claire, took note of Josh's reactions: "What I thought was interesting about that was that Josh didn't see himself as different—he felt he was in the norm of what was being said."[20] Josh, Seth, and Melody all appear to be children who have metabolized their difference positively—they feel confident about themselves and about their relationship with the world.

Some of you may not trust that your children will be so robust in developing a positive sense of difference or so adept in normalizing their experience. You may decide to shield your children from stigma or shame by not telling them how they were conceived. To date, the studies show your children will be as well adjusted as other children. But I just want to alert you to one thing these studies have not measured—the anger and sense of betrayal reported by many donor children who do later discover the truth of their difference.

If they find out this difference, will the difference be damaging? I think we can learn something from the children conceived with a birth other who are inevitably "outed"—children of lesbian and gay families, particularly two-parent gay or lesbian families. Jamie Bergeron grew up in Courtland, New York, with two mothers. In elementary school, she had to put up with her classmates' teasing—they called her "test-tube baby" and referred insultingly to her lesbian mothers. Rather than thinking this experience damaged her, she believes it gave her a stronger sense of her own identity, because she had to identify who she was, what her opinions were, and defend herself and her family.[21] Like Seth, Melody, and Josh, Jamie says knowing she's a donor child has in no way been a liability. At the same time, Jamie had the unfortunate experience of meeting up with a merging of homophobia and what I might label "assisted reproductive technophobia." She didn't hold the privilege that birth-other children from heterosexual families can exercise—to tell or not to tell about her donor roots. If we de-link the technophobia from the homophobia, and focus for a moment just on the technophobia, we have to remember that even when the children normalize their experience, they have to go out into a potentially unfriendly world stamped as different.

Will the World See Me as Different?

This brings me to my last but perhaps most important point about the question of difference—the social context. In 1999, the Donor Conception Support Group of Australia concluded:

> People conceived by donor conception feel different because they joined their families in a nontraditional way. Whether this difference is disturbing to them or integrated into their self-image partly depends on the attitude of those closest to them.[22]

"Difference" is a relative concept. For example, I am different from approximately ninety percent of people in this world because I'm left-handed. In the United States in the twenty-first century this may be an occasional inconvenience, but not a psychological problem for me, because no one casts aspersions on my character because of my difference. But in certain other cultures I would be seen as a pariah and would even have to hide my left-handedness in public. We have not arrived at a time when donor or surrogate conceptions are as well accepted as left-handedness. So, until the culture around them can offer positive support and acceptance, you'll have to remember that your children will need your strong support to feel robust and positive about their difference as children born with the aid of a birth other.

WHOM DO I BELONG TO?

If my dad didn't make me, but he's always been my dad, but my uncle Thomas actually made me, who am I a part of? If my mom carried me inside her, but Aunt Meg gave her the egg so I could be born, who is Aunt Meg to me? And so forth. Given so many players, no matter how carefully you talk to your children, they'll still have to carve their own paths as they sort out their sense of belonging.

Children's Reveries

I want to come back to the "family reverie," a family's shared thoughts about the donor or surrogate, but this time through the lens of the child. The family reverie is not the same as the family romance. The family romance was a concept coined by Sigmund Freud. It's all about another wonderful, make-believe family that exists somewhere and may be the child's real family. In the family romance, the imagined family is typically idealized and romanticized as something far superior to the family the child wakes up to every day and goes to sleep in every night. School-age children use these fantasies to start creating their own independent lives away from their powerful parents, albeit in fantasy. When your child is engaged in family reveries about the donor or surrogate, these are thoughts about real people, not storybook characters. The cast of characters includes mothers and fathers, sisters and brothers, sperm donors, egg donors, surrogates, and possible half siblings. Your child will engage in these fantasies not to separate, but to connect with you.

In Ken Corbett's work with Andy, the seven-year-old son of lesbian mothers, he discovered that not only did the two mothers stop having fantasies about their son's anonymous donor as soon as Andy was born, but in turn, Andy never allowed himself to think about the donor. Andy's anxiety diminished dramatically when both the therapist and his mothers gave him room to have his own fantasies about the donor, along with his moms sharing theirs with him. Now Andy finally had a sense that he belonged.[23]

Sociologist Rosanna Hertz provides us with an illuminating window into these reveries among single mothers and their children in her study of twenty-five single women who used sperm donors to have a child. The mothers craft a father from fantasy. Those who used anonymous donors recast the donor as doing something positive for them and for their children. The mother and child fantasize together about the genetic father.

As time goes on, the mother looks at her child and sees a trait she doesn't recognize—it must have come from someone else, not her. She and her child can only imagine the traits come from the missing piece of the child's genetic make-up—the donor. So they fantasize about this person, how his genes contributed to the child's traits and personality. The mothers and children together engage in imaginary conversations with the donor— what they would say if they could meet him or his family. This is the stuff of family reveries that allows a child to explore whom he or she came from and whom he or she belongs to. The reveries also allow a child true freedom to create a whole person from a vial of sperm, even if just in fantasy.[24]

Maggie Shea Rousseau is just turning eighteen. When she does, she will be able to find out the identity of her donor. In the meantime, she knows that the sperm her mother used came from a man of Czech–German ancestry who stands five feet ten inches and has sandy hair and a medium build. When Maggie thinks of him, she doesn't use the word "Daddy" or "Dad" or even "father". Those terms feel foreign, strange. But she does wonder: "What does he look like? How does his mind work? What parts of her—the eyes, the emotional steadiness, the love of animals—are because of him?"[25]

While the children fill in the blanks to create a whole picture of a person, you parents might, too. A mother of a two-year-old conceived with a "yes" donor has a dream:

> This is my hope: If Sasha wants to find her donor in 16 or 18 years or 25 years, he will want to be found. That he will be a decent human being and, perhaps someday, a compassionate friend. That . . . he has thought of us now and then, as I have thought of him, a familiar stranger standing at one juncture of the grand, glistening web that binds us all.[26]

It may be hard to find the place inside yourselves to encourage these daydreams. You might feel yourself growing anxious about fanning the flames of your children's fantasies, only to have your children feel let down later. Paul is a father who had two children using a "yes" donor. He's worried: "I wouldn't want them to think they'd be immediately accepted if they suddenly show up at the door and say, 'Here I am, Dad!'"[27] As you watch your children have their own reveries, you may feel protective, not wanting them ever to have to experience such rejection. Or you may feel your own sense of rejection as you watch your children generate positive feelings toward the potential interloper in your family. You may find this particularly true if you're in a lesbian and gay family. Your child's search to fill in the missing piece may feel threatening to your own status as a parent, particularly if you're the nonbiological parent, and particularly if you have no legal rights to your child.

Try to hold on to the real significance of these fantasies. Your children's and your participation in these reveries do not mean that your children are on a quest to find a whole, better new family. Rather, these fantasies give your children the space to develop a full sense of who they're connected to and who they belong to. Maggie Rousseau offers reassurance in that regard: "I hope he's a good guy [the donor] and that I'd like him. I want to see what kind of intellectual guy he is. I'd like to meet him, but not in the sense that he's my long-lost father."[28]

Now let's consider the potential letdowns that may indeed occur if the reality does not meet up with the child's fantasy. Let's say your son finally meets his donor and thinks he's a real loser. Rather than being avoided, these letdowns, should they occur, can be negotiated by tender holding on your part and gentle reminders to your child that reveries are just that—dreams we have that may never come true.

Obviously, your family's reveries will be different if your child knows the birth other. That person is not a figment of your family's imagination. He or she is a real person who may be sitting in the living room sipping tea. But even then, both you and your children will need room to play creatively with the place the donor or surrogate holds in your family matrix. Stephen Byrnes, the gay father in a couple who turned to a surrogate to have their daughter, Sammy, muses about Tammi, the surrogate with whom they have continued contact: "I wonder: What will Sammy's relationship with Tammi be? With Tammi's children? Will they attend each other's weddings? How will they introduce themselves? As 'half surrogate siblings'?"[29] In another family, Daisy knows that Byron, a friend of her mother's, is her donor. She's known him since she was born. Now age ten, she has fantasies that maybe her single mom and Byron could "hook up." She imagines what it would be like to have Byron as a father, rather than as the man from across the country that she sees twice a year.

Both Stephen and Daisy are having reveries about people they already know. In Daisy's case, her fantasies may speak to her longing to have a father. But in both cases, Stephen and Daisy serve to benefit from their reveries—not just about what is, but about what could be. If such reveries are foreclosed, your children might grow to believe that certain aspects of your family life are forbidden or dangerous, creating constriction rather than expansion in their sense of belonging and connection to you.

The Birth Other Dreams, Too

There is, of course, one missing player here—the birth other. As you and your children engage in your reveries, so might the birth other. Even if none of these reveries reach the minds of the children, the idea that the birth other might be thinking about the child can affect how the child fares, directly or indirectly.

Xytex, a commercial sperm bank, understood this well. It has encouraged donors to include messages to their unborn offspring about their reasons for becoming a sperm donor, their philosophy of life, and/or their wishes for their offspring.[30] The donors are helping to create a human life, and the sperm bank is inviting them to consider that they are also creating people who may someday want to know about their roots and who they come from.

The image of the callous sperm donor who ejaculates into a cup for a sum of money or the six-foot Harvard beauty who auctions her eggs at a high price are stereotypes that do not match the reported experiences of men and women who have donated their eggs, sperm, or wombs so a child could be born. Many wish for a good life for the children they have created. Others wonder who the children are and what they are doing in their lives. In the words of a thirty-seven-year-old sperm donor, "I hope, as any parent would hope for their own family, that they grow up reasonably unscathed by the rigors of childhood and everything that's out there in the world. . . . And I hope that they hook into something that makes life work for them, something they have a passion for."[31] A forty-eight-year-old man who donated sperm sixteen years previously imagines what he would say to the donor children if he ever met them. He would want to ask them if they have had a good life and invite them to tell him about themselves. He would want them to know "that it wasn't a casual decision to participate in this program. And that over the years they have been on my mind probably every day of my life."[32]

A twenty-year-old woman who was advertising to become a donor only to a religious couple already had fantasies about her relationship with her offspring. She wanted to donate only to a religious couple "because I want to someday see these kids up in Heaven with me. That would be awesome. I probably won't have any contact with them until then, so that will be my first time meeting him or her."[33] Now this may be a pie-in-the-sky fantasy, and more to do with her own narcissistic needs than the children's welfare, but nonetheless she is already carrying beatific fantasies about her offspring's spiritual connection to her.

The dreams, of course, are not always so benevolent. Donors worry their offspring will show up and demand college tuition. They think about the overwhelming experience of having ten or more offspring appear at their doorstep, all looking like the donor. They worry the donor offspring will want to insert themselves into their families. They worry about how their spouses or their children will feel about these other children. They grow anxious that someone somewhere is contemplating them as a possible parent. While parents and children are engaged in their own family-building reveries, we have to consider the possibility that such anxiety-ridden reveries on the part of the birth other may present yet another burden that the children will have to carry in their lives—knowing that someone who made them may be anxious about their existence.

Forget about Dreaming—I Want the Facts

Whether enlivening or burdening, reveries aren't the only thing that solidifies a sense of family belonging. Children also search for some actual information about the donor or surrogate. Some children want to know from the time they can talk. Other children show no curiosity about the donor or surrogate, just as some adopted children are really not that interested in their birth parents. Some only come to a curiosity about the donor or surrogate later in their childhood, typically in adolescence.

You may be a parent who was surprised to find out that your child not only doesn't show an interest in the donor or surrogate but forgot he or she had one. You read the books. You told the stories. Then one day, when your child is about ten or so, you decide to raise the topic again, and your child looks up and says, "What? You never told me that." This, of course, makes no logical sense, as your child not only has been told but has discussed it with you several times in the past. So what is going on? It's a simple case of psychological defenses called up by the child to insulate him- or herself from the information until he or she is emotionally or cognitively ready to use it. The name of the defense: repression. If this should occur, you can accept your child's newfound wonderment or surprise about the information while gently reminding him or her that you've talked about it before. You can also avoid such repression taking hold by keeping the dialogue alive and active in your family life, rather than bringing it up only on rare occasions.

A mother reported to me that she had both an older adopted son and a younger seven-year-old daughter who was an egg-donor baby. Both know about their origins. Her adopted son has wanted to know all about his birth parents, who are known, as it was an open adoption. But she was struck that her daughter, in contrast, shows absolutely no interest in knowing the egg donor. Her daughter just knows that someone else gave her egg so Mommy and Daddy could have a baby. She exhibits no curiosity about the donor. So what's different about these two children in the same family? Developmentally, it is presently easy for her daughter to divorce the egg from any connection to an actual person. Adoption did not offer such sleight of hand to her son, for the narrative is not about eggs and sperm but about whole people, a birth mother and a birth father. It is quite possible that as the daughter grows older her interest will be piqued, certainly by adolescence, as to whom she came from rather than what made her.

Maggie Rousseau indeed did not have much interest in meeting her donor until she reached adolescence. Then it changed: "I'd like to see a picture of him. I'd like to ask him what he's been through in life. . . . I'd like to get to know him with e-mails and letters before I sit down at a coffee shop with him. I'm trying not to hope for too much. I'm not looking for a close relationship. I'd just like to know him for the sake of knowing him."[34] Some people say that our culture inflates the importance of blood ties and makes the assumption that all people want to know their biological roots. They argue that this is simply a cultural construct, rather than an innate need or desire on the part of all human beings. Others, including myself, argue that the search for one's body roots appears to be a cross-cultural phenomenon that slices across all humanity, albeit with wide variations on the theme. Whether innate or socially constructed, it appears that the vast majority of people in our culture maintain that desire, and that includes children born with the aid of a birth other. Some children will go to great lengths to search out the information about their roots, a search that can extend well into adulthood.

Shelley Kreutz found out when she was ten that she was conceived with an anonymous sperm donor. Her very first question when her mother told her was "Can I find out who he is?" Ten years later, as a college student, she was still trying to find out. She received information from her mother's doctor about the donor's hair color and eye color and learned that he was a medical student at a particular hospital. She went to the hospital to look at old photographs of medical students. She went on-line, where she joined a growing donor–offspring community. She plans to send a letter out to all the medical students from the donor's era. She explains, "I just want to know about him. It's like a missing piece of a puzzle, as a lot of us say. It's the part we don't know about."[35]

As the children try to connect, sperm donors who were originally anonymous are now being contacted in increasing numbers to be told that a child is searching for them. One of these donors reported that at first he was bowled over, even suspicious. But then he went and met the young woman searching for him: "Seeing her was very emotional. The profile, the mannerisms, everything was so much like me that it was scary. We had a good time together, and I was relieved that everything went so well." Not just the child, but the donor may be psychologically affected by the discovery of a missing piece mirrored in his or her offspring. However, even if this is so, this donor, now himself the father of a young son, does not want to repeat the experience with other donor offspring if they should contact him.[36]

Now let's turn to the phenomenon of belonging for the child who is never told. As we know, there are some children who are never told but suspect. William Cordray was thirty-seven when he first found out he was a donor-insemination child. But he reports that throughout his childhood he suspected his father was not his genetic father. He could never find common traits between him and his father. He was shy, a reader, liked modern dance, ballet, art history, and theater. His father was an athletic nonreader. At age five he asked his mother if he was adopted. His mother gave a true but sly answer: "No, you're my child." His perceived mismatch with his father persisted, and by adolescence he had developed his own family reverie—his mother had been adulterous, and that's how he was conceived. He searched around among his parents' friends to find out if any were his real dad. He found himself growing isolated and moody. Finally, he found out his nightmare wasn't true; his mother was a sperm-donor recipient, not an adulteress.[37] William Cordray's experience confirms that sometimes children know what's up, and if you don't tell them directly, they might develop their own theories, which may be way off the mark and more fantastic than the truth. Along the way, they may also develop emotional symptoms as they grope to make sense of their uncomfortable feelings of not belonging.

A gap in intellectual functioning that may show up in some families is not only a fact but an experience that may be poignantly felt by the child. A young woman didn't find out until she was twenty-three or twenty-four that she was a sperm-donor baby:

I have never felt connected with my social father. In fact, at times, I would look at him and think to myself when he had done something that seemed to me rather childish, "this person's genes contributed to my being?" We were very much opposites. I was into reading books and creating objets d'art . . . he worked as a baked goods deliveryman and expressed interest in nothing else, except for baseball perhaps. The elementary school I attended suggested to my mother that I attend a program for very advanced students, while my social father couldn't spell what I felt were relatively simple words.[38]

Children can also begin to wonder why they are so different from one of their parents in personality, interests, or physical looks. Sometimes the child feels superior, sometimes just an outsider, with the uneasy sense that something's wrong with this picture. So what does this do to a child's sense of belonging? That child will never have the opportunity to engage in authentic family reveries, reveries that help the child place him- or herself in the family. That child may have a funny feeling somewhere, but no opportunity to find out the true facts of his or her genetic roots. It is understandable to want to seal your child's sense of belonging in the family by sheltering him or her from the fact that he or she didn't come from you. You just need to know the risk—it may backfire if your child feels alienated or different but can't figure out why.

One of my main reasons for advocating disclosure, except under circumstances where it places children under hostile fire or threatens weakened bonds or fragile development, is that I believe children fare best when they have the full opportunity to explore their sense of belonging, to both the parents they've grown up with and the adults who've helped make them. They won't do this alone, but rather in concert with the thoughts, feelings, and actions of everyone who counts as part of the family matrix. Feeling this sense of belonging goes hand in hand with the last developmental task I want to talk about—establishing a sense of identity.

WHO AM I?

As we grow up, we all have to balance our sense of belonging with our discovery of our own unique individuality. According to Erik Erikson's eight stages of development, a good deal of adolescence is devoted to one side of that equation—finding your own identity. Of course, you've already been working on this well before you hit puberty, but nothing like you'll experience it in adolescence. If you fail to find your identity, you're left with a sense of confusion. A child born with a donor or surrogate has some unique challenges in completing Erikson's fourth stage of development, Identity versus Confusion. In Western culture, it's presumed that children will have a better sense of their identity and higher self-esteem if they know their genetic roots. Denied that information—physical, medical, social, psychological, and even educational—they will suffer from genealogical bewilderment. This would apply to both adopted children and birth-other children who don't know who their progenitors are. According to the experts, that genetic void leaves children baffled and bewildered and is not in their best interests.[39]

But you know, when I tried to find studies scientifically documenting this relationship between genealogical bewilderment and weakened self-identity, I found none. So I want to go on record as saying it is our current assumption, rather than our current knowledge, that leads experts to conclude that children will leave adolescence with identity confusion if we deny them full access to their genetic histories. Instead, I would just say that both adopted children and children conceived with a birth other may have a different journey as they sort out the question "Who am I?"

The Hole Inside versus the Missing Puzzle Piece

Some of the children tell us it feels like a "hole inside" as they try to put together a whole picture of themselves. I'm remembering Nadine, an eighteen-year-old adopted young woman who told me she was desperate to find her birth mother and her birth mother's family. Tall, blond, and blue-eyed, she had nothing in common with either of her parents, who were short and dark. Every time she walked into a family party, she looked into a sea of people who looked nothing like her. For once, she wanted to walk into a room and find herself mirrored by people who looked, talked, or acted like her. Christine Whipp is now forty-six years old. She only found out when she was forty that she was the product of donor insemination. She always assumed her mother's family was her gene pool, but now she's all shaken up: "I don't even know who I am anymore. . . . DI [donor insemination] robbed me of half my genetic history, and it robbed my children and grandchildren, too."[40]

Now let's look at the exact opposite challenge—instead of a *missing* piece, *too many* pieces of the puzzle. That's what can happen when your children do know their donors or surrogates and have to piece all that together to sort out "Who am I?" Where are you supposed to put this extra "parent"—if you already have two? And what do you do with the extra piece when you also have a missing piece? I have two mommies, but I don't have a daddy—so what does that make the donor? I have two daddies, but no mommy—so what does that make my surrogate?

Our Families Are Our Mirrors

Our identity is never formed in isolation. We figure out who we are in our relationships with our most intimate others. It's not just how we interact with them; it's also how we think about them, how we feel about them, and how they think about us. Key players in this drama are our mothers and fathers. Identity formation is a challenging task for *any* child. Now imagine the complications when we include in the relationship list (1) a mom who is a child's social and biological parent but not her genetic parent; (2) an aunt who is the child's progenitor, the egg donor who gave her eggs so her sister could have a baby; (3) the child's dad, her genetic parent, who mixed his genes with his sister-in-law's in a dish so he and her mom could have their child. Could we say this might be a fairly daunting identity task for the daughter?

At a very early age, toddlers discover that the little person they see in the mirror is not someone who will come out and play with them but someone who *is* them. This is a great revelation and stimulates hours of exploration and study. In adolescence, children rediscover the mirror. They'll stare into it for hours and hours, looking for both perfection and flaws, but, more important, trying to get a reading of just who they are.

In a more figurative sense, children count on other people to mirror a sense of themselves. Many children who have an anonymous donor lament that they are missing one key person who could be that mirror. We all know the stories about identical twins separated at birth who are reunited in adulthood only to find that they have pursued the exact same career or use the identical toothpaste and cologne or crave the same food or play the same sports or have the same quirky habit of turning around twice before they get into bed at night. By reuniting, they have finally found that mirror, discovering something about themselves as they see it reflected in their genetic double. To complete their identity formation, birth-other children may long for just such a mirror in the image of their genetic donor.

When we live with our mothers and fathers and sisters and brothers, we take such mirroring moments for granted, like the air we breathe. We often don't even think about them, and when we do, it is to figure out self-consciously how we're alike and how we're different from the people we're related to. But if you don't have access to all those people, you have to stretch to imagine what you got from or share with the people you are related to—both by blood and by bonds—that makes you who you are.

Nicky is a young woman who feels she has to compensate for the loss of half her identity by holding on to the hope that someday she will find out who her sperm donor was. In the meantime, she pays scrupulous attention to her only access to blood ties, her mother's side of the family, "always searching for similar personality traits and interests in an attempt to affirm who I am and why I am what I am."[41] She doesn't feel so great about her own sense of identity. She worries that when her mother dies she will have lost her only immediate biological link and feel very alone and solitary. Nicky imagines that her identity conundrums might even be passed down to her own children someday because they'll never be able to know a quarter of their biological heritage. She's not longing to find her sperm donor so she can discover her missing father or complete her family. All she wants to do is find the additional mirror that will reflect to her a sense of who *she* is.

The Family Romance That Helps Shape Identity

This identity search, so fervent in the teenage years, can actually be traced back to the family romance that children often engage in during grade school. Unlike the family reverie, the family romance is a child's solo affair. Your children engage in these fantasies so they can imagine new possibilities for themselves—envisioning their own talents and capabilities separate from their family connections. Not having even reached puberty, they're still too young to go off on their own. Instead, they transport themselves to other fantasized parents far away from home. Typically, children fabricate made-up people to be those imaginary parents. These family romances are often quite grandiose in their storyline, as children elevate themselves to the status of the child of some king or queen.

A child born with a birth other has a bit of a complication in the family romance. Why? Because there's some reality to the fantasized parent. We have found that adopted children can conjure up unknown birth parents as the key players in the family romance.[42] Now we're beginning to see the same thing among children with donors or surrogates. The wonderful birth other who gave the gift of life or half the child's genetic make-up might someday show up on the scene to claim his or her long-lost child. The nice people who so generously give mommies and daddies their eggs, their sperm, or their wombs can easily be transformed into the rich and mighty king or queen who will bring the child fortune and glory.

Ten-year-old Deanna's mom and dad were fighting a lot. They worried about how the fighting was affecting Deanna. Deanna said she didn't care; she loved her parents very much, and she was too busy thinking about other things. Actually, she was busy dreaming about her egg donor, whom she would never know. Deanna's a great basketball player. She bets her egg donor is, too. Her parents certainly aren't. Deanna loves her long, swanlike neck. Both her parents kind of have stumps for necks. She must have her egg donor's neck. She imagines the time she and her donor will meet in a café, falling into each other's arms, overwhelmed with emotion. They won't be able to believe how much they look alike. Deanna will be at Harvard then, studying biology. Her egg donor will already be a well-known scientist. They'll move in together and become a rich and famous duo. All the people from home who ignored Deanna in fifth grade will suddenly be clamoring for her attention. They'll want to meet her famous donor, too.

Deanna's family romance may indeed shield her from her parents' fighting. She might even be using it to get back at them for their fighting, erasing her parents and usurping them with the wonderful donor. But I don't think so. I know Deanna, and it seems clear that she is daydreaming about herself—her first forays away from home showered with grandiose fame and fortune. Her anonymous egg donor becomes the perfect hook to hang her hat on as she shapes her dreams for her own future.

Not all birth-other children are as lucky as Deanna, with her benign donor dream. Occasionally, the family romance turns into the family nightmare. As the time comes to forge their own identity, some children find themselves having to cut down to size the birth other who their parents and the books read to them have always presented in such glowing terms. They may start railing against the so-called nice person who gave the gift of sperm, eggs, or womb. Tyler was eleven when he rolled his eyes at me and pronounced scornfully, "Nice man, yeah, right. I bet you he just did it for the money." The adopted child might have to dismiss his birth father as having just done it for the sex and then abandoning him. But the birth-other child might now have to face a more chilling thought—that the donor or surrogate didn't even do it for fun, but for money. Some gift.

In fantasy, your child may glorify the birth other. Your child may defame the birth other. Your child may simply incorporate the birth other into the family, particularly if that person is an active participant. It doesn't matter which way it goes. That person may play a very active role in your children's fantasy life as they begin to shape their own identity. In my own practice, all the children I have worked with who know they have a donor have shown an interest at one time or another in the person who helped make them. In that way, they're just like adopted children and adults I've worked with. It helps them pin down their own identity. With limited information at their disposal, sometimes they'll feel compelled to construct an actual parent in fantasy. I still hold that it's important to refer to the birth other in terms other than "mother" or "father," but that does not mean the children will do the same. Let's remember that no matter what we label the donor or surrogate, we cannot control a child's inner fantasy life. In the chambers of the family romance, children may still transform "birth other" into "parent." That doesn't mean they're bewildered or confused. They're just fantasizing—playing an identity game like any other child, calling on the imagined birth other as their king or queen.

Occasionally, the romance goes beyond play, and then we have to pay attention. For children with a missing piece, they may need to construct a parent where there was none. I am reminded of Kira, a child born to a single mother with an anonymous donor. At age eight, Kira had taken to adopting all the men in her life as father figures, going so far as calling her next-door neighbor Daddy. At age eleven, she fabricated a tale to her entire school about her father who had traveled with her and her mother to Canada. If pushed to the wall, she would say that she wasn't lying. She has a father. She just doesn't know where he is. So what's a little white lie about going to Canada?

In a culture that assumes all children have both a mother and a father, it is hard to forge an identity without one. So Kira pretends to her whole school that she has one. Her mom, Barbara, handled it in a warm and caring way. She acknowledged to Kira how nice it would be to have a father and how much she knew that Kira wished she had one. At the same time, she got Kira back on good footing in her identity quest by reminding her that all her schoolmates and teachers would support her for who she really is, a vibrant and wonderful girl who has a mom but no dad. A family romance spinning out of control, shared with the world as fact rather than fancy, marks the time for a parent to step in, offering gentle support and understanding but setting the record straight about reality.

Now we come to Annie. Annie knew that she was much smarter than her father. This often caused her great embarrassment when her friends came over because she hung out with the brainy crowd, and they all had mothers and fathers who were intellectual whizzes. She knew that her sperm donor had been a medical student who was now an up-and-coming cancer researcher. Although she would not be able to contact him until she was eighteen, in her fantasies she pressed "delete" for her dad and replaced him with her "real" father, her sperm donor who would take her to medical conferences. In her imaginings, all her friends would be totally impressed with his awards and accomplishments and shower her with compliments. She dealt with the extra piece in her family, the donor, in this way to consolidate her identity as an honor student and future PhD. The only problem was when, like Kira, she put her fantasy into action, telling new people she met that her father was a doctor. Like Barbara, her parents had to set the record straight for her. But her parents also needed some help to understand that Annie's fantasy, as long as it stayed just that, was not delusional or destructive or even repudiating of her own family—it was just Annie trying to work with her extra piece of the puzzle in sorting out who she was.

Children engage in family romances to figure out their own identities: Am I a child with a father (or mother) or not? Am I a child with two fathers, or not? No matter how you craft your story to your children, much of it is out of your hands as your children carry on with their own lives and try to make sense of their full identity in the context of all the people they carry within them. Here, it is the village inside, rather than the village out there, that your children actively engage with as they shape their own identity.

Whose Blood Pulses through Me?

Recall that around age ten children may begin to wonder about who the donor or surrogate is. Sometimes the wish to know explodes in adolescence. Even if they have known the birth other all their lives, that person begins to take on new meaning. Children are rapidly changing both cognitively and emotionally and come to realize the significance of the birth other to their own being. They're now able to envision their future, not in grandiose fantasy but in reality. It dawns on them that if they have a donor, that person will be carried on into their own children's genes someday. By now they are understanding what it means to inherit nearsightedness or allergies from the people who made them. They may feel a new need to know who their siblings are—not just so they don't marry them but so they can meet people of their own generation who carry some of the same genes they do. So the adolescent desire to find out about the donor or surrogate or half siblings is not just a search for belonging. It's also fundamentally a search for the self.

Your children are growing up in a society that still places a great deal of weight on blood ties and genetic origins: parents are the people who make you. Your children are simultaneously growing up with the new consciousness of social parenting: parents include the people who intended to have you and the people who raise you. Our society leaves your children with no choice but to negotiate both concepts of parent—those who make you and those who raise you—as they leave their families and consolidate their sense of who they are and who they came from.

All children conceived with a birth other who have been told about it will need to forge an identity that incorporates the fact that they were not a product of a sexual union between two adults. They will know that they were conceived through a scientific procedure that involved a person who is *not* their parent but who helped bring them into the world. Even "turkey baster" children, born of the simplest form of assisted reproductive technology, will know themselves to be products of science rather than sex, as basic as that scientific method may be. They may self-identify as tubesters. Some have even taken to thinking of themselves as "half-adopted." They're like adopted children because there's a birth someone out there who isn't raising them but who shares their genes and participated in making them. They're *not* like adopted children because there's another birth someone who helped make them and is also right there raising them.[43] That's what makes them only "half."

Children find their own creative ways of incorporating their birth-other origins into their identity. Actually, I have yet to meet a child or to have heard of an individual conceived with a birth other who complained, "I wish my parents had never told me. Why did they have to do that?" Around identity issues, the biggest complaint I've come across is the sadness, resentment, or confusion when someone grew up forging one identity only to have it torn asunder when discovering that the parent he or she thought was his or her genetic parent turned out not to be.

When that happens, a person has to recalibrate his or her identity, whether at age ten, fifteen, thirty, or fifty. First, they'll face the initial disruption, "So who am I anyway?" It's as if the whole world has been temporarily turned topsy-turvy. Then they have to find their footing again, reshaping their identity with the new knowledge that their parent is not their genetic parent and that someone else is responsible for half of their genetic make-up. Amanda Turner, a psychologist in England, studied the cases of sixteen people from the United Kingdom, the United States, Australia, and Canada who had not been told they were donor-insemination babies until they were adults. She found that many experienced shock, feeling their whole identity was threatened. They coped with their identity disruption by developing fantasies about the donors, what we might call a belated family reverie.[44]

If such late discovery should happen to your child, all is not lost. His or her identity will not be permanently shattered. It's just that he or she will have to do some remedial work, to go back and engage in the family reveries with your support and involvement and come forward again with a new answer to "Who am I?"

Does It Matter If You Never Know You Have a Birth Other?

What about the identity issues if your children are never told about their origins? To date, the studies have only followed children who don't know into their adolescence, and none of the studies has directly addressed identity issues. And as these children become adults, they would be a difficult group to study. They themselves do not identify as individuals born with a birth other, so how would we find them to study? But here's what I can surmise from the children we know about. They're no different from any other child who grows up with one or two parents and accepts those parents as the real parents, the ones you take totally for granted. Let's challenge for a moment the traditional notion that blood ties are the cornerstone of identity. If they're not, it shouldn't make any difference at all that these children don't know. They grow up with parents who love them and shepherd them from birth to adulthood, all the while mirroring to them a sense of self from the intimate bonds that are forged. That's the stuff of healthy identity formation.

Yet what about a mom's sudden silence when a passing stranger says, "Oh, what a beautiful child! Where did she ever get those blue eyes?" Or what about the very special relationship that develops between Uncle Bob and little Joey, when Uncle Bob has nine other nephews but no other for whom he, unknown to Joey, is the sperm donor? Recall my notion of the inner village, composed of all the child's internalized relationships within the family matrix—with parents, with the birth others, with the birth others' significant others, with siblings and half siblings. Obviously, when a child isn't told, there will be an empty place where the birth other won't reside because the child has no awareness he or she exists. But those members of the family matrix who do know will be holding that person in their minds. They will also be holding the child in mind as someone who was made with the assistance of a donor or surrogate.

So far, we have no evidence to suggest that these children grow up compromised in their subjective sense of who they are in the world, even if based on incomplete or erroneous knowledge about the self. The only evidence we have at our disposal comes from the people who forged an identity based on not knowing and then had that taken away from them when they later found out. They repeatedly say they always knew something was askew. Maybe they're just imagining it after the fact; maybe they're a select small group— the people who always suspected and go on a search to find out. Others who never suspected may remain content with who they are. I don't have any conclusive data to offer you, but I just want to leave you with one question to think about: Is it possible children have an unconscious way of knowing that defies everyone's intentions not to tell, the unthought known, and that such inner rumbling might end up striking a discordant note in the symphony of your child's identity formation?

INGREDIENTS FOR HEALTH

Everything suggests that children born with the assistance of a donor or surrogate can grow up to become healthy and happy adults. They may even be stronger for their experience. But now you know that there are some key ingredients to ensure your children's success. You need to be ready to hold your child, in every sense of that word, with a commitment to working out your own anxieties so you can think clearly enough to provide your child with the love and the support and guidance he or she will need. Rather than foreclosing fantasy, you'll do best to open it up as much as you can, allowing for both family reveries and family romances to unfold. Childhood is always a work in progress, in which you will need to allow room for the ebb and flow of the experience over time so your children can develop both a strong, positive sense of identity and a clear sense of family belonging. As challenging as it might be, you need to create space for the dark as well as the bright feelings.

Parents, however, are only one piece of the village. Until our society rids itself of reproductive technophobia and makes room for all different kinds of families, your children may suffer. Until the scientific community pays more careful attention to the laboratory manipulations that may compromise a child's healthy development and corrects them wherever possible, your children may suffer. And until the professional community conducts further research and provides more counseling and supportive services to families turning to assisted reproductive technology, both children *and* parents may suffer.

In the meantime, a child grows through us. As your children grow, they may wonder if the donor or surrogate ever thinks about them. The birth other may be wondering about your child. You may be wondering what your child is thinking about the donor or surrogate. You may wonder what your child is thinking about you. As all this goes round and round, your child may be left with gaps. He or she may need to mourn a missing piece or accept extra ones. It is a challenge for a child. Sometimes, it is so much a challenge that parents and a supportive community are not enough to help a child through. If that happens, an empathic and understanding psychotherapist sensitive to the experiences of birth-other families may be able to provide a "room of one's own" for your child to sort through the feelings of being different, establish a sense of belonging, and forge a positive identity based on a complicated inner village. But most of the time, the main thing the child needs is you—to come through. And the mission will always be the same—to raise a whole and healthy child.

When Clear Thinking
Trumps Anxiety

> It's like our whole lives together have been this one big, messy, incredible experiment. And it worked.
>
> —A mother in a lesbian couple with two sperm-donor daughters[1]

W̶e now come to the end of our journey, answering tough questions and figuring out how to build strong families in this fertile new world. Writing a book is always a learning experience. I've learned that what I said at the beginning is right—the terrain is changing so rapidly that it's hard to keep up. It's a little like traversing a fast-moving stream on rolling boulders. It's an exhilarating and exciting experience, as long as you trust your own footing and feel confident you'll make it to the other side. To do it without falling into the water, you have to accept that it moves ever so rapidly and you have to believe you can keep up. You also have to train yourself to cross moving boulders. We could say that parenthood with a birth other is the fast-moving stream you are crossing and the moving boulders are all the new tough questions that keep popping up as you step across the water. Your training involves replacing anxiety with clear thinking so you can raise robust children prepared to step out into their own futures.

Just in the short span of time from striking the first key in Chapter 1 to writing the first words of this final chapter, brand new boulders have cropped up. As the millennium rolled in, a new reproductive technique, in which doctors mix DNA material from three different people, was beginning to be used to make babies before we had enough research on the safety or effectiveness of this new technique.[2] *The Wall Street Journal* alerted us, "Hold on to your fig leaves. Scientists are working on a cloning technique that could help make babies in ways Adam and Eve never imagined."[3] In this procedure, called *haploidization*, an adult skin cell is substituted for a sperm or an egg, meaning two women together or two men together could hypothetically create a baby genetically related to both of them. From the cover of *Time* magazine came a clarion call: "Human cloning is closer than you think— For couples who can't have a child—or who have lost one—the unthinkable may soon be possible."[4] And then, in the next few years, there was even more to come. To outdo cloning, a study was released announcing that mouse stem cells, both male and female, had been turned into egg cells. These unfertilized eggs seem capable of developing parthenogenically—that is, without the help of sperm—into embryos. In other words, babies could theoretically be conceived as easily as you make yogurt—with a little starter material. So fathers could make their own eggs, and children could be biologically created by only one person—a mom *or* a dad, the purest form of a single-parent family.[5] Indeed, in 2004, Japanese scientists produced live mice with two mothers and no father. These are the first mammals to be born through a form of parthenogenesis.[6] In China, the same year, doctors were able to impregnate an infertile woman by creating a hybrid egg, removing the nucleus from the infertile woman's egg and transferring it into the egg of a woman whose nucleus had been removed, a technique known as "nuclear transfer." It allows a couple to have their own genetic child using the shell of another woman's egg, a whole new way of being a birth other.[7] Fertility clinics have developed advanced methods to select the most robust embryos in the petri dish, increasing the odds of a viable pregnancy and decreasing the number of multiple births because fewer embryos need to be implanted in the uterus.[8] Women can now freeze their eggs for later use, negating the need for egg donors in older women who can no longer produce viable eggs.[9] Women can now set up an egg market account for the future, as men have already been doing with their sperm. Donor insemination has already been replaced by the injection of a single sperm from the man into a woman's egg among many heterosexual couples, allowing the couple to have a child genetically related to both of them following male infertility. Indeed, birth others could end up being a thing of the past.

As new options flourish, so do parents' questions. I sat at lunch with a young woman who had been my student, someone I care about deeply. As we ate, she shared with me her thoughts about having her second baby using a gestational carrier. She does not suffer from infertility, and her own womb works fine except that her body had a strong reaction to being pregnant. She contracted a rare and debilitating condition during her first pregnancy—nothing fatal, but temporarily impairing. It took her several months to regain her health, and she still has some health fallout from the illness. The odds of its happening again if she gets pregnant are quite high. She didn't know if she could subject her body to that experience twice, and she also worried for her beloved daughter, who would lose her mother to serious sickness for nine months and more. So she wondered, what are the downsides of using a surrogate? How would a surrogate feel about offering her womb when there wasn't any infertility and my friend had a working womb of her own? Would she be better off adopting? Should she just tough it out and get pregnant again? How does she take the best care of the little girl she already has? How would it be for her daughter to be born from her and have a sibling born from a surrogate? How would it be for the sibling? These were all the questions swimming through her head.

A colleague who is an expert in the field of gamete donorship shared with me her distress. She had been counseling a fifty-nine-year-old woman and a sixty-three-year-old man who were exploring the possibility of an egg-donor baby. All she could envision was the birth of a future orphan.

More and more people are thinking about creative ways to have babies. And we still all have so many questions and feelings about the experience, whether we are parents, children, professionals, or community members. I've anticipated that at one point or another as you've read what I've written, you may have taken issue with a particular thing I said or with a phrase I used. I know that anytime we put our ideas into words, such reactions are inevitable, but I think maybe even more so because of the intensity of our thoughts, feelings, and attitudes about babies made with the help of birth others or with the help of any form of assisted reproductive technology. Each of you may also have had your own unique experience, different from any addressed in these last chapters. So I welcome your thoughts and experiences and hope that in addition to providing a map for raising a child born with a surrogate or donor, I have also opened up a forum so that our differences or disagreements can become a creative dialogue among all of us as we work together to make room for the new families of the twenty-first century.

Our task was to walk together through the experience of having a child with a birth other so we could harness our feelings to our thoughts and allow clear thinking to trump anxiety. Now I want to tell you a story so we can test our skills. This is the true story of a fifty-two-year-old single mother, Susan Buchweitz. Susan gave birth to a baby boy using a donated egg and sperm. Her intent was to purchase an embryo produced by anonymous donors from a local fertility clinic. Ten months after the baby's birth, the fertility clinic contacted her to tell her they had made a mistake—they had implanted her with the wrong embryo. That embryo belonged to a couple who had used an egg donor and the husband's sperm. It was intended to become that couple's child. The fertility clinic contacted the couple as well, to tell them about the mistake. Now the couple want their baby back. The husband is suing for full custody of the child Susan has borne and raised as her own since 2001. A family court in California has awarded him twice-weekly visitation. Susan has only been awarded temporary custody. The couple gave birth to their own baby girl. The fertility doctor knew immediately after the implantation that there had been an embryo mix-up, but at that time he chose not to reveal this either to Susan or to the couple to whom the embryo belonged. Worried that the disclosure might cause Susan to want to terminate her pregnancy, he chose instead to "leave it in God's hands."

Susan's story touches every major theme we have explored together over the past nine chapters. Susan is a single woman with a strong desire to have a child. In fact, three years of trying to conceive with her fiancé led to the breakup of their relationship but not to the breakdown of her strong wish to become a mother. With access to assisted reproductive technology, she persevered until she got her wish, which came well after her fiftieth birthday. Then we have strange bedfellows, an older single mother and a heterosexual couple faced with infertility coming together at the same fertility clinic. The tension between the power to create and the fear of creation culminated in the thing we all fear—someone made a mistake. I do not know the doctor who caught the mistake, but I can certainly speculate that anxiety trumped clear thinking in his initial decision not to tell both Susan and the couple about the mix-up that had happened. Now comes the issue of possession: to whom does this baby belong, the woman who gave birth to him or the man who provided his sperm with the intent, along with his wife, of rearing the baby that was conceived? What about the attachments that have unfolded over the first three-plus years of this baby's life? And most important, in the words of a mother who clearly loves her child, Susan ponders, "My biggest concern right now is the future. How will he be told his story in a positive way so that he feels really good about himself?"[10] What would you do in this situation—if you were Susan, if you were the father, if you were the wife in the couple, if you were a mental health professional asked to weigh in on the best interests of the child and the parents' rights, if you were the judge making a decision about custody?

I'll answer for myself. As a mother and a trained developmental psychologist, common sense tells me that I would keep this baby with the only mother he has ever known. I'm assuming here that he has already established a strong and positive bond to Susan and she to him. I would think about including the father in the child's life, but as his genitor, not his pater. Just as known donors often become involved with the children they've helped conceive, so could this man become a vital part of this child's family matrix, but not his daddy. And someday this little boy will need a very clear narrative about his origins, one that is both truthful and helps him sort out the complicated relationships with the man he comes from, that man's wife, his half siblings, and whoever else might enter into the matrix as he grows. And all of the adults would need to work closely together if they are to ensure the best interests of this little boy. That's what I would do.

Assisted reproductive technology is all about becoming parents, and as soon as we become parents, we learn a very humbling fact of life. We no longer come first; our children do. No matter how your baby is made, embracing parenthood is about ensuring the best interests of your child, even when those interests work against your own. It's not so easy to do when you're feeling too anxious. And it's much easier to do when you feel calm and assured. If you have had your child with the help of a donor or surrogate, I hope I have helped you find that sense of calm in the midst of your unique experience. Your children are not the direct product of a sexual union. They may be the product of erotic love and passion, but not of sexual intercourse. They are born of science, not of sex. Besides you, there is a someone else in their lives, a donor or surrogate. If you neither ignore, shrink from, nor deny the significance of that uniqueness, but rather acknowledge it and think very carefully about how to integrate it into your family's experience, you stand to ensure your children's resilience and well-being. It takes mindfulness, creativity, and authenticity. And both joy and sorrow.

Decidedly, you are all raising your children in a society so rapidly changing in its reproductive possibilities that today becomes obsolete by tomorrow. Even our religious texts have had to be reinterpreted to accommodate this fertile new world. An infertile Jewish couple asked Rabbi Moishe Heinemann, an international expert on Jewish law, whether their child would be Jewish if they used a surrogate mother who wasn't, for by law a child is Jewish only if he or she is born to a Jewish mother. He ruled that their child would indeed be Jewish, as the host mother would simply be an incubator. Rabbi Heinemann also developed an Orthodox procedure for ensuring the paternity and maternity of a baby conceived in a test tube: An Orthodox Jew must be on hand to collect the sperm and the egg and to seal the contents of the test tube.[11]

Every day we face a new challenge in rethinking family when a birth other is involved. Someday your families may no longer be unique. Imagine your own children as grandparents, sitting their grandchildren on their knee and telling them about the circumstances of their own births, how it happened in the old days with in vitro fertilization, donor insemination, donor eggs, surrogacy, and so forth. Think about their grandchildren looking at them, eyes wide, and exclaiming, "No way! Why didn't they just _____?" (Readers, I'll leave it to your imagination to fill in the blank.) But for right now, having a donor or a surrogate or a petri dish conception is still rather radical.

In this fertile new world, we are at the cutting edge, but also in the infant stages of providing a supportive environment to help the children grow. A recent highly publicized court case of two women and two babies that I made reference to earlier brings home how young we still are as a society in our ability to keep our eyes on the prize—the best interests of the children.

To review. E.G. and K.M. were a lesbian couple. K.M. donated her eggs, and E.G. was the gestational mother. They used an anonymous sperm donor. E.G. gave birth to twin girls. For the first five years of the girls' life, they raised the children together, although by California law E.G., the birth mother, is the only assigned legal mother. K.M., the genetic mother, would have had to do a second-parent adoption. Instead, she signed a document waiving her rights to parenthood when she donated her eggs at the clinic, a common procedure designed to secure the rights of the intended parent in egg-donor situations and based on a model of heterosexual parenting rather than lesbian couples. But for those first five years the twins had two biological mothers, one their gestational mother and the other their egg mother. The couple then separated. As often happens after a divorce, each remembers their shared history very differently. K.M. always considered herself the twins' mother. E.G. said she didn't. She says her daughters have only one mother, E.G. K.M. says they have two. Before the separation, the twins referred to K.M. as Mama K. and E.G. as Mama E. In a court battle full custody was awarded to the gestational and legal mother, E.G. K.M., the genetic mother, was denied any rights, even visitation. E.G.'s lawyer likened K.M. to a stepparent and nothing more. She argued that giving K.M. shared custody would be trampling on E.G.'s rights and giving K.M. more rights than stepparents have. One of the children in particular is said to look strikingly like K.M. The twins know they came from K.M.'s eggs.

So now let's step back and look at this situation, guided by our principle of allowing clear thinking to trump anxiety and informed by our premise that family building in birth-other families should always put the best interests of the child first. The twins have a parent who raised them for five years. She is their genetic mother. They know this. But because she, perhaps unwittingly, signed a piece of paper at a fertility clinic so she and her partner could go forward with their plan to have a child, in a court of law she is not recognized as their mother. Although the court admitted in its decision that this ruling presented "harsh consequences for the children," the decision was intended to protect the rights of parents against claims of romantic partners who are temporarily involved in the children's lives.[12]

I hope we have learned from our own answers to the tough questions that the gestational mother's arguments, her lawyer's position, and the court's decision are all clear examples of unclear thinking. Let's project into the future. The children may yearn for their lost mother, their genetic mom, out of their sense of belonging and their quest to establish their own identities. K.M. was not just an anonymous or even a known egg donor. K.M. was the woman who harvested her eggs so they could be born, raised them with her partner for the first five-plus years of their lives, and then fought for her right to be their parent. How does she not qualify as a mother? And what will the twins think of their birth mother, or womb mother, for denying them access both to their genetic heritage and to their other mother? And what about the anonymous sperm donor—will E.G. ever allow the girls space for the family reveries that will help strengthen their family ties and give them the opportunity to explore fully who they are? And what narrative will E.G. provide them about their family—who's in it and why? How will E.G. end up feeling about denying her children their birthrights? How will K.M. feel if she permanently loses her children? Already, she hates "waking up in the middle of the night, but the one consoling part is that it's the only time when I know exactly what they're doing. I know they're sound asleep."[13]

If clear thinking were to take hold, the courts would get it that stepparents have nothing to do with lesbian co-parents. Judges and lawyers would be educated to understand the hurdles that lesbians may have to go through to receive assisted reproductive services so they can have families of their own. If the children were to have had all the supports they need to grow robust and healthy, these supports would have been in place way before they were ever born. Fertility clinics would have separate procedures for each of the members of the cohort that might show up for services—infertile couples, single women, single men, lesbian families, gay families. E.G. and K.M. would have received in-depth legal and psychological counseling before they ever embarked on their journey into parenthood. They would have drawn up a written co-parenting agreement, if indeed their intent was to raise children together. Laws would be in place to assure the children access to both their mothers throughout their childhoods—the mother whose eggs they came from and the mother who birthed them. As I write these words, E.G. and K.M.'s case is presently being brought before the California Supreme Court. One only hopes that clear thinking will prevail in that court to give the children what they really need—their mommies.

Unclear thinking about the best interests of a birth-other child is equally prevalent among heterosexual families. Diandra Douglas, actor Michael Douglas's ex-wife, and Zack Hampton Bacon III have been involved in a nasty and ongoing custody battle. Although never married, they tried to have a baby, with every intention of raising the child together. When their fifth attempt at in vitro fertilization failed, they turned to a surrogate, who delivered twin girls who sadly did not survive. Finally, they found another surrogate who gave birth to twin boys, using Mr. Bacon's sperm and the surrogate's eggs. Their relationship broke up, and Mr. Bacon has retained his residence in New York, while Ms. Douglas returned to California. Presently, Ms. Douglas is suing for full custody of the children, whom she wants raised in California, and Mr. Bacon is fighting for joint custody. Ms. Douglas isn't the twins' genetic mother, nor is she their gestational mother, but she's legally recognized as their mother based on the new principle, intent to parent. Ms. Douglas seems to have fallen into the trap of immaculate deception, denying her children access to their genetic father, whose intention was not to be a sperm donor but a parent. Not only could the children lose a dad, they could lose access to the only genetic parent in their lives—Mr. Bacon, the man who will later become a significant mirror in their identity quest. At this moment I do not know how this case will resolve. Mr. Bacon says whatever happens, he wants his sons to know that he fought hard to have them.[14] And wouldn't clear thinking tell us that these twins need exactly what E.G. and K.M.'s twins need—their parents?

All of you who have built your families with the help of a birth other have learned just that—you are your children's parents, and they need you. Each year society seems a bit more accepting of the new ways of making babies. And each year the number of children born with the assistance of a birth other goes up. Raising your children has not only afforded you the opportunity to build a family with the aid of a surrogate or donor and help your children grow, but you have helped us all rethink family. Who's a mommy? Who's a daddy? What is a family? How do birth others fit into the picture? A family can be people who are biologically related to each other or not. A family can have a daddy or not. A family can have a mommy or not. A family can have two mommies or two daddies. A family can be a hybrid with biological and nonbiological parents—like stepfamilies, like birth-other families. A hybrid family can be any family where only some of the members are biologically related but everyone lives together as a family, like foster parents who take in sisters and brothers as their foster children. You are all challenging us to reexamine our assumptions and attitudes and open ourselves up to the changes in family, where bonds are just as thick as blood.

You have also helped us rethink childhood. There is no child without all the people who make the child and all the people who raise the child. To that we all owe you great thanks. So thank you. And what a wonderful world it will be when you have nothing more to teach us, for then, at last, we will all be family.

Resources

Alternative Reproductive Resources
2000 North Racine
Chicago, IL 60614
Phone: 773-327-7315
website: www.arr1.com
e-mail: arrinfo@arr1.com

American Society for Reproductive Medicine
1209 Montgomery Highway
Birmingham, AL 35216
Phone: 205-978-5000
website: www.asrm.org
e-mail: asrm@asrm.org

The American Surrogacy Center
website: www.surrogacy.com
e-mail: tasc@surrogacy.com

Centers for Disease Control and Prevention
Division of Reproductive Health
4770 Buford Highway, NE, Mail Stop K-20
Atlanta, GA 30341
Phone: 770-488-5200
website: www.cdc.gov/nccdphp/drh/art.htm
e-mail: ccdinfo@cdc.gov

Donor Conception Network
P.O. Box 7471
Nottingham NG3 6ZR, United Kingdom
Phone: 44-620-8245-4369
website: www.dcnetwork.org
e-mail: enquiries@dcnetwork.org

Donor Conception Support Group of Australia
P.O. Box 53
Georges Hall NSW 2198, Australia
Phone: 61-2-9793-9335
website: members.optushome.com.au/dcsg/
e-mail: dcsg@optushome.com.au

Fertility Choice Surrogacy Center
website: www.fertilitychoice.com

FertilityPlus
website: www.fertilityplus.org

Growing Generations
5757 Wilshire Boulevard, Suite 601
Los Angeles, CA 90036
Phone: 323-965-7500
website: www.growinggenerations.com
e-mail: family@GrowingGenerations.com

International Consumer Support for Infertility
P.O. Box 959
Parramatta NSW 2124, Australia
Phone: 61-2-9670-2380
website: www.icsi.ws
e-mail: infor@icsi.ws

Law Offices of Theresa M. Erickson
10616 Scripps Summit Court, Suite 240
San Diego, CA 92131
Phone: 858-795-7450
website: surrogacylawyer.net
e-mail: Terickson@Ericksonlaw.net

Organization of Parents through Surrogacy
P.O. Box 611
Gurnee, IL 60031
Phone: 847-782-0224
website: www.opts.com

Rainbow Flag Health Services and Sperm Bank
933 Central Avenue
Alameda, CA 94501
Phone: 510-521-7737
website: www.gayspermbank.com
e-mail: Leland@gayspermbank.com

RESOLVE: The National Infertility Association
1310 Broadway
Somerville, MA 02144
Phone: 617-623-1156
Helpline: 888-623-0744
website: www.resolve.org
e-mail: info@resolve.org

Single Mothers by Choice
P.O. Box 1642
New York, NY 10028
Phone: 212-988-0993
website: www.singlemothersbychoice.com
e-mail: mattes@pipeline.com

The Sperm Bank of California
2115 Milvia Street, 2nd floor
Berkeley, CA 94704
Phone: 510-841-1858
website: www.thespermbankofca.org
e-mail: info@thespermbankofca.org

Notes

CHAPTER ONE

1. As reported by Ken Corbett (2001, p. 603).

2. Susan L. Cooper and Ellen S. Glazer (1994).

3. See Rebecca Mead (1999).

4. Bob Shacochis, "Missing Children," in Jill Bialosky and Helen Schulman (1998, p. 56).

5. See cover of *Time*, August 28, 2000 issue.

6. Story of a single mother to her five-year-old-son, quoted in Tammerlin Drummond (2000).

7. Sometimes a woman will contract with a man to have sex with him in order to have a baby, and both parties will agree in advance that the man will have no paternal responsibilities for the child so conceived. Some think of these situations as a creative and inexpensive form of donor insemination. Others take moral issue with these actions, seeing them as inappropriate sexual activity or exploitation of sexual unions for the purpose of parenthood.

CHAPTER TWO

1. Barbara Jones, "Heedless Love," in Jill Bialosky and Helen Schulman (1998, p. 13).

2. Agnes Rossi, "In Vitro," in Jill Bialosky and Helen Schulman (1998, p. 61).

3. As quoted in Harbour Fraser Hodder (1997, p. 56).

4. Adam Pertman (2000) writes about this same phenomenon in his book, *Adoption Nation*: "Infertile couples seldom fully accept the notion that they'll never have children. Often they try sophisticated and expensive medical interventions, sometimes they turn to sperm or egg donors (a misnomer, since the men and women 'donors' are usually paid), occasionally they employ a surrogate mother. Invariably, they fantasize about somehow defying physiological reality and getting pregnant" (p. 28).

5. Personal conversation with Dr. Shana Millstein, psychologist and senior researcher at the University of California, San Francisco, September 13, 2002.

6. To elaborate on each of the three stories: Athena was the daughter of Zeus. No mother bore her. Zeus pursued Athena's mother, Metis, until he caught her and got her with child. Zeus, warned by an oracle that Metis was carrying a female child but would then bear a son who was fated to depose him, took swift action to protect himself. He coaxed Metis to a couch with honeyed words and then swallowed her whole. That was the end of Metis, except that she continued to give him advice from within his belly. In the due course of time, Zeus was suddenly hit with an unbearable headache and howled with rage. With the aid of Hermes, who recognized the screams as labor pains, Zeus's skull was cracked open and out popped Athena, fully grown and fully armed. Some think of Athena's birth as a strange form of parthenogenesis, the conception and birthing of a child by one single parent. But in actuality, by mythical account, Zeus was the first gestational carrier (see Robert Graves, *The Greek Myths* vol. 1, New York: Penguin, 1986, p. 46, for an account of Athena's birth).

Then comes the Old Testament story of Abraham, Sarah, Hagar, Ishmael, and Isaac in the Book of Genesis. Abraham was in his eighties. His wife, Sarah, could not conceive. Sarah offered up her Egyptian handmaid, Hagar, to bear a child with Abraham, on Sarah's behalf. Hagar indeed conceived, after which she was reported to have turned on Sarah: "when she [Hagar] saw that she had conceived, her mistress [Sarah] was despised in her eyes." Sarah was then harsh with Hagar, and Hagar fled from her. Hagar bore Abraham a son, Ishmael, when Abraham was eighty-six years old. Thirteen years later, when Abraham was the ripe old age of ninety-nine, God appeared and announced that He would grant Abraham a second son, this time with Sarah. Sarah was ninety years old when Abraham's and her son, Isaac, was born. The original handmaid's tale, Hagar is the icon of the first surrogate birth, and Sarah's miraculous birthing is the foreshadowing of the twenty-first-century revolutionary reproductive possibilities of postmenopausal motherhood (see Book of Genesis: 16, 17, in *The Holy Scriptures*, Philadelphia: Jewish Publication Society of America, 1959, for an account of Abraham, Sarah, Hagar, Ishmael, and Isaac).

Finally, we can turn to the New Testament and the story of the birth of Jesus, looked at through the lens of historical document and metaphor, rather than religious doctrine. Mary is a virgin who becomes pregnant. An angel comes to announce to her that God is the genetic father of her child-to-be. How this occurred scientifically is left to our imagination, but we are told that neither Joseph's sperm nor his sexual union with Mary was involved. In essence, we have the first written account of a sperm-donor birth: an archetypal image of the divine genetic father and the social father left to pursue his life as a carpenter and carry out the everyday tasks of raising his child (see Diane Ehrensaft, 2000, for a full account of this interpretation of Jesus as the archetype of the sperm-donor baby).

7. To quote directly from Bob Shacochis, "For a man, history's answer, unlike technology's, has been brutally simple: Choose between the barren woman and your unborn children. But science has rolled the dilemma between its magician's fingers and come up with another option" ("Missing Children," in Jill Bialosky and Helen Schulman, 1998, p. 54).

8. In January 2005 Adrianna Illescu, a sixty-six-year-old Romanian professor and single woman, gave birth to a baby girl, Eliza Maria, born six weeks premature and conceived through in vitro fertilization using sperm and egg from anonymous donors. Maria's twin died in the womb. As of early 2005, Professor Illescu is the world's oldest new mom. Her daughter's birth has sparked debates in Romania over the ethics of a woman beyond the age of fertility having babies.

The sixty-three-year-old mother, Rosanna Della Cortes, gave birth in 1994. She was assisted in her pregnancy by Dr. Severino Antinori, an Italian gynecologist and embryologist. He has also been in the center of an international controversy about human cloning. He claims to have created cloned human embryos. He and his colleague, Dr. Panayiotis Zavos, have argued in favor of human cloning as an opportunity for infertile couples.

9. As quoted in Davy Rothbart (2003).

10. Stephen Byrnes, "Scenes from a Surrogacy," in Jill Bialosky and Helen Schulman (1998, p. 187).

11. In reflecting on our culture's present unease about cloning, Robin Mrantz Henig, author of *Pandora's Baby*, a history of in vitro fertilization research, had the same thought about the future obsoleteness of our attitudes: ". . . some of this new century's most far-fetched techniques may eventually become so commonplace as to offer no apparent need for deliberation or debate. Ultimately, some of this genetic gerrymandering may become, as with in-vitro fertilization, just another part of the landscape in the strange terrain of genomes, genes and generation" (as quoted in Robin Mrantz Henig, 2002).

12. For a full discussion of these studies, see Michele Hansen, Jen-

nifer J. Kurinczuk, Carol Bower, and Sandra Webb (2002); Laura A. Schieve, Susan F. Meikle, Cynthia Ferre, Herbert Peterson, Gary Jeng, and Lynne Wilco (2002); and Rick Weiss (2002).

13. Karen Springen and David Noonan (2003).

14. Sophie Cabot Black, "The Boys," in Jill Bialosky and Helen Schulman (1998, p. 32).

15. As quoted in Rebecca Mead (1999, p. 62).

16. As reported in Claudia Kalb (1999).

17. See Diane Ehrensaft (1997) for a full discussion of the phenomenon of the quest for the perfect child amid the fears of imperfection and a description of the elevated status of childhood where life revolves around the child rather than the child accommodating to the life around him or her.

18. See Diane Ehrensaft (1997) for a full discussion of expectable parental narcissism.

19. As quoted in Lori B. Andrews (1999, pp. 136–138). See especially Chapter 8, "The X Vials," for an extensive discussion of the designer baby syndrome.

20. For accounts of the Fasanos' experience, see "You're Carrying Someone Else's Child" (1999); Jim Yardley (1999); and Michael Grunwald (1999).

CHAPTER THREE

1. Mary Ann Thompson (2002, pp. 29, 62).

2. As described in Mary Ann Thompson (2002, p. 38).

3. Jody Messler Davies (1998, p. 805).

4. Susan L. Cooper and Ellen S. Glazer (1994, p. 154).

5. Agnes Rossi "In Vitro," in Jill Bialosky and Helen Schulman (1998, pp. 61–62).

6. Susan L. Cooper and Ellen S. Glazer (1994, p. 154).

7. Mary Ann Thompson (2002, pp. 29, 60).

8. Ronny Diamond, David Kezur, Mimi Meyers, Constance N. Scharf, and Margot Wienshel (1999, p. 147).

9. Bob Shacochis, "Missing Children," in Jill Bialosky and Helen Schulman (1998, p. 56).

10. Susan L. Cooper and Ellen S. Glazer (1994, p. 233).

11. For a discussion of the surrogate husband's experience, see Susan L. Cooper and Ellen S. Glazer (1994, Chapter 7, "Surrogacy").

12. Adam Pertman (2000), who confronted this reality with his wife, describes the pain with poignant clarity: "No one who hasn't confronted infertility can fully grasp the raw brutality of being deprived of something so fundamental as the ability to reproduce. Any biologist will tell you we were built to do

it. Every culture glorifies it. Whatever power put us here secured its command-ing role in life by making it a compelling instinct and an ecstatic experience" (p. 173).

13. Agnes Rossi, "In Vitro," in Jill Bialosky and Helen Schulman (1998, p. 62).

14. Harbour Fraser Hodder (1997, p. 56).

15. The same phenomenon is true for the infertile woman who turns to adoption as a means to satisfy her burning desire for a child. She will be plagued by the ease with which the birth mother has been able to have sex and perhaps without even trying to conceive a child who she will then give up as if the child had no personal meaning to her.

16. Susan L. Cooper and Ellen S. Glazer (1994) speak to this jeal-ousy: "Sarah [of the Bible] was the first, but by no means the last, woman to find that she had unanticipated reactions of jealousy and resentment to the pregnancy and childbirth experience of another woman, even one who was bearing a child for her" (p. 261).

17. Mary Ann Thompson (2002, p. 144).

18. P. C. Vey, *The New Yorker*, September 29, 2003, p. 80.

19. Throughout the experience of reproduction with a birth other, class issues will continue to surface. It is not only about the medical student with both vi-rility and advanced degrees under his belt. It is also about working-class women who rent their wombs so wealthier women can have babies of their own. It is about families with lesser means who cannot afford the cost of sophisticated reproductive techniques. It boils down to tensions between haves and have-nots, either fecundity or funds.

20. Stephen Byrnes, "Scenes from a Surrogacy," in Jill Bialosky and Helen Schulman (1998, p. 189).

21. Marsha Levy-Warren, "A Clinical Look at Knowing and Telling: Secrets, Lies, and Disillusionments," in Vivian B. Shapiro, Janet R. Shapiro, and Isabel H. Paret (2001, pp. 256, 258).

22. Mary Ann Thompson (2002, p. 48).

23. Jane T. Schnitter (1995).

24. Rosanna Hertz, personal communication, January 28, 1998, and February 3, 1998.

CHAPTER FOUR

1. Oxenhandler describes it like this: "Our children have been 'placed' with us—the very word we use for foster care. When I peered into the wicker laun-dry basket during those first nights of my daughter's life, it was not only to see if she was breathing, but to make sure that she had not been placed elsewhere by whatever

divine agency—as quixotic as any bureaucrat—had placed her with me" (Noelle Oxenhandler, 2001, p. 193).

2. Sarah Lyall (2003).

3. Although not a solution to the genetic asymmetry, this creative solution allows both mothers to have a biological connection to their child, and the child will have two biological mothers, one gestational and the other genetic.

4. Karen Springen and David Noonan (2003).

5. Sophie Cabot Black, "The Boys," in Jill Bialosky and Helen Schulman (1998, p. 32).

6. Susan L. Cooper and Ellen S. Glazer (1994, p. 251).

7. As reported in Annette Baran and Reuben Pannor (1989).

8. Emma Scrimgeour, "The Story of Seth's Egg," in Jane Haynes and Juliet Miller (2003, pp. 105–108); Flora Scrimgeour, "Seth," in Jane Haynes and Juliet Miller (2003, pp. 109–119).

9. Sam McManis (2003).

10. By known donor here I am not referring to donors or surrogates known only by name, address, and identifying information, but to donors who already are and will continue to be known personally by the family. All other donors, both known or anonymous, should also be afforded counseling before proceeding as a donor, not as a part of the family matrix but as a component of their participation in a clinic or sperm or egg bank, just as is already being offered routinely to potential surrogates.

11. *The American College Dictionary*, New York: Random House, 1962.

12. Susan L. Cooper and Ellen S. Glazer (1994).

13. Their precise arguments to the higher court were as follows: "The couple argues that they are being denied the right to be parents of their children from the moment of their birth and they will incur financial expense and suffer emotional pain if they are forced to go through an adoption process. They also contend 'Melissa' (the surrogate) never possessed parental rights and is being forced to take the role of mother that she does not want" (as quoted in Pamela Ferdinand, 2001).

14. Cheryl Saban (1993, p. 243).

15. Case reported in Susan L. Cooper and Ellen S. Glazer (1994, Chapter 6, "Ovum Donation").

16. Sheri Glucoft-Wong, personal communication, May 8, 2003.

CHAPTER FIVE

1. Hillary Rodham Clinton, *It Takes a Village*, New York: Simon & Schuster, 1996, p. 50.

2. D. W. Winnicott, *Talking to Parents*, Reading, MA: Addison-Wesley, 1993, pp. 132–133.

3. Agnes Rossi, "In Vitro," in Jill Bialosky and Helen Schulman (1998, p. 68).

4. As Oxenhandler explains, for parents the snatching stranger "can appear both as punishment for the failure to properly value a child and as an expression of the extreme valuation of that same child" (Noelle Oxenhandler, 2001, p. 190).

5. Joan Raphael-Leff, a British psychoanalyst who specializes in reproductive issues, recognizes this potential when she explains that for the parents the "donor is a further stranger in their midst, invoking mythical or paranoid ideas about the source of the biological contribution. The necessary sperm or egg donor/surrogate may be disavowed or, alternatively, elaborate fantasies may be constructed around their omnipotent qualities" (Joan Raphael-Leff, "Eros and ART," in Jane Haynes and Juliet Miller, 2003, p. 41).

6. According to Oxenhandler, "when we understand the intimate link between the evil stranger and the Eros of parenthood, we can to some degree defuse the terror that he inspires. For when we look him in the eye, we will see that though he does, alas, exist as a matter of fact he also exists as an inner figure. . . . As such, he is a repository not only for negative feelings, but for others—including the sense of the undeserved arrival of our children into our lives, of the slender thread of ownership, and of the extravagant and risky nature of our love" (Noelle Oxenhandler, 2001, p. 194).

7. Mary Swick coined the term "ghost mother" in her discussion of birth mothers and open adoption (see Mary Swick, "The Ghost Mother," in Jill Bialosky and Helen Schulman, 1998). I am extending this term to "ghost parent" and applying it to birth others in alternative-to-the-stork families.

8. Mary Swick, "The Ghost Mother," in Jill Bialosky and Helen Schulman (1998, p. 130).

9. Calvin Calarusso (1987, p. 227).

10. Germaine Greer, "Afterword," in Jane Haynes and Juliet Miller (2003, p. 210).

11. Ken Corbett (2001, pp. 599–624).

12. Bruno Bettelheim, *A Good Enough Parent: A Book on Child-Rearing*, New York: Vintage, 1988, p. 377.

13. Adam Pertman (2000).

14. Stephen Byrnes, "Scenes from a Surrogacy," in Jill Bialosky and Helen Schulman (1998, p. 190).

15. Marsha Levy-Warren, "A Clinical Look at Knowing and Telling," in Vivian B. Shapiro et al. (2001, pp. 252, 267).

16. Marsha Levy-Warren, "A Clinical Look at Knowing and Telling," in Vivian B. Shapiro et al. (2001, pp. 268–269).

17. Sue Stuart-Smith, "Egg Donation: The Mission to Have a Child," in Jane Haynes and Juliet Miller (2003, p. 177).

18. Dr. Corbett explains the effects on the two mothers, Ellen and R.J.: "As opposed to their fears that their fantasies would prove overstimulating or would separate them as a family, they were able to entertain the possibility of the opposite—the possibility of minds opening onto and into their collective fantasies in such a way as to bring them together as a family" (Ken Corbett, 2001, p. 610).

19. Stephen Byrnes, "Scenes from a Surrogacy," in Jill Bialosky and Helen Schulman (1998, p. 194).

20. Jill Smolowe and Natasha Stoynoff, (2003, pp. 88, 94).

21. F. Van Balen (1996).

CHAPTER SIX

1. As Susan L. Cooper and Ellen S. Glazer (1994) teach us in their book *Beyond Infertility*, "many couples attempting to decide about openness vs. secrecy in using donor gametes think about how they would explain the process to their children, when they would tell them, and how they might get across the idea that the information, though not a secret, is private and should be shared discriminately. Couples deciding to be open need a game plan—a rough idea about how they might handle the telling—in order to feel more comfortable with their decision. Feeling comfortable with [gamete donation or surrogacy] is essential before embarking on the process" (p. 174).

2. Ethics Committee of the American Society for Reproductive Medicine (2004, p. 527).

3. "Inhabitants of the modern Western world are well aware that each child has one biological father and one only. We know that, in sexually reproducing organisms, only one sperm fertilizes the egg, and we know this rule holds for people as well as penguins. The doctrine of single paternity, as a folk belief, goes so far back in Western history and is so extended through our social and legal institutions that it is difficult for us to imagine that anyone would entertain any other view of biological paternity" (Stephen Beckerman and Paul Valentine, 2002, p. 1).

4. Susan L. Cooper and Ellen S. Glazer (1994) document this phenomenon: "Physicians implied, or stated outright, that secrecy was the only reasonable option—the choice of informed well-adjusted, and reasonable couples; revealing the secret would cause the child to be stigmatized—rejected by friends

and family. Furthermore, telling the child about how he or she was conceived would do psychological harm" (p. 162).

5. Carole Lieber Wilkins (2003) echoes this affirmation of the benefits of disclosure in her publications for Resolve: "With very few exceptions, the best interests of the children and their families are served by children growing up with the knowledge that they are not genetically related to one of their parents."

6. Annette Baran and Reuben Pannor (1989, p. 61).

7. Christopher Bollas, *The Shadow of the Object: Psychoanalysis of the Unthought Known*. London: Free Association Press, 1987.

8. Marsha Levy-Warren, "A Clinical Look at Knowing and Telling: Secrets, Lies, and Disillusionments," in Vivian B. Shapiro et al. (2001, pp. 251–275).

9. See M. Brown (1994) and Peggy Orenstein (1995).

10. Annette Baran and Reuben Pannor (1989, p. 77).

11. Annette Baran and Reuben Pannor (1989, p. 67).

12. Susan Klock and Donald Meier (1991).

13. According to Jane Haynes, a British psychologist who interpreted these data: "This would suggest that protection of the father and fears that his infertility—which may be perceived as synonymous with a lack of potency—will be unmasked, take precedence over a balanced consideration of a child's subsequent need to understand his or her origins" (Jane Haynes, "Donor Insemination amongst Lesbian Women," in Jane Haynes and Juliet Miller, 2003, p. 164).

14. Susan Golombok and Fiona MacCallum (2003).

15. Annette Baran and Reuben Pannor (1989).

16. Anna Mulrine (2004).

17. Marsha Levy-Warren, "A Clinical Look at Knowing and Telling: Secrets, Lies, and Disillusionments," in Vivian B. Shapiro et al. (2001, pp. 257–258).

18. Annette Baran and Reuben Pannor (1989).

19. Robert D. Nachtigall and Gay Becker (2002).

20. Ask Dr. Gayle, 1999.

21. Annette Baran and Reuben Pannor (1989, p. 64).

CHAPTER SEVEN

1. Anndee Hochman (2002, p. 228).

2. Antonio Regalado (2004).

3. Joan Raphael-Leff, "Eros and ART," in Jane Haynes and Juliet Miller (2003, p. 44).

4. International Consumer Support for Infertility (2001).

5. Carol Lieber Wilkins (2003).

6. Dr. Anne Bernstein (1994) points out that before even figuring out what and when to tell a child, "parents' own emotional acceptance of how their family was formed is the first and most important step in preparing to talk with children" (p. 169).

7. Anne C. Bernstein (1994, p. 180).

8. Carole Lieber Wilkins (2003, pp. 3–6).

9. Kate Bourne (2002, p. 23).

10. David Scott Levin, *Developmental Experiences: Treatment of Developmental Disorders in Children*, New York: Jason Aronson, 1985.

11. Vivian B. Shapiro et al. (2001, p. 190).

12. Adam Pertman (2000).

13. Jane T. Schnitter (1995, pp. 11, 15).

14. "How to Tell Your Kids about Egg and Sperm Donation" (2003).

15. Sigmund Freud, *The Sexual Enlightenment of Children*, New York: Collier Books, 1963.

16. Annette Baran and Reuben Pannor (1989, p. 69).

17. Annette Baran and Reuben Pannor (1989).

18. Speaking specifically about donor insemination, Susan L. Cooper and Ellen S. Glazer (1994) explain: "Although professionals disagree to some extent about what is the best age to explain donor insemination to children, virtually all agree that adolescence is not the time to tell. This is the time when teenagers struggle on many levels with identity issues. They need to feel that they fit in and are not different from peers. It is also a time of many physical and emotional changes. Introducing DI during the adolescent years could precipitate an emotional trauma" (p. 175).

19. Erik Erikson, *Identity, Youth, and Crisis*, New York: Norton, 1968.

20. Marsha Levy-Warren, "A Clinical Look at Knowing and Telling," in Vivian B. Shapiro et al. (2001, pp. 251–275).

21. As reported in David Noonan and Karen Springer (2001, p. 47).

CHAPTER EIGHT

1. Anndee Hochman (2003).

2. Anne C. Bernstein (1994, p. 21).

3. A. R. Radcliffe-Brown and D. Forde, Eds., *African Systems of Kinship and Marriage*, Oxford: Oxford University Press, 1950.

4. Indeed, the legal status, particularly in surrogacy families, makes this distinction even more complicated. By law in most states, the birth mother is

the legal mother. Therefore, in families using a surrogate, the mother may have to go through the procedure of "adopting" her child from the surrogate, who until such adoption takes place, is the "mother" of the child in the eyes of the law.

5. Joyce Sukamp Friedman (1996).

6. Kate Bourne (2002, p. 23).

7. American Infertility Association (2003, p. 6).

8. See Anne C. Bernstein (1994) for more discussion about the developmental progression of children's thoughts and ideas about conception and birth.

9. Sue Stuart-Smith, a British psychologist writing about egg donation, points out that we still know very little about the role of the uterine environment and that the woman who carries the child is creating a physical environment for the child and providing the basic materials from which the fetus grows and develops (Sue Stuart-Miller, "Egg Donation: The Mission to Have a Child," in Jane Haynes and Juliet Miller, 2003, pp. 166–178).

10. Razan Nathalie, *Our Beautiful Work of A.R.T.* (2002), *A Part Was Given* (2002), and *From Out of My Body . . .* (2002).

11. Elaine R. Gordon (1992, pp. 13, 14).

12. Elaine R. Gordon (1992, p. 20).

13. Elaine R. Gordon (1992, p. 22).

14. Kate Bourne (2002, p. 11).

15. Joyce Sukamp Friedman (1996, p. 28).

16. Joyce Sukamp Friedman, (1996, p. 29).

17. Sheri Glucoft-Wong, personal communication, February 26, 2004.

18. Annette Baran and Reuben Pannor (1989, pp. 82–83).

19. Melodie Ward Leslie, "Private Business," in *Let the Offspring Speak* (1997, pp. 39–42).

20. Jane Haynes, "Donor Insemination among Lesbian Women," in Jane Haynes and Juliet Miller (2003, pp. 143–165).

21. Marsha Levy-Warren speaks to the importance of paying attention to what the children are really asking of us about their birth-other origins, especially when they haven't yet been told: "We must be attuned to the developmental readiness of children to hear the unrevealed truths that surround them in their families. We have to try to listen to the actual questions of children and their preconscious derivatives and not read into these questions what we as adults may sense is more deeply motivating them unconsciously" (Marsha Levy-Warren, "A Clinical Look at Knowing and Telling: Secrets, Lies, and Disillusionments," in Vivian B. Shapiro et al. (2001, p. 273).

22. Anne C. Bernstein (1994, p. 182).

CHAPTER NINE

1. In this study, conducted by Professor Christina Bergh at Sahlgrenska University Hospital in Sweden, hospital admissions were higher in IVF and ICSI children and the rate of birth defects was 6.2 percent for ICSI children, 4.1 percent for IVF babies, compared to 2.4 percent for the naturally conceived children. As reported in BBC On-line News, Martin Hutchinson, "Public Reassured of IVF Safety," July 2, 2003.

2. Michele Hansen et al (2002).

3. Laura A. Schieve et al. (2002).

4. As reported in Rick Weiss (2002).

5. Rosie Mestel (2003).

6. Susan Golombok and Fiona MacCallum (2003).

7. Paolo Serafini (2001).

8. Susan Golombok, F. Tasker, and C. Murray (1997). In this study both teachers and parents assessed the children, and the children all had knowledge of their donor-insemination roots.

9. A. Brewaeys, S. Golombok, J. K. Naaktgeboren, and E. V. van Hall (1997).

10. Using comparison groups of adopted children and naturally conceived children, Golombok et al. now have findings through adolescence. Based on questionnaires and standardized interview measures, the results showed that any differences found in parent–child relationships had more to do with a history of infertility than with the mode of conception. Mothers who had experienced infertility showed lower levels of sensitive responding than did mothers with a naturally conceived child, and there was less reasoning between mother and child and between father and child in families where parents had experienced infertility than in families of naturally conceived children. A particularly interesting finding was that parents' affection for their children was higher for parents who used in vitro procedures than for parents who turned to adoption. This suggests that a genetic link between the parents and the child may be related to greater affection toward a child. Whether this finding will be replicated in families where only one parent is genetically linked to the child remains to be seen, but it does speak to genetic ties priming the pump for parental affection. In this respect, children conceived with birth others may be different than their peers who are adopted and more like children who are naturally conceived. The authors concluded their study with the following quote: "the concerns that have been raised about the negative psychological consequences that may result from conception by IVF remain unfounded as these young people entered their adolescent years . . . it appears from the current results that conceiving a child by

IVF does not have a deleterious effect on parenting or on the psychological development of the adolescent child" (Susan Golombok, Fiona MacCalllum, and Emma Goodman, 2001, p. 607).

11. F. Van Balen (1996).

12. Diane Finiello Zervos, "Dark Reflections: The Shadow Side of Assisted Reproductive Techniques," in Jane Haynes and Juliet Miller (2003, p. 190).

13. Jane Haynes, "Donor-Insemination among Lesbian Women," In Jane Haynes and Juliet Miller (2003, p.163).

14. "My Daddy Was a Donor" (2002).

15. Linda Villarosa (2002).

16. Kathryn Trueblood (1998, p. 95).

17. *Let the Offspring Speak* (1997, p. 167).

18. Emma Scrimgeour, "The Story of Seth's Egg," in Jane Haynes and Juliet Miller (2003, p. 108).

19. Flora Scrimgeour, "Seth," in Jane Haynes and Juliet Miller (2003, pp. 118–119).

20. Jane Haynes, "Donor Insemination among Lesbian Women," in Jane Haynes and Juliet Miller (2003, p. 151).

21. Erica Goode (2001).

22. Michael Dudley and Gaire Neave, "Issues for Families and Children Where Conception Was Achieved Using Donor Gametes," in *Let the Offspring Speak* (1997, p. 134).

23. Ken Corbett (2001, pp. 609, 610).

24. To quote from Hertz, "Mothers, and then mothers and their children create stories about who those men are to help the children develop self-feelings that help them 'pin down the self.'" Hertz argues that, by engaging in such mental play the mothers give the children a sense of unity over their physical self, solidifying where all the different parts come from. In doing so, the mothers also reflect to the children the role of the donor in their development, particularly as the child grows to be more and more like the donor (more obvious in known-donor situations). Her underlying premise is that the child's self emerges in relation to significant others, the search to know these people is deep, donors and surrogates are included in those significant others, and parents can help a child in the search by allowing "family reveries" to unfold (Rosanna Hertz, 2002, p. 3).

25. Anndee Hochman (2002, p. 230).

26. Anndee Hochman (2003, p. 66).

27. Peggy Orenstein (1995).

28. Anndee Hochman (2002, p. 230).

29. Stephen Byrnes, "Scenes from a Surrogacy," in Jill Bialosky and Helen Schulman (1998, p. 193).

30. Susan L. Cooper and Ellen S. Glazer (1994).

31. Peggy Orenstein (1995).

32. Anndee Hochman (2003, p. 64).

33. Rebecca Mead (1999, p. 60).

34. Anndee Hochman (2002, p. 241).

35. David Noonan and Karen Springen (2001, p. 47).

36. Linda Villarosa (2002, p. D5).

37. William Cordray, "The Need for a Sense of Self-Identity," in *Let the Offspring Speak* (1997, pp. 35–38).

38. Ellen Coe, "My Father Was Not My Father," in *Let the Offspring Speak* (1997, p. 47).

39. According to Susan L. Cooper and Ellen S. Glazer (1994), "children who have no knowledge of their genetic history must live with a sense of bafflement about how they came to be and bewilderment about who they are. Our current understanding about human nature and the psychological development of human beings indicates that a genetic void is not in the best psychological interest of a person" (p. 351).

40. "My Daddy was a Donor" (2002).

41. Nicky, "To Whom It May Concern," in *Let the Offspring Speak* (1997, p. 30).

42. L. L. Warner, "Family Romance Fantasy Resolution in George Eliot's *Daniel Deronda*," *Psychoanalytic Study of the Child*, vol. 48 (1993): 379–397.

43. See Rosanna Hertz (2002) for a discussion of the concept of half-adopted and its meaning to children and their single mothers in donor-insemination families.

44. BBC News (2000).

CHAPTER TEN

1. As quoted in Susan Dominus (2004, p. 144).

2. Leila Abboud (2002).

3. Antonio Regalado (2002).

4. *Time* magazine cover, February 19, 2001.

5. As reported in Rick Weiss (2003) and Nicholas Wade (2003).

6. Carl T. Hall (2004).

7. Denis Grady (2003).

8. Amy Dockser Marcus (2004).

9. Claudia Calb (2004) and Diana Kapp (2003).

10. Harriet Chiang (2004).

11. Nicholas Zamiska (2004).

12. See Peggy Orenstein (2004) [and Patricia R. Olsen (2003)] for a discussion of the case of E. G. and K. M..

13. Quoted in Peggy Orenstein (2004, p. 29).

14. Leslie Eaton (2004).

Bibliography

Abboud, Leila. "FDA Interrupts Some Fertility Treatments." *The Wall Street Journal*, October 7, 2002: A4.

Adams, Jane Meredith. "One Pregnancy, Four Mothers, Two Fathers, and an Army of Lawyers." *O, The Oprah Magazine*, December 2002: 181–186.

American Infertility Association. *Out of the Dish: Talking to Children about Their IVF Origins*, 2003.

Andrews, Lori B. *The Clone Age: Adventures in the New World of Reproductive Technology*. New York: Henry Holt, 1999.

Andrews, Lori B. *Future Perfect: Confronting Decisions about Genetics*. New York: Columbia University Press, 2001.

Ask Dr. Gayle. "'Artificial Insemination': Tell Children the Truth?" www.askdr gayle.com, August 29, 1999.

BBC News, "'Shock' of Sperm Donor Babies." August 31, 2000, news.bbc.co.uk.

Baran, Annette, and Pannor, Reuben. *Lethal Secrets: The Psychology of Donor Insemination*. New York: Amistad, 1989.

Bartholet, Elizabeth. *Family Bonds: Adoption, Infertility, and the New World of Child Production*. Boston: Beacon Press, 1999.

Beckerman, Stephen, and Valentine, Paul. *Cultures of Multiple Fathers*. Gainesville, FL: University of Florida Press, 2002.

Bernstein, Anne C. *The Flight of the Stork*. Indianapolis: Perspectives Press, 1994.

Bialosky, Jill, and Schulman, Helen, Eds. *Wanting a Child*. New York: Farrar, Straus & Giroux, 1998.

Bourne, Kate. *Sometimes It Takes Three to Make a Baby: Explaining Egg Donor Conception to Young Children.* Melbourne: Melbourne IVF, 2002.

Brewaeys, A., Golombok, S., Naaktgeboren, J. K., and van Hall, E. V. "Donor Insemination: Dutch Parents' Opinions about Confidentiality and Donor Anonymity and the Emotional Adjustment of Their Children." *Human Reproduction,* vol. 12 (1997): 1591–1597.

Brown, M. "Whose Eyes Are These, Whose Nose?" *Newsweek,* March 7, 1994: 12.

Calarusso, Calvin. "Mother, Is That You?" *Psychoanalytic Study of the Child,* vol. 42 (1987): 223–237.

Calb, Claudia. "Fertility and the Freezer." *Newsweek,* August 2, 2004: 52.

Chiang, Harriet. "Mom Awarded $1 Million over Embryo Mix-up." *San Francisco Chronicle,* August 4, 2004: B2.

Cooper, Susan L., and Glazer, Ellen S. *Beyond Infertility: The New Paths to Parenthood.* New York: Lexington Books, 1994.

Cooper, Susan L., and Glazer, Ellen S. *Choosing Assisted Reproduction: Social, Emotional, and Ethical Considerations.* Indianapolis: Perspectives Press, 1998.

Corbett, Ken. "Nontraditional Family Romance." *Psychoanalytic Quarterly,* vol. 52 (2001): 599–624.

Davies, Jody Messier. "Thoughts on the Nature of Desires: The Ambiguous, the Transitional, and the Poetic. Reply to Commentaries [on 'Between the Disclosure and Foreclosure of Erotic Transference–Counter Transfereence']." *Psychoanalytic Dialogues,* vol. 8, no. 6 (1998): 805–823.

Diamond, Ronny, Kezur, David, Meyers, Mimi, Scharf, Constance N., and Weishel, Margot. *Couple Therapy for Infertility.* New York: Guilford Press, 1999.

Dominus, Susan. "Growing Up with Mom and Mom." *The New York Times Magazine,* October 24, 2004: 68–75, 84, 143–144.

Drummond, Tammerlin. "Mom on Her Own." *Time,* August 28, 2000: 54.

Dutton, Gail. *A Matter of Trust: The Guide to Gestational Surrogacy.* Irvine, CA: Clouds Publishing, 1997.

Eaton, Leslie. "Parenthood is Redefined, but Custody Battles Remain Ugly." *The New York Times,* June 12, 2004: A13.

Ehrensaft, Diane. "Alternatives to the Stork: Fatherhood Fantasies in Donor Insemination Families." *Studies in Gender and Sexuality,* vol. 1, no. 4 (2000): 371–397.

Ehrensaft, Diane. *Spoiling Childhood: How Well-Meaning Parents Are Giving Children Too Much but Not What They Need.* New York: Guilford Press, 1997.

Ethics Committee of the American Society for Reproductive Medicine. "Informing

Offspring of Their Conception by Gamete Donation." *Fertility and Sterility*, vol. 81, no. 3 (2004): 527–531.

Ferdinand, Pamela. "Massachusetts Case Tests Legal Standing of Surrogate, Genetic Mothers—Procedure for Placing Name on Birth Certificate Is at Issue." *The Washington Post*, September 6, 2001: A6.

Freilicher, Liza, and Scheu, Jennifer, with Wetanson, Suzanne. *Conceiving Luc.* New York: William Morrow, 1999.

Friedman, Joyce Sukamp. *Building Your Family through Egg Donation.* Fort Thomas, KY: Jolance Press, 1996.

Golombok, Susan, and MacCallum, Fiona. "Practitioner Review: Outcomes for Parents and Children Following Non-traditional Conception: What Do Clinicians Need to Know?" *Journal of Child Psychology and Psychiatry*, vol. 44, no. 3 (2003): 303–315.

Golombok, Susan, MacCallum, Fiona, and Goodman, Emma. "The 'Test-Tube' Generation: Parent–Child Relationships and the Psychological Well-Being of In Vitro Fertilization Children at Adolescence." *Child Development*, vol. 72, no. 2 (2001): 599–608.

Golombok, Susan, Murray, Clare, Brinsden, Peter, and Abdalla, Hossam. "Social versus Biological Parenting: Family Functioning and the Socio-emotional Development of Children Conceived by Egg or Sperm Donation." *Journal of Child Psychology and Psychiatry*, vol. 40, no. 4 (1999): 519 527.

Golombok, Susan, Tasker, F., and Murray, C. "Children Raised in Fatherless Families from Infancy: Family Relationships and the Socio-emotional Development of Children of Lesbian and Single Heterosexual Mothers." *Journal of Child Psychology and Psychiatry*, vol. 38 (1997): 783–791.

Goode, Erica. "A Rainbow of Differences in Gays' Children." *The New York Times*, July 17, 2001: D1, D7.

Gordon, Elaine R. *Mommy, Did I Grow in Your Tummy?: Where Some Babies Come From.* Santa Monica, CA: EM Greenberg Press, 1992.

Gosden, Roger. *Designing Babies: The Brave New World of Reproductive Technology*, New York: W. H. Freeman, 1999.

Grady, Denis. "Pregnancy Created Using Egg Nucleus of Infertile Woman." *The New York Times*, October 14, 2003: A1, A18.

Grunwald, Michael. "Embryo Mix-Up is Double Trouble." *San Francisco Chronicle*, March 31, 1999: A2.

Hall, Carl T. "Look Moms: No Dad!" *San Francisco Chronicle*, April 22, 2004: A1, A18.

Hansen, Michele, Kurinczuk, Jennifer J., Bower, Carol, and Webb, Sandra. "The Risk of Major Birth Defects after Intracytoplasmic Sperm Injection and In Vitro Fertilization." *The New England Journal of Medicine*, vol. 346, no. 10 (March 7, 2002): 725–730.

Haynes, Jane, and Miller, Juliet, Eds. *Inconceivable Conceptions*. New York: Brunner-Routledge, 2003.

Henig, Robin Mrantz. "Adapting to Our Own Engineering." *The New York Times*, December 17, 2002: A35.

Hertz, Rosanna. "The Father as an Idea: A Challenge to Kinship Boundaries by Single Mothers." *Symbolic Interaction*, vol. 25, no. 1 (2002): 1–31.

Hochman, Anndee. "Whose Sperm Is It, Anyway?" *O, The Oprah Magazine*, December 2002: 228–231, 239–241.

Hochman, Anndee. "Sperm Search." *Out*, March 2003: 60, 62, 64, 66.

Hodder, Harbour Fraser. "The New Fertility." *Harvard Magazine*, November–December 1997: 54–64, 97–99.

Holmes, Helen Bequart, Ed. *Issues in Reproductive Technology*. New York: New York University Press, 1994.

"How to Tell Your Kids about Egg and Sperm Donation," *Internet News*, May 22, 2003: 2.

International Consumer Support for Infertility. *Building Your Family with the Help of Assisted Reproductive Technologies (ART)* Fact Sheet. 2001.

Kalb, Claudia. "Baby Boom: The $50,000 Egg." *Newsweek*, March 15, 1999: 84.

Kapp, Diana. "Forever Fertile." *San Francisco Magazine*, October 2003: 68–77.

Klasker, Judith N., and Borg, Susan. *In Search of Parenthood: Coping with Infertility and High-Tech Conception*. Boston: Beacon Press, 1987.

Klock, Susan, and Meier, Donald. "Psychological Factors Related to Donor Insemination." *Fertility and Sterility*, vol. 5 (1991): 484–495.

Let the Offspring Speak: Discussions on Donor Conception. New South Wales, Australia: The Donor Conception Support Group of Australia, 1997.

Lyall, Sarah. "British Judge Rules Sperm Donor Is Legal Father in Mix-Up Case." *The New York Times*, February 27, 2003: A5.

Marcus, Amy Dockser. "Progress in the Search for a Better Embryo." *The Wall Street Journal*, May 11, 2004: D1, D6.

Martin, April. *The Lesbian and Gay Parenting Handbook*. New York: Harper-Perennial, 1993.

McGee, Glenn. *The Perfect Baby: Parenthood in the New World of Cloning and Genetics*. Lanham, MD: Rowan & Littlefield, 2000.

McManis, Sam. "Midlife Mommy." *San Francisco Chronicle*, May 11, 2003: E1, E4–5.

Mead, Rebecca. "Annals of Reproduction, Eggs for Sale." *The New Yorker*, August 9, 1999: 56–65.

Mestel, Rosie. "Some Studies See Ills for In Vitro Children." *Los Angeles Times*, January 24, 2003: A1, A14.

Mulrine, Anna. "Making Babies." *U.S. News & World Report*, September 27, 2004: 61–67.

"My Daddy Was a Donor." *Observer*, January 20, 2002: Online News.

Nachtigall, Robert D., and Becker, Gay. "Secrecy: The Unresolved Dilemma of Donor Insemination." *Resolve*, Disclosure Issues, Fact Sheet 61A, August 2002: 1–3.

Nathalie, Razaan. *From Out of My Body Your Soul Did Grow*. Edina, MN: Beaver's Pond Press, 2002.

Nathalie, Razaan. *Our Beautiful Work of A.R.T.* Edina, MN: Beaver's Pond Press, 2002.

Nathalie, Razaan. *A Part Was Given and an Angel Was Born*. Edina, MN: Beaver's Pond Press, 2002.

Noonan, David, and Springen, Karen. "When Daddy Is a Donor." *Newsweek*, August 13, 2001: 46–47.

Olsen, Patricia R. "Who's the Real Mom?" *San Francisco Chronicle Magazine*, June 22, 2003: 14–17.

Orenstein, Peggy. "Looking for a Donor to Call Dad." *The New York Times Magazine*, June 18, 1995: 28–35, 42, 50, 58.

Orenstein, Peggy. "The Other Mother." *The New York Times Magazine*, July 25, 2004: 24–29.

Oxenhandler, Noelle. *The Eros of Parenthood*. New York: St. Martin's Press, 2001.

Pertman, Adam. *Adoption Nation: How the Adoption Revolution Is Transforming America*. New York: Basic Books, 2000.

Ragone, Helena. *Surrogate Motherhood: Conception in the Heart*. Boulder, CO: Westview Press, 1994.

Regalado, Antonio. "Cancer Patients Get New Hope for Having Kids." *The Wall Street Journal*, March 9, 2004: D1, D3.

Regalado, Antonio. "Could a Skin Cell Someday Replace Sperm or Egg?" *The Wall Street Journal*, October 17, 2002: B1.

Rothbart, Davy. "Scavengers of Other People's Lives." *San Francisco Chronicle*, January 5, 2003: D3.

Saban, Cheryl. *Miracle Child: Genetic Mother, Surrogate Womb*. Far Hills, NJ: New Horizon Press, 1993.

Schieve, Laura A., Meikle, Susan F., Ferre, Cynthia, Peterson, Herbert, Jeng, Gary, and Wilco, Lynne. "Low and Very Low Birth Weight in Infants Conceived with Use of Assisted Reproductive Technology." *The New England Journal of Medicine*, vol. 346, no. 10 (March 7, 2002): 731–737

Schnitter, Jane T. *Let Me Explain: A Story About Donor Insemination*. Indianapolis: Perspectives Press, 1995.

Serafini, Paolo. "Outcome and Follow-up of Children Born after In Vitro Fertilization Surrogacy (IVF Surrogacy)." *Human Reproductive Update*, vol. 17 (2001): 23–27.

Shanley, Mary Lyndon. *Making Babies, Making Families*. Boston: Beacon Press, 2001.

Shapiro, Vivian B., Shapiro, Janet R., and Paret, Isabel H., Eds. *Complex Adoption and Assisted Reproductive Technology*. New York: Guilford Press, 2001.

Silver, Lee M. *Remaking Eden: How Genetic Engineering and Cloning Will Transform the American Family*. New York: Avon Books, 1998.

Smolowe, Jill, and Stoynoff, Natasha. "Teaming with Love." *People*, March 10, 2003: 88, 94.

Springen, Karen, and Noonan, David. "Sperm Banks Go On-Line." *Newsweek*, April 21, 2003: E14–E15.

Tasker, Fiona L., and Golombok, Susan. *Growing Up in a Lesbian Family: Effects on Child Development*. New York: Guilford Press, 1997.

Thompson, Mary Ann. *The Gift of a Child*. Maui: Inner Ocean Publishing, 2002.

Trueblood, Kathryn. *The Sperm Donor's Daughter*. Sag Harbor, NY: Permanent Press, 1998.

Van Balen, F. "Child Rearing Following In-Vitro Fertilization." *Journal of Child Psychology and Psychiatry*, vol. 37 (1996): 687–693.

Vercollone, Carol Frost, Moss, Heidi, and Moss, Robert. *Helping the Stork: The Choices and Challenges of Donor Insemination*. New York: Macmillan, 1997.

Villarosa, Linda. "Once-Invisible Sperm Donors Get to Meet the Family." *The New York Times*, May 21, 2002: D10.

Wade, Nicholas. "Pennsylvania Researchers Turn Stem Cells to Egg Cells." *The New York Times*, May 21, 2003: A29.

Weiss, Rick. "In Vitro Children Likely to Have Higher Rate of Complications." *San Francisco Chronicle*, February 12, 2002: A4.

Weiss, Rick. "Mouse Stem Cells Turned into Egg Cells." *San Francisco Chronicle*, May 21, 2003: A9.

Wilkins, Carol Lieber. "To Tell or Not To Tell: Issues of Disclosure in Donor Conception." Disclosure Issues: Fact Sheet 61 A, Resolve: The National Infertility Association, Somerville, MA, 2002.

Wong, B. D. *Following Foo*. New York: Harper Entertainment, 2003.

Yardley, Jim. "Investigators Say Embryologist Knew He Erred in Egg Mix-Up." *The New York Times*, April 17, 1999: A13.

"You're Carrying Someone Else's Child," *Newsweek*, April 12, 1999: 61.

Zamiska, Nicholas. "Ruling Guides Orthodox Sites' Sabbath Sales." *The Wall Street Journal*, August 17, 2004: B1, B4.

Index

About the Author

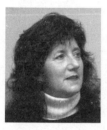

Diane Ehrensaft, PhD, a noted developmental and clinical psychologist in the San Francisco Bay area, Oakland, California, specializes in psychotherapy and consultation with parents and children in families formed with the help of assisted reproductive technology. A faculty member of The Wright Institute, Berkeley, California, since 1981 and a member of the mental health professional group of the American Society for Reproductive Medicine, she publishes and lectures internationally on issues of raising children and strengthening families, and is also the author of *Spoiling Childhood: How Well-Meaning Parents Are Giving Children Too Much, but Not What They Need*. She has watched her two children and now one grandchild grow up in this fertile new world.